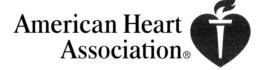

American Heart
Association®

Learn and Live SM

BLS for Healthcare Providers

Edward R. Stapleton, EMT-P, BLS Science Editor
Tom P. Aufderheide, MD, BLS Science Editor
Mary Fran Hazinski, RN, MSN, Senior ECC Science Editor
Richard O. Cummins, MD, MPH, MSc, Senior ECC Science Editor

Contributors
John M. Field, MD, ACLS Science Editor
Vinay M. Nadkarni, MD, Pediatric Science Editor
Arno Zaritsky, MD, Pediatric Science Editor
Robert A. Berg, MD
Louis Gonzales, BS, NREMT-P
Robert W. Hickey, MD
Ahamed H. Idris, MD
Graham Nichol, MD, MPH
Eric Niegelberg, EMT-P
John Kattwinkel, MD
Richard E. Kerber, MD
Rashmi U. Kothari, MD
Peter J. Kudenchuk, MD
Susan Niermeyer, MD
Charles L. Schleien, MD
Mark E. Swanson, MD
Roger D. White, MD

International Contributors
Vic Callanan, MD
Anthony J. Handley, MD
Walter G.J. Kloeck, MD, BCh
David A. Zideman, MD

ISBN 0-87493-318-8
© 2001 American Heart Association

Acknowledgment

We gratefully acknowledge the many contributions of our editor, F.G. Stoddard. The high quality of our publications is due in large part to his sharp eye, dedication to excellence, and sense of style.

Strongest minds are often those of whom the noisy world hears least.

— William Wordsworth, *The Excursion*

Contents

Chapter 6
Adult CPR

Contents

Chapter 9
Pediatric Basic Life Support

Chapter 10
Safety During CPR Training and Actual Rescue

Chapter 11
Special Resuscitation Situations

Chapter 12
CPR and Defibrillation: The Human Dimension

Appendix A
Comparison Across Age Groups of Resuscitation Interventions

Appendix B
Skills Performance Sheets

Glossary

Index

Preface

The AHA offers a variety of courses on basic life support (BLS) and cardiopulmonary resuscitation (CPR) for healthcare providers. With the knowledge and skills you learn in these courses, you can save the life of a family member, a friend, a coworker, a citizen in your community, or a patient in the hospital or clinic where you work.

The BLS for Healthcare Providers Course is intended for participants who must have a credential (a card) documenting successful completion of a course in CPR and BLS for healthcare professionals. Such credentials are typically required for people who provide healthcare to patients in a wide variety of settings, both in-hospital and outside the hospital.

This course will teach you how to recognize and respond to life-threatening emergencies such as cardiac arrest, respiratory arrest, and foreign-body airway obstruction (choking). You will learn to recognize heart attack and stroke in adults and breathing difficulty in children. This course teaches the skills needed to respond to the emergencies you identify. You will learn the skills of CPR for victims of all ages (including ventilation with barrier devices and bag-mask devices), use of an automated external defibrillator (AED), and relief of foreign-body airway obstruction. These skills will enable you to recognize emergencies and provide the first three links in either the AHA adult Chain of Survival or the pediatric Chain of Survival. With these skills you may save the life of a patient, a member of your community, or a loved one.

Participants in this course will use one of two manuals, *Fundamentals of BLS for Healthcare Providers,* or this manual, *BLS for Healthcare Providers.*

BLS for Healthcare Providers is intended for use by licensed and certified healthcare professionals. It assumes that the reader has a healthcare education, and it contains a stronger emphasis on anatomy and physiology and on scientific rationale for actions and recommendations than is included in *Fundamentals of BLS.* You will also find information about reducing risk of heart disease and injury prevention that you may wish to use for patient education.

This manual is designed to provide information that will be useful to you before, during and after the BLS for Healthcare Providers Course. It contains several features designed to help you learn CPR, ventilation with a barrier device and a bag-mask device, and use of an AED. Each chapter includes *learning objectives*, a *learning checklist,* and *review questions.* These features will make learning easier. At the start of each chapter, carefully read the learning objectives. Reading them carefully will help you focus on the essential information. When you finish reading the chapter, review the learning checklist. Then answer the review questions. If you cannot answer a question or if you choose the wrong answer, review the parts of the chapter related to that question.

Throughout the manual you will see colored boxes. These boxes highlight important and useful information. **Critical Concepts** presents essential information for mastering the knowledge and skills taught in this course. Critical signs and symptoms included in these boxes and in the text are called **red flags. A red flag** says "Warning! This is vital information about critical signs and symptoms."

Foundation Facts further explains the recommended actions and provide important supportive information.

FYI boxes present background material for your information only. These boxes contain information about various topics, such as different types of 911 systems, that may be useful or interesting to some participants. You are *not required* to know the information presented in FYI boxes to fulfill the core learning objectives.

The skills performance sheets ("Performance Criteria") in the appendix of this manual list the skills you will practice in class. To obtain a course completion card, you must satisfactorily demonstrate the skills listed on each sheet to your instructor, and you must score at least 84% on a written examination. Review each skill, read each chapter in this manual, pay attention to the details, and practice carefully. It is easy to forget some CPR skills, so practice the skills and reread this manual after you complete the course.

The appendix also contains case scenarios. These scenarios will help you learn to apply your knowledge of CPR to realistic situations. Take advantage of this learning opportunity. It will do more than prepare you for the course. It will prepare you to save a life.

To obtain more information about ways to reduce the risk of heart disease, stroke, and injury and updated information on CPR, visit the AHA website at www. americanheart.org/cpr. This site also contains links to other sites with useful information.

We wish you success as you learn CPR. When you complete the course, you will be prepared to recognize emergencies in adults, to prevent many causes of cardiac arrest in infants and children, and to respond to emergencies using the skills of CPR.

Edward R. Stapleton, EMT-P

Tom P. Aufderheide, MD

Mary Fran Hazinski, RN, MSN

A 58-year-old man collapses at home immediately after eating dinner with his wife and 2 grown children. His wife runs to his side and finds him unresponsive to voice and painful stimuli. She tells their son to call 911 while she begins to evaluate the ABCs. She opens her husband's airway with the head tilt–chin lift maneuver and discovers that he is not breathing. After she provides 2 rescue breaths, her husband has no signs of circulation (that is, no normal breathing, coughing, or movement): he is in cardiopulmonary arrest. The woman continues CPR and asks her daughter to meet the ambulance in front of their home.

The 911 dispatcher collects the information from the victim's son and immediately sends a police car and a paramedic unit to the scene. The police arrive 4 minutes after the collapse, carrying an AED. After verifying that the victim has no response, no breathing, and no signs of circulation, a police officer attaches the AED. The device advises a shock 2 times in succession. The officer delivers 2 shocks. The device then advises "no shock indicated." The officer reassesses the victim and finds that he has signs of circulation (he is moving) but is still in respiratory arrest.

The police officer continues rescue breathing, using a pocket mask with supplemental oxygen, until the EMS unit arrives 2 minutes later. The paramedics attach a monitor and insert a tracheal tube in the victim's airway. His heart rate is 42 bpm, and his blood pressure is very low — 70/40 mm Hg. The paramedics immediately start an IV and administer atropine sulfate to increase the heart rate. His heart rate rises to 78 bpm, and his blood pressure increases to 110/60 mm Hg.

The victim is transported to a nearby hospital, where he is diagnosed as having an acute myocardial infarction. He is treated with fibrinolytics (clotbuster medications) to clear the blocked coronary arteries in his heart. The treatment reopens the blocked arteries and restores blood flow to his heart. The man returns home to his wife and children with a renewed interest in engaging in a heart-healthy lifestyle and with a profound appreciation for a strong community Chain of Survival.

Basic Life Support in Perspective

Overview

Cardiovascular disease is the leading cause of death in the United States for both men and women. In 1997 cardiovascular disease claimed 953 110 lives in the United States (see Figure 1).[1] This year approximately 2 million people in the United States will be diagnosed as having an acute coronary syndrome (ACS). More than one half million of these patients will be hospitalized with a diagnosis of unstable angina,[2] and 1.5 million will experience an acute myocardial infarction (AMI).[3]

Of the 1.5 million patients with AMI, approximately one half million will die, and 50% of these deaths will be sudden, occurring within the first hour of the onset of symptoms.[4] When out-of-hospital mortality is included, the fatality rate for the first prolonged attack of ischemic pain is 34%. In 17% of these patients, ischemic pain is their first, last, and only symptom.[5]

Current management of AMI contrasts dramatically with the expectant waiting and retrospective diagnosis of 2 decades ago. Fibrinolytic agents (clot-dissolving medications) and percutaneous coronary interventions (PCIs) reopen the blocked coronary vessels that cause myocardial ischemia, saving lives and improving quality of life.[6-13] These interventions, however, must be administered within the first few hours of symptom onset to be most effective.

Sudden cardiac death is the major complication of cardiovascular disease. In the United States approximately 250 000 people die from sudden cardiac death each year. The most frequent initial rhythm documented in witnessed sudden cardiac arrest is ventricular fibrillation (VF). The most effective treatment for VF is automated external defibrillation. Defibrillation, however, is another intervention with time-limited success. The probability of successful defibrillation decreases by approximately 7% to 10%

Learning Objectives

After reading this chapter and participating in the introductory portion of the BLS for Healthcare Providers Course you should be able to

1. Name the links in the AHA adult Chain of Survival and state the importance of each link

2. Define emergency cardiovascular care

3. Distinguish between the actions of basic life support and those of advanced cardiovascular life support

4. Discuss the value of Utstein-style reporting when maintaining a cardiac arrest database

for every minute defibrillation is delayed, and VF tends to convert to asystole within a few minutes if left untreated.[14-24]

Stroke is the third leading cause of death in the United States and the leading cause of brain injury in adults. In the United States approximately 500 000 persons suffer a stroke each year, and nearly a quarter of those die.[1]

Until recently care of the stroke patient was largely supportive, with therapy focused on treating complications.[25] In the past no treatment was available to alter the course of the stroke itself, so there was no need to rapidly identify, transport, or manage stroke victims.[25]

Now fibrinolytic therapy offers the opportunity to limit brain damage and improve outcome in selected patients with acute ischemic stroke.[26-29] For eligible patients, fibrinolytic therapy reduces disability and death from stroke.[26-29] Furthermore, these drugs improve the quality of life of stroke victims and are cost-effective: treated patients are more likely to be discharged home and less likely to be discharged to a nursing home.[30,31]

For these reasons, intravenous fibrinolytic therapy should be considered for all patients presenting to the hospital within 3 hours of the onset of signs and symptoms consistent with acute ischemic stroke[26,29,30,32] (Class I Recommendation).

The need for new cardiovascular interventions is not limited to adults with ACS and stroke. Many victims of trauma, drowning, electrocution, suffocation, airway obstruction, drug intoxication, and the like may be saved by prompt initiation of access to the emergency medical services (EMS) system, cardiopulmonary resuscitation (CPR), and use of the automated external defibrillator (AED).

Respiratory failure, congenital anomalies, or perinatal asphyxia may require resuscitation at birth. Trauma, a leading cause of disability and death in children and young adults,[33,34] requires prompt intervention with basic life support (BLS) and advanced life support not only to save lives but also to help avoid devastating brain damage that may result in long-term suffering and economic hardship.

The Purpose of This Manual

This manual is designed to meet the needs of healthcare providers who respond to cardiovascular and respiratory emergencies and others who aspire to serve as BLS instructors in the American Heart Association Training Network. The manual covers

- The role of the healthcare provider and the community in the total emergency cardiovascular care (ECC) system and the Chain of Survival

- A brief review of the anatomy and physiology of the respiratory, cardiovascular, and cerebrovascular systems

- The pathophysiology, recognition, and treatment of heart disease and stroke and the concept of prudent heart living

- The information and techniques needed for adult and pediatric CPR and special rescue situations

- The information needed to treat VF with an AED

- The pathophysiology, recognition, treatment, and prevention of foreign-body airway obstruction

- Injury prevention in the pediatric age group

- Safety factors in training and actual rescue

- Understanding the human dimension of CPR, including the psychology of resuscitation and stress management through critical incident stress debriefing (CISD)

- Ethical and legal considerations in CPR

In writing this manual we have tried to keep in mind the diversity of those who participate in the Healthcare Provider Course (for example, doctors, nurses, emergency medical technicians [EMTs], and public school teachers). Accordingly we have tried to respect the reader's knowledge without making assumptions about the reader's clinical experience in emergency cardiovascular care.

For the physician and nurse, some sections of this manual will serve as a basic review (anatomy and physiology, signs and symptoms of heart attack). For the lay rescuer, some sections will enrich existing knowledge or serve as "nice-to-know" information (advanced care and reference to medications).

Sidebars and Algorithms

We have used sidebars to present 3 types of material:

- Critical Concepts, such as the signs and symptoms of stroke

- Foundation Facts, which present the rationale for performing a procedure

- FYI (For Your Information), which presents material that may enrich a reader's understanding of a topic

When appropriate we have included algorithms that summarize the approach to a particular condition. Because the roles of the lay rescuer and EMT-basic are critical to BLS, these algorithms are based on prehospital care, but they can easily be adapted to many clinical situations in-hospital, outside the hospital, and in other settings.

The Purpose of This Chapter

This chapter reviews the lifesaving potential of BLS and advanced cardiovascular life support (ACLS), explains the importance of a community-wide EMS system, and defines the role of BLS and ACLS in emergency cardiovascular care. This chapter also presents the structural components of the Chain of Survival needed to save the lives of victims of cardiac arrest.

The Community as the Ultimate Coronary Care Unit

Public education and training are crucial aspects of any effort to reduce sudden cardiac death. Because the majority of sudden deaths caused by cardiac arrest occur outside the hospital, it is clear that the community must be recognized as "the ultimate coronary care unit."[35]

The CPR-ECC programs described in this chapter have been and will continue to be valuable forums for educating the community about its responsibility. Optimally the focus of any course or community program should be on both lifesaving techniques and prevention through reduction of risk factors.

Community training programs should incorporate education in primary prevention, which includes risk-factor detection and modification and awareness of the signals of an impending cardiovascular event.

Information should also be presented about secondary prevention, or prevention of myocardial infarction and sudden cardiac death in patients known to have coronary artery disease. It is clear that coronary artery disease, stroke, and other forms of atherosclerotic vascular disease are affected by community nutritional patterns, prosmoking messages delivered to children, and cultural and social pressures that mold unhealthy behaviors and lifestyles.

FIGURE 1. Community-based emergency cardiovascular care.

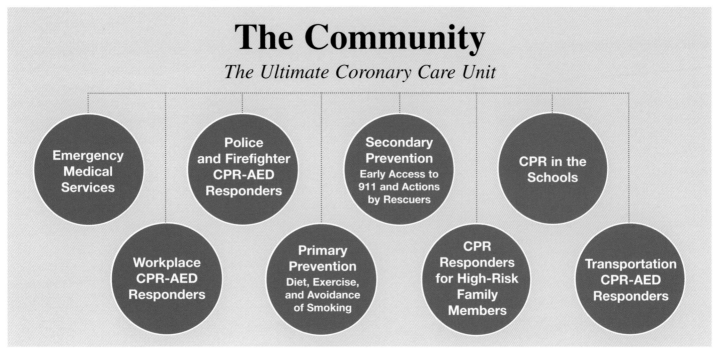

The Community
The Ultimate Coronary Care Unit

Emergency Medical Services

Police and Firefighter CPR-AED Responders

Secondary Prevention
Early Access to 911 and Actions by Rescuers

CPR in the Schools

Workplace CPR-AED Responders

Primary Prevention
Diet, Exercise, and Avoidance of Smoking

CPR Responders for High-Risk Family Members

Transportation CPR-AED Responders

Training laypersons in CPR and the use of AEDs saves lives that might otherwise be lost due to cardiac arrest. Communities with a high number of laypersons trained in lifesaving techniques such as CPR and use of an AED may achieve resuscitation rates as high as 49% for patients with documented out-of-hospital VF (a chaotic, uncoordinated quivering of the heart muscle).[36,37]

Training in CPR and use of an AED can take many forms. Emergency first responders such as police officers and firefighters should be trained in both adult and pediatric CPR and use of the AED so that early CPR and defibrillation can be offered throughout the community (including public transportation such as airplanes, trains, and ferries).

Training in CPR and AED use can also be provided to the general public through programs in the schools and the workplace, and programs for family members of persons considered to be at high risk for sudden cardiac arrest (certain newborns and patients with heart disease or chronic and dangerous arrhythmias). Take a moment to review the matrix (Figure 1) that illustrates the concept of community-based ECC.

Emergency Cardiovascular Care

ECC includes all responses (prehospital and in-hospital) needed to stabilize the victim or patient who develops sudden and often life-threatening events affecting the cardiovascular, cerebrovascular, and pulmonary systems. Acute ischemic coronary syndromes (angina and AMI) and stroke are by far the most frequent causes of these potentially catastrophic events. The ultimate goal of ECC is to maximize the outcome for all victims or patients.

In relation to cardiovascular and cerebrovascular diseases, ECC specifically includes

■ Recognition of the early warning signs of heart attack and stroke and activation of the EMS system, efforts to prevent complications, reassurance of the victim, and prompt availability of monitoring equipment

■ Provision of immediate CPR and use of the AED at the scene for victims of sudden cardiac arrest

■ Provision of ACLS at the scene and stabilization of the victim before transport

■ Transfer of the stabilized victim to an appropriate hospital where definitive cardiovascular care can be provided

The term *emergency cardiovascular care* in this context extends to the care of other life-threatening catastrophic events that may not initially involve the heart or brain, such as an obstruction of the airway by a foreign object, submersion/near-drowning, electrocution, trauma, and hypothermia. Pediatric and neonatal resuscitation are also included, even though in most instances in this age group the primary event does not occur in the heart or brain.

Emergency transportation without life support is not emergency cardiovascular care. Although transportation is an important aspect of ECC, the major emphasis of ECC is on early provision of definitive care, including CPR and use of an AED, advanced airway management, drug and electrical therapy, and stabilization of the victim of other life-threatening emergencies (for example, control of hemorrhage). Unnecessary delays at the scene must be avoided, but defibrillation when necessary and stabilization to the extent possible should be achieved before and during transport of the victim to the site of continuing care.

Basic Life Support

The 2 components of emergency cardio-vascular care are BLS and ACLS. BLS includes those interventions that can be rapidly performed by trained laypersons to ensure recognition of common emergencies, early access to ACLS, adequate airway, breathing, and oxygenation, and adequate circulation.

If BLS is performed correctly, (1) cardiac arrest may be prevented by rapid transport or initiation of skills that prevent cardiac arrest (for example, rescue breathing); (2) cardiorespiratory function may be restored by use of an AED; or (3) brain viability may be maintained by performance of CPR until advanced life support is provided.

BLS skills can be quickly mastered and performed anywhere by lay and professional rescuers alike. Because BLS skills may be lifesaving, they should be taught to everyone who is capable of learning them.

CPR is a critical component of BLS. Prompt bystander CPR is crucial to all resuscitative efforts.[38,39] In the absence of prompt bystander CPR, successful resuscitation of the out-of-hospital cardiac arrest victim is unlikely, despite the availability of a well-trained team of paramedics with a rapid response time.[38,39] AEDs are also an important part of BLS for lay responders and healthcare providers. The early delivery of an electric shock to a victim of sudden cardiac death can be lifesaving. Relief of foreign-body airway obstruction by providing 1 or more abdominal thrusts can restore adequate breathing and prevent death.[40] These are all examples of the value of early BLS.

All persons trained in CPR and use of an AED should have a well-formulated plan of action for use in an emergency, based on local community resources and the EMS system. When symptoms that sug-gest profound circulatory collapse and imminent cardiac arrest occur, a mobile life support unit should be summoned. This should reduce elapsed time from onset of symptoms to entry into the EMS system. In the absence of such a system, the victim should be brought without delay to an Emergency Department or other facility with 24-hour life support capability.

BLS should be initiated by any person present when cardiac or respiratory arrest occurs. To be successful, ECC depends on the layperson's understanding of the importance of early activation of the EMS system and his or her willingness and ability to initiate prompt, effective CPR. Accordingly, providing lifesaving BLS at this level can be considered primarily a public or community responsibility. The healthcare community, however, is responsible for providing leadership in educating the public and supporting community education and training.

Advanced Life Support

ACLS includes BLS plus the use of adjunctive equipment to support ventilation, establishment of intravenous access, administration of drugs, use of cardiac monitoring, defibrillation or other control of arrhythmias, and care after resuscitation. It also includes the establishment of communication necessary to ensure continued care. A physician must supervise and direct ACLS efforts in 1 of 3 ways: (1) in person at the scene, (2) by direct communication such as over the telephone, or (3) by a previously defined alternative mechanism such as standing orders or protocols.

Community-wide EMS

ECC should be an integral part of a community-wide EMS system. Each system should be based on local needs for patient care and available resources and should follow regional, state, and national guidelines. The success of such a system requires participation and planning to ensure operational and equipment compatibility within the system and between adjacent systems. The community must be willing both to fund the program and to monitor its effectiveness.

The initial planning for a community-wide EMS system should be handled by a local advisory council on emergency services charged with assessing community needs, defining priorities, and managing available resources to meet those needs. Critical evaluation of operating policies, procedures, statistics, and case reports must be the continuing responsibility of the medical director.

Operational activities must be evaluated against adopted protocols and reported outcomes. Skills evaluation of trained personnel, whether based in or out of the hospital, must be conducted on a regular basis. Ongoing educational programs, such as mock codes, must be developed to enhance skills retention.

The ECC segment of a community-wide emergency system is best provided through a trilevel system of coronary care. At level 1 are the ECC units, which include basic and advanced fixed ECC units and basic and advanced mobile units capable of defibrillation.[41,42] At level 2 are the emergency care units, coronary care units, and intermediate care units capable of providing fibrino-lytic therapy[43,44] and intensive care. At level 3 are the tertiary care centers capable of coronary revascularization and other necessary interventions.

The Expanding Role of BLS

As new technology develops, the distinction between BLS and ACLS becomes more blurred. Many techniques traditionally considered in the realm of ACLS have become routine BLS interventions. For example, the need to use a barrier device to reduce the chances of transmitting an infectious disease has become a critical issue for many BLS providers and is an essential component of any system in which lay responders (police and firefighters) participate. Lay

FIGURE 2. The AHA adult Chain of Survival. The 4 links or actions in the chain are (1) phone 911, (2) CPR, (3) early defibrillation, and (4) advanced care.

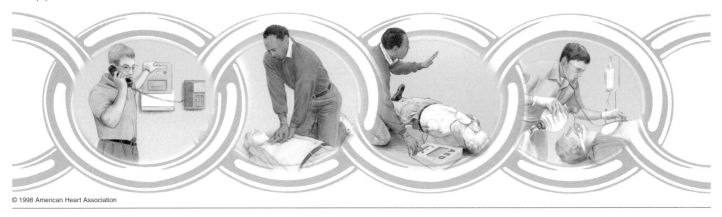

responders now commonly use basic adjuncts such as the pocket mask, bag-mask system, and laryngeal mask airway to provide positive-pressure ventilation. Some lay responders also administer supplemental oxygen to victims of myocardial infarction and stroke.

Emergency cardiovascular care and the relationship of BLS and ACLS are summarized in Figure 2.

The Chain of Survival

In recent years many clinicians, administrators, and researchers have recognized the need to improve the total community ECC system to optimize patient survival. Communities must identify weaknesses in the ECC system, implement modifications to strengthen the system, and optimize treatment for these critical patients.

The central question to be answered is whether the community ECC system results in optimal patient survival for out-of-hospital cardiac arrest. What is optimal in one community may not be possible in all communities. Early reports of high survival rates in mid-sized cities provided the EMS prototype adopted by most communities.[14,45] It is now clear, however, that provision of EMS care in rural and large metropolitan areas presents different challenges to EMS systems.[46] Each community must examine and devise its own mechanisms to achieve optimal patient survival rates.

Survival from cardiac arrest depends on a series of critical interventions. If any of these critical actions is neglected or delayed, survival is unlikely. The AHA has adopted and supported the ECC systems concept for many years.[47,48]

The term Chain of Survival[41] provides a useful metaphor for the elements of the ECC systems concept (see Figure 2). The ECC systems concept summarizes the present understanding of the best approach to the treatment of persons with sudden cardiac death. The 4 links in the adult Chain of Survival are

- Early access to the EMS system

- Early CPR

- Early defibrillation

- Early advanced cardiovascular care

Epidemiological and clinical research have established that effective ECC, whether prehospital or in-hospital, depends on these strong links, which are closely interdependent.[41] The Chain of Survival concept underscores several important principles:

- If any one link in the chain is weak or missing, survival rates will be poor. Weakness in system components is the main explanation for the variability in survival rates reported during the past 20 years.[45]

- All links must be strong to ensure rapid defibrillation. Unfortunately,

long 911 call–to-defibrillation intervals are common. Shorter intervals are necessary to improve survival rates.[41]

- Because the Chain of Survival has many links, evaluation of a single link will not measure the effectiveness of the system. Rather, the whole system must be tested. The survival-to-discharge rate has emerged as the gold standard for assessing the effectiveness of the treatment of cardiac arrest.

Recently considerable progress has been made toward providing clear methodological guidelines for study design, uniform terminology, and reporting of results.[45,49,50] This progress should facilitate future research on CPR and implementation of the Chain of Survival in each community.

The First Link: Early Access

Early access encompasses the events initiated after the patient's collapse until the arrival of EMS personnel prepared to provide care. Recognition of early warning signs, such as chest pain and shortness of breath, that encourages victims or rescuers to call 911 before collapse is key to the effectiveness of this link. With a cardiac arrest the following major events must occur rapidly:

- Early identification of patient collapse by a person who can activate the EMS system

- Recognition of lack of response

- Rapid notification (usually by telephone) of the EMS dispatcher before CPR is begun for an adult and after approximately 1 minute of rescue support for an infant or a child

- Rapid recognition by the dispatcher of a potential cardiac arrest

- Rapid dispatch of first responders (police and firefighters) and EMS responders to bring defibrillation and ACLS capabilities to the scene (Note: Many public areas may have AEDs at the scene.)

- Rapid arrival of first responders and EMS responders at the scene

- Arrival of EMS responders at the victim's side with all necessary equipment

- Identification of arrest

Each event is a vital part of the early access link. In most communities responsibility for these events rests with the 911 telephone system, the EMS dispatch system, and the EMS responder system.

The 911 Telephone System

In the United States widespread use of 911 has simplified and expedited emergency assistance. Nevertheless, many US communities do not have 911 service. A more recent development is the implementation of enhanced 911 in many communities. This option automatically provides dispatchers with the caller's address and telephone number. Obtaining 911 service—preferably enhanced 911—should be a top priority for all communities.

The EMS Dispatch System

Rapid emergency medical dispatch has emerged as a vital part of the early access link.[51-58] Although the organization, structure, and protocols of emergency medical dispatch (EMD) may vary from one EMS system to another, most EMD functions are the same across systems.

A new responsibility for EMS dispatchers is the provision of dispatcher-directed instructions, including how to perform

CPR, to 911 callers. Dispatchers may offer to provide instructions to the caller on how to perform CPR until EMS responders arrive. In controlled trials this method has been shown to be feasible and effective.[51]

All EMD systems should be able to immediately answer all emergency medical calls, quickly determine the nature of the call, identify the closest and most appropriate EMS responder unit(s), dispatch the unit to the scene on average in less than 1 minute, provide critical information to EMS responders about the type of emergency, and offer telephone-assisted CPR instructions.

The EMS Responder System

The EMS responder system is typically composed of responders trained in both BLS and ACLS.[59] The system may be structured for either a 1-tier or a multi-tier level of response. Most 1-tier systems use ACLS-trained (paramedic) responders, although some 1-tier systems use only BLS providers.

Two-tier systems usually provide first-responder units staffed with BLS-prepared EMTs or firefighters close to the scene,[59] followed by the second tier of ACLS responders. Two-tier systems in which first responders are trained in early defibrillation (BLS-D or EMT-D) are most effective in providing rapid defibrillation.[14]

Once dispatched, EMS responders must quickly reach the scene of the cardiac arrest, locate the patient, and arrive at the patient's side with all necessary equipment.

The Second Link: Early CPR

CPR is most effective when it is started immediately after the victim's collapse. Bystander CPR has been consistently shown to have a significant positive effect on survival.[19-21] The one possible exception is a situation in which the call-to-defibrillation interval is extremely short.[59] Bystander CPR is the best treat-

ment that a cardiac arrest patient can receive until the arrival of a defibrillator and ACLS care.[60,61]

Training in basic CPR has an additional effect on improving survival from out-of-hospital cardiac arrest. The CPR course also teaches citizens how to gain access to the EMS system more efficiently, thus shortening the time to the EMS call and defibrillation.

Bystander CPR rarely causes significant injury to victims, even when provided inappropriately for people not in cardiac arrest.[41]

Community-wide CPR programs should be developed wherever possible, including schools, military bases, housing complexes, workplaces, and public buildings. Communities need to remove psychological barriers that discourage citizens from learning and performing CPR.

Although bystander CPR is clearly of value, it is only temporizing and loses its value if the next links (early defibrillation and early ACLS) do not rapidly follow. Therefore, for an adult victim the bystander should establish that the victim is unresponsive, phone 911 for help, and then start CPR. Communities must target groups most likely to observe cardiac arrest or have the opportunity to perform bystander CPR. They should also place a priority on activation of the EMS system. The dispatcher should be told "CPR is in progress."

A lone, unassisted rescuer with an adult victim should activate the EMS system after establishing that the victim is unresponsive. In a pediatric arrest or special situations of adult arrest in which the most likely cause of arrest is respiratory (for example, trauma, submersion/near-drowning, or drug overdose), the EMS system should be activated after the trained rescuer provides approximately 1 minute of rescue support. This delay in EMS activation is appropriate to provide immediate ventilation when the likelihood of VF is low and the probability of respiratory arrest is high.

FIGURE 3. Emergency cardiovascular care: BLS and ACLS.

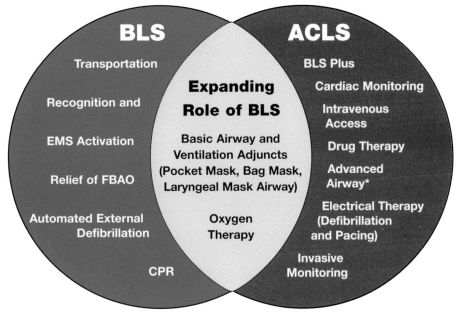

Emergency Cardiovascular Care

BLS
- Transportation
- Recognition and
- EMS Activation
- Relief of FBAO
- Automated External Defibrillation
- CPR

Expanding Role of BLS
- Basic Airway and Ventilation Adjuncts (Pocket Mask, Bag Mask, Laryngeal Mask Airway)
- Oxygen Therapy

ACLS
- BLS Plus
- Cardiac Monitoring
- Intravenous Access
- Drug Therapy
- Advanced Airway*
- Electrical Therapy (Defibrillation and Pacing)
- Invasive Monitoring

FBAO indicates foreign-body airway obstruction.
*Advanced airway management includes multiple techniques for establishing a patent airway, including tracheal intubation, surgical airway maneuvers, and suctioning.

The Third Link: Early Defibrillation

Early defibrillation is the link in the Chain of Survival that is most likely to improve survival rates (see Table 1).[14-24] The placement of AEDs in the hands of large numbers of trained rescuers may be the key intervention for increasing survival from out-of-hospital cardiac arrest.[62,63] The AHA strongly recommends that every emergency vehicle that may transport cardiac arrest patients be equipped with a defibrillator and that emergency personnel be trained to use and permitted to operate this device.[42]

Public Access Defibrillation

Time to defibrillation (the interval between collapse and defibrillation) is the critical variable for successful conversion from VF to a normal rhythm. Every minute that passes can reduce the chance for successful conversion by 7% to 10%.[64] The time to first shock can be shortened by placing AEDs in public buildings, stadiums, public transportation, condominiums, the workplace, and other locations where large numbers of people gather. Public access defibrillation (PAD) should result in increased return of spontaneous circulation, which should ultimately translate into increased survival. The PAD concept encompasses many CPR-AED responders. Take the time to review the FYI box to better understand how responders and response systems may be organized.

To permit and encourage the use of AEDs by the lay public, nearly all states have enacted facilitating legislation. In addition, the Cardiac Arrest Survival Act provides immunity for lay rescuers who use AEDs and for businesses or other entities or individuals who purchase AEDs for public access defibrillation.

This type of legislation serves 3 main purposes. First, it expands current "Good Samaritan" coverage of nontraditional responders or laypeople to include the use of AEDs. Second, it encourages the use of AEDs by providing immunity for the key players in the PAD program. State legislation may specify those to whom immunity is extended, specifically owners of AEDs, users of AEDs, and instructors and medical directors of PAD programs. Third, in many states PAD legislation defines the structural components of the PAD program, including involvement with the local EMS system, training requirements, and maintenance of AEDs. The structure of AED legislation varies from state to state. You should become familiar with the legislation in your state.

As AEDs become more common, physicians, nurses, and EMS personnel may find themselves in Good Samaritan circumstances in which an AED may be available.

Every medical professional should be familiar with the basic operation of an AED. This is why the AHA has made AED training an integral part of the Healthcare Provider Course. The details of PAD systems are covered in greater detail in Chapter 7 of this manual.

The Fourth Link: Early Advanced Care

Early advanced care provided by paramedics at the scene is another critical link in the management of cardiac arrest. ACLS brings equipment to support ventilation, establishes intravenous access, administers drugs, controls arrhythmias, and stabilizes the victim for transport. ACLS serves 3 primary purposes in the treatment of cardiac arrest:

1. It is designed to prevent cardiac arrest through the use of advanced airway management, administration of medications, and other interventions.

2. It includes therapies that may help resuscitate victims of cardiac arrest who are not in VF or who are not responding to defibrillation.

3. It can provide defibrillation if VF develops and prevent refibrillation and help stabilize the patient after resuscitation.

ACLS also includes numerous assessments and interventions that are used to treat noncardiac causes of respiratory and cardiac arrest.

EMS System Evaluation

The best way to evaluate the strength of the Chain of Survival is to assess the survival rates achieved by the system. The

---

FYI: Public Access Defibrillation

The AHA promotes the fastest possible defibrillation of victims of cardiac arrest. The public health initiative Public Access Defibrillation (PAD) is designed to place AEDs throughout the community in the hands of trained, nontraditional rescuers. These include police, security guards, and family members of patients at high risk for cardiac arrest.

PAD programs place AEDs in homes, police cars, worksites, and public gathering places under the supervision of licensed physicians. PAD rescuers must be trained in CPR and use of an AED. When AEDs are readily available, rescuers can provide defibrillation within the first few minutes of out-of-hospital cardiac arrest, dramatically increasing the victim's chances of survival.

The AHA has developed the Heartsaver AED Course to support the PAD movement and specific PAD programs. The course is designed to help rescuers learn how to perform CPR and use a pocket mask and an AED. These skills are essential in caring for the victim of cardiac arrest.

---

cost of data collection for a system may be significant. However, it is only through evaluation that systems can routinely improve their services. All ECC systems should assess their performance through an ongoing evaluation process. For evaluation data to be meaningful, it is necessary to compare EMS systems. This, in turn, requires the use of standardized definitions and terms of reference (see Table 2). Until recently, uniform terminology has not been available, producing a cardiac arrest Tower of Babel.[35] Reported survival rates in the literature range from 0% to 44%. It is not yet understood whether these profound variations are due to differences in population, treatment protocol, system organization, rescuer skills, or reporting practices.

There is now international consensus on the importance of using standard terminology and methods to evaluate survival from cardiac arrest and the Chain of Survival (Utstein style).[50] Clear, unambiguous international terminology has been created, a uniform method of reporting data has been established, and methods for cardiac arrest research have been improved.[50] These Utstein reporting definitions and criteria are now also available for pediatric arrest,[65] laboratory animal research,[66] and in-hospital arrest.[67]

Improving the ECC system, however, first requires an accurate measurement of the baseline survival rate for each community.

TABLE 1. Effectiveness of Early Defibrillation Programs

Location	Before early defibrillation	After early defibrillation	Odds ratio for improved survival
King County, Washington	7 (4/56)	26 (10/38)	3.7
Iowa	3 (1/31)	19 (12/64)	6.3
SE Minnesota	4 (1/27)	17 (6/36)	4.3
NE Minnesota	2 (3/118)	10 (8/81)	5.0
Wisconsin	4 (32/893)	11 (33/304)	3.3

Values are percent surviving and, in parentheses, how many patients had VF. From Reference 64.

This can be achieved by implementing the following recommendations:

1. Develop an evaluation process in every ECC system.

2. Include an accurate assessment of survival rates using standardized nomenclature and reporting methods. In assessments of survival, integrate into EMS systems evolving concepts of consensus terminology, data collection, system description, and CPR research methods.

3. Set goals to improve the survival rate. The goals established should be feasible, given the structure and demographic characteristics of the local system. To identify these goals, it will be necessary to evaluate current performance (including the survival rate) and identify weak links in the Chain of Survival.

4. Develop an ongoing program of quality improvement. Review survival rates, identify gaps between goals and current performance, identify strategies to improve system performance, and evaluate whether performance improves with these modifications.

5. Design the evaluation specifically to benefit the local community. As a secondary interest, information should be shared regionally and nationally to help other communities develop optimal systems.

Role of the AHA in the Community Chain of Survival

The AHA is the world's largest volunteer health organization. The AHA mission is to reduce disability and death from cardiovascular diseases and stroke.

In 1963 the AHA established a Committee on Cardiopulmonary Resuscitation. The committee was expanded in 1971 to include ECC and became the Committee on Emergency Cardiac Care. A working group on pediatric resuscitation was added in 1978. In 1989 the ECC subcommittee gained committee status, and the working groups were elevated to subcommittees.

In 1997 the term *cardiac* was replaced with the word *cardiovascular* to reflect the increased emphasis on early management of stroke. Today the Emergency Cardiovascular Care Committee provides leadership to a training network of more than 200 000 instructors of BLS, ACLS, and pediatric life support.

The goal of the AHA CPR-ECC programs is to increase the number of persons who are knowledgeable about prevention of heart disease and arrest and to educate the lay public and healthcare professionals about the emergency treatment of cardiopulmonary arrest. The AHA provides support for prevention and treatment of cardiovascular disease through research, education, and community service programs. The ECC training network is an effective structure for dissemination of educational programs that allows people in the community to participate in a variety of ways.

Many opportunities exist for volunteers to serve the AHA in the areas of development, communications, and program, including ECC. To help the AHA achieve its mission, contact your local AHA.

Summary of Basic Life Support

Basic life support includes the first 3 links in the Chain of Survival: early access to 911, early CPR, and early defibrillation. When connected with the fourth link, early advanced life support, BLS maximizes the chances of survival of victims of heart attack, stroke, and sudden cardiac arrest. Healthcare providers play an essential role in the development of ECC systems, education of the public, and performance of BLS in clinical situations.

Summary of Key Concepts

Take the time to review the key concepts covered in this chapter:

- Cardiovascular disease is the leading cause of death in the United States.

- Ventricular fibrillation is the most common cardiac arrest rhythm; it is treated with early defibrillation.

- BLS and ACLS are components of emergency cardiovascular care.

- The Chain of Survival represents the interventions needed to save victims of sudden cardiac arrest and includes early access to 911, early CPR, early defibrillation, and early advanced care.

- Every minute that passes reduces the chances of conversion from VF to a normal rhythm.

- Public access defibrillation is an AHA initiative that places AEDs throughout the community in the hands of laypersons to decrease the time interval from cardiac arrest to defibrillation.

- A universal, enhanced 911 system is essential to reduce time from EMS notification to arrival of EMS personnel.

- A standard process and nomenclature (Utstein style) is essential to evaluate the effectiveness of ECC and EMS systems.

TABLE 2. Definitions and Terminology in ECC[67]

Cardiac arrest — Cardiac arrest is the cessation of cardiac mechanical activity. It is a clinical diagnosis, confirmed by unresponsiveness, absence of detectable pulse, and apnea (or agonal respirations).

Cardiopulmonary resuscitation (CPR) — CPR is an attempt to restore spontaneous circulation through any of a broad range of maneuvers and techniques.

Basic CPR — Basic CPR is the attempt to restore spontaneous circulation by using chest wall compressions and pulmonary ventilation.

Bystander CPR, layperson CPR, or citizen CPR — These terms are synonymous; however, *bystander CPR* is preferred. Bystander CPR is an attempt to provide basic CPR by a person not at that moment part of the organized emergency response system.

Basic life support (BLS) — BLS is the phase of ECC that includes recognition of cardiac arrest, access to the EMS system, and basic CPR. It may also refer to the educational program in these subjects.

Advanced CPR or advanced cardiovascular life support (ACLS) — These terms refer to attempts to restore spontaneous circulation with basic CPR plus advanced airway management, tracheal intubation, defibrillation, and intravenous medications. ACLS may also refer to the educational program that provides guidelines for these techniques.

Emergency medical services (EMS) or emergency personnel — persons who respond to medical emergencies in an official capacity are emergency (or EMS) personnel. The EMS system has 2 major divisions: EMS dispatchers and EMS responders.

> *EMS dispatchers* — EMS personnel responsible for dispatching EMS responders to the scene of medical emergencies and providing telephone instructions to bystanders at the scene while professionals are en route.

> *EMS responders* — EMS personnel who respond to medical emergencies by going to the scene in an emergency vehicle. They may be first, second, or third responders, depending on the EMS system. They may be trained in ACLS or BLS. All should be capable of performing defibrillation. *Emergency medical technician (EMT)* usually denotes BLS training. *Paramedic or EMT-P* usually denotes ACLS training.

ECC system — The ECC system refers to all aspects of ECC, including that rendered by emergency personnel. The extended ECC system also includes bystander CPR, rapid activation of the EMS system, Emergency Departments, intensive care units, cardiac rehabilitation, cardiac prevention programs, BLS and ACLS training programs, and citizen defibrillation.

Chain of Survival — The Chain of Survival is a metaphor to communicate the interdependence of a community's emergency response to cardiac arrest. This response is composed of 4 links: early access, early CPR, early defibrillation, and early ACLS. If a link is weak or missing, the result will be poor survival despite excellence in the rest of the ECC system.

Presumed cardiac cause — Cardiac arrest due to presumed cardiac cause is the major focus of ECC. When reporting cardiac outcome data, studies of cardiac arrest should exclude arrests due to obvious noncardiac causes. Because of practical considerations (lack of autopsy information, cost), all arrests are considered to be of cardiac cause unless an obvious noncardiac cause can be identified. Common noncardiac diagnoses that should be separated during analysis of cardiac arrest outcome include sudden infant death syndrome, drug overdose, suicide, drowning, trauma, exsanguination, and terminal illness.

Time intervals — The Utstein recommendations have provided a rational nomenclature for important time intervals. Time intervals should be reported as the A-to-B interval, which represents the period that begins at time point A and ends at time point B. These are more informative than imprecise terms like *downtime* or *response time*. The following terms, for example, are suggested:

> *911-call–to-dispatch interval* — The interval from the time the call for help is first received by the 911 center until the time the emergency vehicle leaves for the scene.

> *Vehicle-dispatch–to-scene interval* — The interval beginning when the emergency vehicle departs for the scene and ending when EMS responders indicate the vehicle has stopped at the scene or address. This does not include the time interval until emergency personnel arrive at the patient's side or the interval until defibrillation occurs.

> *Vehicle-at-scene–to–patient-access interval* — The interval from when the emergency response vehicle stops moving at the scene or address until EMS responders are at the patient's side.

> *Call-to-defibrillation interval* — The interval from receipt of the call at the emergency response system center until the patient receives the first shock.

Review Questions

1. While walking down the street you see a 50-year-old man collapse. He is unresponsive, and you send a bystander to phone 911. You begin CPR immediately, using a pocket mask. The police arrive with an AED. The defibrillator delivers a shock to the patient. A normal heart rhythm returns, and paramedics administer drugs to stabilize the heart rhythm. These actions *collectively* best describe

   a. basic life support

   b. the Chain of Survival

   c. the entire ECC system

   d. CPR

2. In the case above, what specific action is exclusively an ACLS intervention?

   a. EMS activation

   b. use of the AED

   c. performance of CPR

   d. administration of drugs

3. You are asked by the administrators of your hospital to set up a cardiac arrest survival database and reporting system. You must select a structure based on 3 criteria: (1) it must represent an international standard; (2) it must use standardized terminology; and (3) it must use standard definitions of response intervals. What style reporting system would meet these criteria?

   a. Hazinski

   b. Aufderheide

   c. Cummins

   d. Utstein

4. You have been performing CPR on a patient who collapsed 4 minutes ago. The police arrive with an AED and deliver shocks to the victim at the beginning of the fifth minute after collapse. When defibrillation is provided approximately 5 minutes after collapse with VF cardiac arrest, what is the *approximate* statistical probability that this victim will survive?

   a. 10%

   b. 20%

   c. 30%

   d. 50%

How did you do?

Answers: **1**, b; **2**, d; **3**, d; **4**, d.

References

1. *Heart and Stroke Facts: 2000 Statistical Update*. Dallas, Tex: American Heart Association; 1999.

2. Graves EJ. National hospital discharge survey, 1991. *Vital Health Statistics,* vol 13. Hyattsville, Md: US Dept of Health and Human Services; 1993.

3. *Heart and Stroke Facts: 1996 Statistical Supplement*. Dallas, Tex: American Heart Association; 1995.

4. Gillum RF. Trends in acute myocardial infarction and coronary heart disease death in the United States. *J Am Coll Cardiol.* 1994;23: 1273-1277.

5. Kannel WB, Schatzkin A. Sudden death: lessons from subsets in population studies. *J Am Coll Cardiol.* 1985;5(suppl):141B-149B.

6. Brouwer MA, Martin JS, Maynard C, Wirkus M, Litwin PE, Verheugt FW, Weaver WD. Influence of early prehospital thrombolysis on mortality and event-free survival (the Myocardial Infarction Triage and Intervention [MITI] Randomized Trial). MITI Project Investigators. *Am J Cardiol.* 1996;78:497-502.

7. Raitt MH, Maynard C, Wagner GS, Cerqueira MD, Selvester RH, Weaver WD. Relation between symptom duration before thrombolytic therapy and final myocardial infarct size. *Circulation.* 1996;93:48-53.

8. Wackers FJ, Terrin ML, Kayden DS, Knatterud G, Forman S, Braunwald E, Zaret BL. Quantitative radionuclide assessment of regional ventricular function after thrombolytic therapy for acute myocardial infarction: results of phase I Thrombolysis in Myocardial Infarction (TIMI) trial. *J Am Coll Cardiol.* 1989;13:998-1005.

9. Res JC, Simoons ML, van der Wall EE, van Eenige MJ, Vermeer F, Verheugt FW, Wijns W, Braat S, Remme WJ, Serruys PW, et al. Long term improvement in global left ventricular function after early thrombolytic treatment in acute myocardial infarction. Report of a randomised multicentre trial of intracoronary streptokinase in acute myocardial infarction. *Br Heart J.* 1986;56:414-421.

10. Mathey DG, Sheehan FH, Schofer J, Dodge HT. Time from onset of symptoms to thrombolytic therapy: a major determinant of myocardial salvage in patients with acute transmural infarction. *J Am Coll Cardiol.* 1985;6:518-525.

11. Serruys PW, Simoons ML, Suryapranata H, Vermeer F, Wijns W, van den Brand M, Bar F, Zwaan C, Krauss XH, Remme WJ, et al. Preservation of global and regional left ventricular function after early thrombolysis in acute myocardial infarction. *J Am Coll Cardiol.* 1986;7:729-742.

12. Newby LK, Rutsch WR, Califf RM, Simoons ML, Aylward PE, Armstrong PW, Woodlief LH, Lee KL, Topol EJ, Van de Werf F. Time from symptom onset to treatment and outcomes after thrombolytic therapy. GUSTO-1 Investigators. *J Am Coll Cardiol*. 1996;27: 1646-1655.

13. Anderson JL, Karagounis LA, Califf RM. Metaanalysis of five reported studies on the relation of early coronary patency grades with mortality and outcomes after acute myocardial infarction. *Am J Cardiol*. 1996;78:1-8.

14. Eisenberg MS, Horwood BT, Cummins RO, Reynolds-Haertle R, Hearne TR. Cardiac arrest and resuscitation: a tale of 29 cities. *Ann Emerg Med*. 1990;19:179-186.

15. Emergency Cardiovascular Care Committee, American Heart Association. *Heartsaver ABC*. Dallas, Tex: American Heart Association; 1999.

16. Emergency Cardiovascular Care Committee, American Heart Association. *Heartsaver CPR in Schools*. Dallas, Tex: American Heart Association; 1999.

17. Bayes de Luna A, Coumel P, Leclercq JF. Ambulatory sudden cardiac death: mechanisms of production of fatal arrhythmia on the basis of data from 157 cases. *Am Heart J*. 1989;117:151-159.

18. Weaver WD, Hill D, Fahrenbruch CE, Copass MK, Martin JS, Cobb LA, Hallstrom AP. Use of the automatic external defibrillator in the management of out-of-hospital cardiac arrest. *N Engl J Med*. 1988;319:661-666.

19. Cummins RO, Graves JR. Critical results of standard CPR: prehospital and inhospital. In: Kaye W, Bircher N, eds. *Cardiopulmonary Resuscitation. Clinics in Critical Care Medicine*. New York, NY: Churchill-Livingstone; 1989.

20. Cummins RO, Eisenberg MS. Prehospital cardiopulmonary resuscitation: is it effective? *JAMA*. 1985;253:2408-2412.

21. Cummins RO, Eisenberg MS, Hallstrom AP, Litwin PE. Survival of out-of-hospital cardiac arrest with early initiation of cardiopulmonary resuscitation. *Am J Emerg Med*. 1985;3: 114-119.

22. Ladwig KH, Schoefinius A, Danner R, Gurtler R, Herman R, Koeppel A, Hauber P. Effects of early defibrillation by ambulance personnel on short- and long-term outcome of cardiac arrest survival: the Munich experiment. *Chest*. 1997;112:1584-1591.

23. Sweeney TA, Runge JW, Gibbs MA, Raymond JM, Schafermeyer RW, Norton HJ, Boyle-Whitesel MJ. EMT defibrillation does not increase survival from sudden cardiac death in a two-tiered urban-suburban EMS system. *Ann Emerg Med*. 1998;31:234-240.

24. Kellermann AL, Hackman BB, Somes G, Kreth TK, Nail L, Dobyns P. Impact of first-responder defibrillation in an urban

25. Easton JD, Hart RG, Sherman DG, Kaste M. Diagnosis and management of ischemic stroke, part I: threatened stroke and its management. *Curr Probl Cardiol*. 1983;8:1-76.

26. The National Institute of Neurological Disorders and Stroke rt-PA Stroke Study Group. Tissue plasminogen activator for acute ischemic stroke. *N Engl J Med*. 1995; 33:1581-1587.

27. del Zoppo GJ, Higashida RT, Furlan AJ, Pessin MS, Rowley HA, Gent M. PROACT: a phase II randomized trial of recombinant prourokinase by direct arterial delivery in acute middle cerebral artery stroke. PROACT Investigators. Prolyse in Acute Cerebral Thromboembolism. *Stroke*. 1998;29:4-11.

28. Bendszus M, Urbach H, Ries F, Solymosi L. Outcome after local intra-arterial fibrinolysis compared with the natural course of patients with a dense middle cerebral artery on early CT. *Neuroradiology*. 1998;40:54-58.

29. Wardlaw JM, del Zoppo G, Yamaguchi T. Thrombolysis for acute ischaemic stroke. *Cochrane Database of Systematic Reviews*. 4th issue. 1999.

30. Kwiatkowski TG, Libman RB, Frankel M, Tilley BC, Morgenstern LB, Lu M, Broderick JP, Lewandowski CA, Marler JR, Levine SR, Brott T, for the NINDS rt-PA Stroke Study Group. Effects of tissue plasminogen activator for acute ischemic stroke at one year. *N Engl J Med*. 1999;340:1781-1787.

31. Fagan SC, Morgenstern LB, Petitta A, Ward RE, Tilley BC, Marler JR, Levine SR, Broderick JP, Kwiatkowski TG, Frankel M, Brott TG, Walker MD, the NINDS rt-PA Study Group. Cost-effectiveness of tissue plasminogen activator for acute ischemic stroke. *Neurology*. 1998;50:883-890.

32. Furlan A, Higashida R, Wechsler L, Gent M, Rowley H, Kase C, Pessin M, Ahuja A, Callahan F, Clark WM, Silver F, Rivera F. Intra-arterial Prourokinase for acute ischemic stroke. The PROACT II Study: a randomized controlled trial. *JAMA*. 1999;282:2003-2011.

33. Division of Injury Control, Center for Environmental Health and Injury Control, Centers for Disease Control. Childhood injuries in the United States. *Am J Dis Child*. 1990;144:627-646.

34. Guyer B, Ellers B. Childhood injuries in the United States: mortality, morbidity, and cost. *Am J Dis Child*. 1990;144:649-652.

35. McIntyre KM. Cardiopulmonary resuscitation and the ultimate coronary care unit. *JAMA*. 1980;244:510-511.

36. White RD, Asplin BR, Bugliosi TF, Hankins DG. High discharge survival rate after out-of-hospital ventricular fibrillation with rapid

defibrillation by police and paramedics. *Ann Emerg Med*. 1996;28:480-485.

37. White RD, Hankins DG, Bugliosi TF. Seven years' experience with early defibrillation by police and paramedics in an emergency medical services system. *Resuscitation*. 1998;39: 145-151.

38. Larsen MP, Eisenberg MS, Cummins RO, Hallstrom AP. Predicting survival from out-of-hospital cardiac arrest: a graphic model. *Ann Emerg Med*. 1993;22:1652-1658.

39. Swor RA, Jackson RE, Cynar M, Sadler E, Basse E, Boji B, Rivera-Rivera EJ, Maher A, Grubb W, Jacobson R, et al. Bystander CPR, ventricular fibrillation, and survival in witnessed, unmonitored out-of-hospital cardiac arrest. *Ann Emerg Med*. 1995;25:780-784.

40. Heimlich HJ. A life-saving maneuver to prevent food-choking. *JAMA*. 1975;234: 398-401.

41. Cummins RO, Ornato JP, Thies WH, Pepe PE. Improving survival from sudden cardiac arrest: the "chain of survival" concept. A statement for health professionals from the Advanced Cardiac Life Support Subcommittee and the Emergency Cardiac Care Committee, American Heart Association. *Circulation*. 1991;83:1832-1847.

42. Kerber RE. Statement on early defibrillation from the Emergency Cardiac Care Committee, American Heart Association. *Circulation*. 1991;83:2233.

43. Gunnar RM, Bourdillon PD, Dixon DW, Fuster V, Karp RB, Kennedy JW, Klocke FJ, Passamani ER, Pitt B, Rapaport E, et al. ACC/AHA guidelines for the early management of patients with acute myocardial infarction. A report of the American College of Cardiology/American Heart Association Task Force on Assessment of Diagnostic and Therapeutic Cardiovascular Procedures (subcommittee to develop guidelines for the early management of patients with acute myocardial infarction). *Circulation*. 1990;82:664-707.

44. ACC/AHA guidelines for the early management of patients with acute myocardial infarction: a report of the American College of Cardiology/American Heart Association Task Force. Special report. *J Am Coll Cardiol*. 1990;16:249-292.

45. Eisenberg MS, Cummins RO, Damon S, Larsen MP, Hearne TR. Survival rates from out-of-hospital cardiac arrest: recommendations for uniform definitions and data to report. *Ann Emerg Med*. 1990;19:1249-1259.

46. Becker LB, Ostrander MP, Barrett J, Kondos GT, CPR Chicago. Outcome of CPR in a large metropolitan area: where are the survivors? *Ann Emerg Med*. 1991;20:355-361.

47. Atkins JM. Emergency medical service systems in acute cardiac care: state of the art. *Circulation*. 1986;74(suppl IV): IV-4-IV-8.

48. American Heart Association. Standards and guidelines for cardiopulmonary resuscitation (CPR) and emergency cardiac care (ECC). *JAMA*. 1980;244:453-509.

49. Jastremski MS. In-hospital cardiac arrest. *Ann Emerg Med*. 1993;22:113-117.

50. Cummins RO, Chamberlain DA, Abramson NS, Allen M, Baskett PJ, Becker L, Bossaert L, Delooz HH, Dick WF, Eisenberg MS, Evans TR, Holmberg S, Kerber R, Mullie A, Ornato JP, Sandoe E, Skulberg A, Tunstall-Pedoe H, Swanson R, Thies WH. Recommended guidelines for uniform reporting of data from out-of-hospital cardiac arrest: the Utstein style. A statement for health professionals from a task force of the American Heart Association, the European Resuscitation Council, the Heart and Stroke Foundation of Canada, and the Australian Resuscitation Council. *Circulation*. 1991;84:960-975.

51. Bang A, Biber B, Isaksson L, Lindqvist J, Herlitz J. Evaluation of dispatcher-assisted cardiopulmonary resuscitation. *Eur J Emerg Med*. 1999;6:175-183.

52. National Association of EMS Physicians. Emergency medical dispatching. *Prehosp Disaster Med*. 1989;4:163-166.

53. Nordberg M. NAEMD (National Academy of Emergency Medical Dispatch) strives for universal certification. *Emerg Med Serv*. 1999;28:45-46.

54. Clawson JJ, Sinclair B. "Medical Miranda" — improved emergency medical dispatch information from police officers. *Prehosp Disaster Med*. 1999;14:93-96.

55. National Heart Attack Alert Program Coordinating Committee Access to Care Subcommittee. Emergency medical dispatching: rapid identification and treatment of acute myocardial infarction. *Am J Emerg Med*. 1995;13: 67-73.

56. Porteous GH, Corry MD, Smith WS. Emergency medical services dispatcher identification of stroke and transient ischemic attack. *Prehosp Emerg Care*. 1999;3:211-216.

57. *Standard Practice for Emergency Medical Dispatch*. Philadelphia, Pa: American Society for Testing and Materials; 1990. Publication F1258-90.

58. Pepe PE, Almaguer DR. Emergency medical services personnel and ground transport vehicles. *Probl Crit Care*. 1990;4:470-476.

59. Troiano P, Masaryk J, Stueven HA, Olson D, Barthell E, Waite EM. The effect of bystander CPR on neurologic outcome in survivors of prehospital cardiac arrests. *Resuscitation*. 1989;17:91-98.

60. Ritter G, Wolfe RA, Goldstein S, Landis JR, Vasu CM, Acheson A, Leighton R, Medendrop SV. The effect of bystander CPR on survival of out-of-hospital cardiac arrest victims. *Am Heart J*. 1985;110:932-937.

61. Bossaert L, Van Hoeyweghen R. Bystander cardiopulmonary resuscitation (CPR) in out-of-hospital cardiac arrest. The Cerebral Resuscitation Study Group. *Resuscitation*. 1989;17(suppl):S55-S69.

62. Cobb LA, Eliastam M, Kerber RE, Melker R, Moss AJ, Newell L, Paraskos JA, Weaver WD, Weil M, Weisfeldt ML. Report of the American Heart Association Task Force on the Future of Cardiopulmonary Resuscitation. *Circulation*. 1992;85:2346-2355.

63. Weisfeldt ML, Kerber RE, McGoldrick RP, Moss AJ, Nichol G, Ornato JP, Palmer DG, Riegel B, Smith SC. Public access defibrillation: a statement for healthcare professionals from the American Heart Association Task Force on Automatic External Defibrillation. *Circulation*. 1995;92:2763.

64. Cummins RO. From concept to standard-of-care? Review of the clinical experience with automated external defibrillators. *Ann Emerg Med*. 1989;18:1269-1275.

65. Zaritsky A, Nadkarni V, Hazinski MF, Foltin G, Quan L, Wright J, Fiser D, Zideman D, O'Malley P, Chameides L, Cummins RO. Recommended guidelines for uniform reporting of pediatric advanced life support: the pediatric Utstein style. A statement for healthcare professionals from a task force of the American Academy of Pediatrics, the American Heart Association, and the European Resuscitation Council Writing Group. *Circulation*. 1995;92:2006-2020.

66. Idris AH, Becker LB, Ornato JP, Hedges JR, Bircher NG, Chandra NC, Cummins RO, Dick W, Ebmeyer U, Halperin HR, Hazinski MF, Kerber RE, Kern KB, Safar P, Steen PA, Swindle MM, Tsitlik JE, von Planta I, von Planta M, Wears RL, Weil MH. Utstein-style guidelines for uniform reporting of laboratory CPR research. A statement for healthcare professionals from a task force of the American Heart Association, the American College of Emergency Physicians, the American College of Cardiology, the European Resuscitation Council, the Heart and Stroke Foundation of Canada, the Institute of Critical Care Medicine, the Safar Center for Resuscitation Research, and the Society for Academic Emergency Medicine. *Circulation*. 1996;94:2324-2336.

67. Cummins RO, Chamberlain D, Hazinski MF, Nadkarni V, et al. Recommended guidelines for reviewing, reporting and conducting research on in-hospital resuscitation: the in-hospital "Utstein style": a statement for healthcare professionals from the American Heart Association, the European Resuscitation Council, the Heart and Stroke Foundation of Canada, the Australian Resuscitation Council, and the Resuscitation Councils of Southern Africa. *Circulation*. 1997;95:2213-2239.

You are a healthcare provider on the medical-surgical floor of a hospital. You enter a room and note that a 50-year-old female patient has collapsed on the floor next to her bed. You check her and find that she is unresponsive. A nursing student responds to your shout for help, and you ask him to call a code 99 (cardiac arrest; may be called code blue). You open the patient's airway and check for breathing. You observe only weak and irregular gasping breaths, and you note that the woman's skin is becoming increasingly cyanotic.

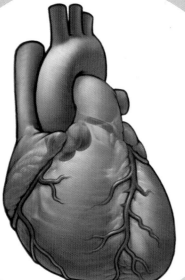

As you prepare to give 2 slow breaths with a mouth-to-mask device, several healthcare providers arrive in the room and begin to set up resuscitation equipment. One of them suggests that rescue breathing is unnecessary because the patient is already breathing. You disregard these comments and immediately provide 2 slow breaths and check for signs of circulation. The patient begins moving her arms but is still taking only gasping breaths. You continue rescue breathing (now using a bag and mask with supplemental oxygen) for about 2 minutes and she begins to respond.

Your colleague asks, "Why did you provide rescue breaths to someone who was breathing?" You explain that the patient was exhibiting "agonal" respirations that were inadequate to maintain oxygenation and ventilation. You further explain that victims of respiratory and cardiac arrest often exhibit this breathing pattern and still require rescue breathing. The victim returns home 1 week later, grateful for your immediate and confident actions.

Anatomy and Physiology of the Respiratory, Cardiovascular, and Cerebrovascular Systems

Overview

The detection of cardiovascular emergencies and effective performance of CPR and relief of foreign-body airway obstruction require a basic understanding of the anatomy and physiology of the respiratory, cardiovascular, and cerebrovascular systems. This chapter will provide a basic review of these 3 critical systems and lay the foundation for the discussion that follows in later chapters.

The Respiratory System

Anatomy of the Respiratory System

The respiratory system (Figure 1) has 4 components: (1) the airways that conduct air from the outside to the inside of the body, (2) the alveoli — small air sacs in the lungs where gas exchange occurs, (3) a neuromuscular component, and (4) the arteries, capillaries, and veins themselves.

The airway is divided into 2 parts, the upper and the lower airway. The upper airway comprises the nose and mouth, the pharynx (behind the tongue), and the larynx (or voice box). The lower airway comprises the trachea (or windpipe), bronchi (1 bronchus to the right lung and 1 to the left lung), and bronchioles (branches of the bronchi that terminate in the alveoli).

The neuromuscular component of the respiratory system is composed of the respiratory center in the brain, the nerves to and from the muscles of respiration, and the muscles of respiration. The chest (thoracic) cage is composed of the ribs, which are attached in back to the spine and in front to the sternum. The major muscles of respiration are (1) the large, sheetlike diaphragm, which is attached to the margin of the lower ribs, which extends from front to back and separates the chest cavity from the abdominal cavity; (2) the muscles between the ribs (the intercostal muscles); and (3) some muscles of the neck and shoulder girdle.

Learning Objectives

After reading this chapter you should be able to

1. Describe the anatomy and physiology of the respiratory system

2. Define respiratory arrest and respiratory insufficiency

3. Name the most common cause of airway obstruction

4. Describe the anatomy and physiology of the cardiovascular system

5. Describe the anatomy and physiology of the cerebrovascular system

The alveoli are tiny air sacs that receive fresh inspired gas (which contains 21% oxygen [or more if supplementary oxygen is used]) from the airways and take up carbon dioxide from the blood. The alveoli are lined by a thin layer of cells. On the other side of this layer lies a fine network of capillaries. The alveoli and associated capillaries are the basic lung units.

The pulmonary arteries carry blood with low oxygen content from the right side of the heart through the pulmonary circulation into the capillaries surrounding the alveoli. The capillaries carry blood to the alveoli to pick up oxygen and eliminate carbon dioxide. The pulmonary veins carry blood with high oxygen content from the lungs back to the left side of the heart.

Physiology of the Respiratory System

The function of the respiratory system is to bring oxygen from the air into the blood and to eliminate carbon dioxide from the body. All body cells need a continuous supply of oxygen to function. During metabolism carbon dioxide is produced and must be eliminated. If oxygen delivery to the cells is inadequate or carbon dioxide elimination is reduced, acidosis can develop.

The function of the cardiovascular system is to transport oxygenated blood from the lungs to the cells of the body and to transport blood containing carbon

FIGURE 1. Anatomy of the respiratory system.

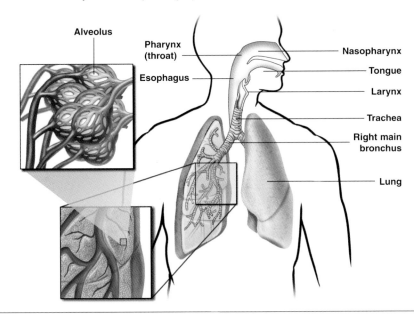

Inspiration (breathing in) is an active process. The diaphragm is the chief muscle of inspiration. It contracts and descends toward the abdominal cavity, increasing intrathoracic volume (volume inside the chest). At the same time the intercostal muscles contract and lift the rib cage, further increasing intrathoracic volume. When the intrathoracic volume increases, intrathoracic pressure and the pressure within the lungs falls below atmospheric pressure. The difference in pressure between the atmosphere and the lungs draws air into the lungs.

Expiration (or exhalation) is generally a passive process. As the muscles relax, the ribs descend and the diaphragm rises, reducing the volume of the chest cavity. The elastic lung passively becomes smaller, and the air inside the lung moves out.

Respiratory Arrest and Insufficiency

Respiratory arrest refers to the absence of breathing. Respiratory insufficiency implies that although breathing may be present, it is inadequate to maintain normal levels of oxygen and carbon dioxide in the blood. Patients in respiratory arrest will require positive-pressure ventilation by mouth-to-mouth, mouth-to-mask, or bag-mask ventilation. Patients with respiratory insufficiency may need positive-pressure ventilation or supplemental oxygen to ensure adequate oxygenation of tissues.

Airway Obstruction

Airway obstruction, particularly foreign-body airway obstruction (FBAO), is presented in detail in Chapter 8. The most common cause of airway obstruction is occlusion by upper airway structures, such as the tongue and epiglottis (a fingerlike structure at the base of the tongue near the back of the throat). Any condition that leads to unresponsiveness or loss of tone in the muscles of the jaw can cause the tongue (or epiglottis) to fall toward the back of the throat and obstruct the airway (see Figure 2).

dioxide from the cells of the body to the lungs. If oxygenation of the blood in the lungs is reduced by respiratory insufficiency or failure or if the delivery of blood (cardiac output) is reduced by poor cardiovascular function, oxygen delivery to the cells will decrease and tissue hypoxia will develop. At this point cells must switch from aerobic (oxygen-requiring) metabolic pathways to anaerobic pathways, which generate lactic and other acids, so that the patient will develop metabolic acidosis.

If respiratory function is impaired, elimination of carbon dioxide may be reduced, resulting in hypercarbia (a high level of carbon dioxide in the blood). If hypercarbia is acute, it will create respiratory acidosis. If hypercarbia is chronic (lasting longer than 24 to 28 hours), renal compensation may retain bicarbonate to buffer the acidosis, partially correcting the acidosis.

In most healthy people the levels of oxygen and carbon dioxide in the blood remain relatively constant. The stimulus to breathe comes from the respiratory center in the brain, and the primary stimulus for altering the depth and rate of breaths is the level of carbon dioxide in the arterial blood near this part of the brain. When the level of carbon dioxide rises, the respiratory center in the brain sends an increasing number of signals through the nerves to the muscles of respiration. Breathing rate and depth increase until the level of carbon dioxide falls. When the level of carbon dioxide in the blood falls, the signals sent by the respiratory center in the brain should decrease and the breathing rate slow. A feedback loop normally maintains a constant (linear) relationship between the carbon dioxide level and the rate and depth of respiration. Thus, the blood level of carbon dioxide is maintained in a narrow range.

In the alveoli, oxygen from the air passes through the alveolar and capillary walls into the blood. Carbon dioxide passes in the opposite direction. Blood leaving the alveolus to return to the left heart should contain high concentrations of oxygen.

Atmospheric air contains about 21% oxygen and 79% nitrogen. Because only about a quarter of the oxygen in inhaled air is taken up by the blood in the lungs during respiration, exhaled air still contains a significant concentration (about 16%) of oxygen as well as a small amount (5%) of added carbon dioxide and water vapor. In rescue breathing the air exhaled by the rescuer and delivered to the victim contains a sufficient amount of oxygen to support oxygenation of the victim.

Death caused by foreign-body airway obstruction is relatively uncommon (1.2

deaths per 100 000) in the United States.[1-4] However, the need for proper emergency airway management in cases of foreign-body obstruction is of key importance for safety at home, in restaurants, and in other public places.

Central Respiratory Arrest

The respiratory center in the brain must function for breathing to occur and for breathing rate and depth to remain adequate to control carbon dioxide levels in the blood. The respiratory center can be severely affected by inadequate blood flow to the brain resulting from stroke (a condition caused by interruption of the blood supply to an area of the brain), shock, or cardiac arrest. Within a few seconds after the heart ceases to beat, respiration will cease. In fact, many conditions that severely reduce oxygenation of blood can lead to respiratory arrest even if the amount of blood flowing to the brain is normal. In these instances respiratory arrest may be complete or the victim may exhibit ineffective "gasping" breathing efforts ("agonal" respirations) often associated with contraction of arm and leg muscles.[5-7] When determining the need for rescue breathing or chest compressions, do not confuse agonal breathing with effective respirations.

Drug overdose, use of narcotics and barbiturates, head trauma, and diseases or injuries that reduce brain function or interfere with normal contraction of the muscles of respiration can also cause respiratory arrest.

The Cardiovascular System

Anatomy of the Cardiovascular System

The cardiovascular system comprises the heart, arteries, capillaries, and veins. The heart of an adult is not much larger than a fist. It lies in the center of the chest, behind the breastbone (sternum), in front of the backbone (thoracic spine), and above the diaphragm. Except for the area against the spine and a small strip down the center of the front of the heart, the heart is surrounded by lung (Figure 3).

The heart is a hollow organ whose chambers are lined by thin, strong endocardium. The tough, muscular wall of the heart is called the myocardium. The heart is surrounded by a sac, or the pericardium.

The heart is divided into 4 sections, consisting of 2 upper chambers (the atria) and 2 lower chambers (the ventricles). The upper chamber (atrium) and lower chamber (ventricle) on the right side of the heart receive blood from the body. The right ventricle pumps this blood into the pulmonary artery for delivery to the lungs. The atrium and ventricle on the left side of the heart receive oxygenated blood from the lungs. The left ventricle pumps this oxygenated blood into the aorta, supplying the body. Valves between the atria and ventricles and between the ventricles and the 2 major arteries (the pulmonary artery and the aorta) carry blood away from the heart. These valves help maintain the forward flow of blood through the heart chambers and into the pulmonary artery or the aorta.

The heart has its own blood supply. The coronary arteries are the first branches of the aorta, and they supply the myocardium and endocardium with oxygenated blood. The 2 main arteries, the left coronary artery and the right coronary artery (Figure 4), branch into a complex network of arteries that supply all areas of the heart.

Physiology of the Heart

The function of the heart is to pump blood to the lungs and body. Arteries and veins carry the blood between the tissues of the body and the heart. In the tissues, oxygen and carbon dioxide are exchanged between the blood and cells. This process occurs in the lungs, the rest of the body, and the heart muscle itself.

All body cells require a continuous supply of oxygen to carry out normal functions. In addition, carbon dioxide, the waste product of the metabolism, must be eliminated from the body through the lungs.

The heart is actually a double pump. One pump (the right side of the heart) receives blood that has returned from the body after delivering oxygen to body tissues. The heart pumps this dark, bluish-red blood to the lungs, where the blood rids itself of carbon dioxide and picks up a supply of oxygen, which turns it a bright red again. The second pump (the left side of the heart) receives the oxygenated blood from the lungs and ejects blood through the great trunk artery (aorta) and into the smaller arteries, which distribute it to all parts of the body.

The adult heart at rest pumps 60 to 100 times per minute. Each time the adult heart beats, it ejects about 2½ ounces of blood (approximately 70 milliliters). At rest the heart pumps about 5 quarts (approximately 5 liters) of blood per minute. During exercise the heart can pump up to 37 quarts (35 liters) per minute. The total blood volume of a person weighing 150 pounds is about 6 quarts (approximately 6 liters).

FIGURE 2. Airway obstruction in unresponsive victim.

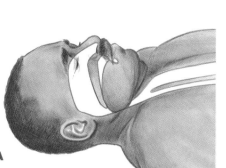

A

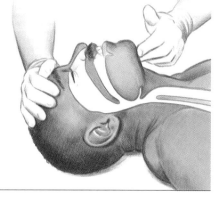

B

FIGURE 3. The heart in relation to other components of the chest.

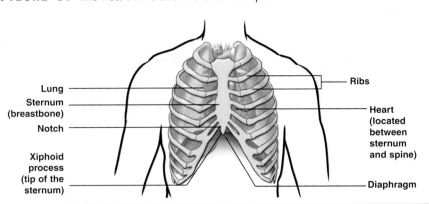

Each contraction of the cardiac muscle, or heartbeat, is initiated by an electrical impulse that arises from the natural pacemaker of the heart and is transmitted to the heart muscle by a specialized conduction system. The heart muscle contracts after it is stimulated by this electrical impulse. The contraction is followed by a period during which the electrical system and the heart muscle are recharged and made ready for the next beat. The heart has its own electrical pacemaker. Heart rate, however, can be altered either by nerve impulses from the brain or by various substances in the blood that influence the pacemaker and the conduction system.

Pathophysiology of the Heart

Blockage of a coronary artery caused by atherosclerosis or a blood clot prevents blood supplied by that artery from

reaching the myocardium. When blood flow through a coronary artery is blocked, any one of a group of conditions called acute coronary syndromes (ACS) may develop. These conditions include what is commonly known as angina and acute myocardial infarction (AMI), or heart attack. Angina is the pain that develops when the heart muscle is deprived of oxygen. AMI occurs when the heart muscle actually starts to die. The size of a myocardial infarction is often defined by the location of the arterial blockage and the amount of heart muscle served by the artery beyond the blockage (Chapter 3, Figure 1).

The management of ACS has improved significantly over the last 2 decades. Fibrinolytic agents ("clotbuster" medications) and percutaneous coronary interventions (PCIs, including angioplasty and possible stent placement) can reopen

blocked coronary vessels, saving lives and improving quality of life.[8-15] Early diagnosis and treatment of AMI significantly reduce mortality,[8] decrease the size of the AMI,[9] improve left ventricular function,[10-13] and decrease the incidence of heart failure.[14,15] These interventions, however, must be administered within the first few hours of symptom onset to be most effective.[14,15]

Some victims of AMI may suffer an electrical complication called ventricular fibrillation (VF). this abnormal and chaotic rhythm causes useless quivering of the heart and cessation of circulation — the heart stops pumping blood. VF is the most frequent initial heart rhythm in witnessed sudden cardiac arrest. It must be treated rapidly with electrical defibrillation to resuscitate the victim. The probability of successfully converting VF to a perfusing rhythm (defibrillation) diminishes rapidly over time; untreated VF changes to asystole (flatline) within a few minutes.[16-25] Once asystole develops, the likelihood of successful resuscitation is extremely low. Early defibrillation is discussed in detail in Chapter 7.

The Cerebrovascular System
Anatomy of the Brain

The central nervous system is composed of the brain and spinal cord (Figure 5). The largest portion of the brain is the *cerebrum*, where nerve centers that regulate all sensory and motor activities of the body are located. The cerebrum is divided into right and left halves, or *hemispheres*, each containing a complete set of sensory and motor centers. Generally the right hemisphere controls the left side of the body and the left hemisphere controls the right side of the body.

The cerebral hemispheres are further subdivided into *lobes*, or sections with specific, distinct functions. Lack of blood supply to brain tissue in a specific area can therefore result in distinct and limited loss of the specific function controlled by that area of the brain.

FIGURE 4. The coronary arteries.

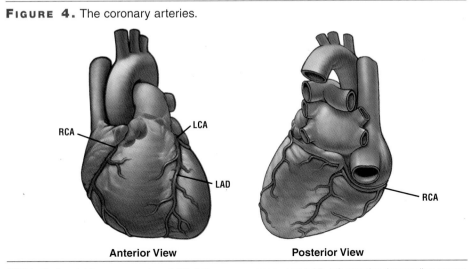

Anterior View   **Posterior View**

RCA indicates right coronary artery; LCA, left coronary artery; and LAD, left anterior descending artery.

The brain stem, or the lower part of the brain (Figure 5), is made up of bundles and tracts of nerves that travel down to the spinal cord from the cerebrum. The brain stem has distinct centers as well. The most important of these monitor and control respiratory and circulatory function.

Circulation of the Brain

The brain requires a constant flow of oxygenated blood; if blood flow to the brain is interrupted, brain damage or death can result. Most of the blood supply to the brain (80%) is provided by the 2 large arteries (right and left) in the front of the neck, called *the carotid arteries* (Figure 6). The rest of the blood flow in the brain comes from 2 arteries (right and left) in the back of the neck, the vertebral arteries, which supply blood to the brain stem. These 2 arteries then join the carotid arteries to form a network that supplies blood to the rest of the brain.

FIGURE 5. Sagittal section of the brain.

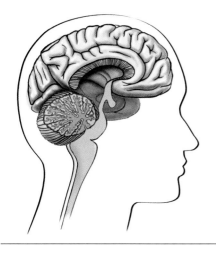

Classification of Stroke. Strokes may be classified in several ways. One method classifies the stroke according to the portion of the brain circulation that is affected. This classification divides strokes into those involving the carotid (anterior) circulation and those that involve the vertebrobasilar (posterior) circulation.

After the carotid and vertebral arteries meet, arteries branch off to supply specific portions of the brain. This specificity of blood supply explains why the obstruction of a single artery branch results in the loss of a specific brain function (stroke), such as weakness and sensory loss in the arm and leg on one side of the body. Lack of blood supply or loss of function of the nerve centers in the brain stem can result in respiratory arrest or cardiovascular collapse.

Pathophysiology of the Brain

Injuries or insults to the brain that damage discrete areas can result in loss of specific functions while other parts of the nervous system continue to function normally. For example, the sudden disruption or blockage of blood supply in an artery that supplies a particular area of the brain (stroke) can result in loss of movement or sensation to one side of the body while the patient remains alert and is able to move the other side of the body normally. Because each hemisphere of the brain controls function on the opposite side of the body, stroke victims usually have weakness and loss of sensation in the arm and leg on the side of the body opposite the side of the brain affected by stroke. Additional symptoms such as slurred speech or visual disruptions may be present, depending on the location of the stroke within the brain.

Major insults to the brain may cause more diffuse brain injury, with loss of responsiveness and reduced functions of the brain. For example, severe head injury or severe hemorrhagic stroke may lead to altered mental status.

Metabolic abnormalities affect all brain cells. A common example is hypoxia (lack of oxygen) during a cardiac arrest. The victim loses consciousness, does not respond to stimuli such as pain, has no ability to move, and loses control of vital functions such as breathing. When cardiac arrest develops, all cells in the body are affected, although the brain may sustain the most significant and immediate insult.

FIGURE 6. Brain circulation.

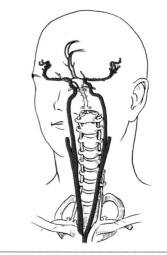

Interaction of Respiratory, Cardiac, and Brain Functions

The major goal of emergency cardiovascular care is to maintain oxygen delivery to vital organs to preserve vital organ function, including brain viability. The heart, lungs, and brain function interdependently. The lungs oxygenate the blood, and the heart delivers oxygenated blood to the brain. Respiratory or cardiac arrest will deprive the brain and other vital organs of oxygen. Sudden obstruction of blood flow or hemorrhage (bleeding) within the brain — the condition we call stroke — will deprive a portion of the brain of oxygen, leading to loss of brain function.

Brain function also affects cardiac and respiratory function, which are regulated by specialized centers in the brain. Because the brain is the controlling center for other vital organ systems, brain dysfunction, such as that which may develop after a stroke, may contribute to cardiopulmonary failure and death.

Summary of Anatomy and Physiology

Knowledge of anatomy and physiology is the foundation for understanding heart disease, stroke, and sudden cardiac death. It also provides the rationale for implementation of the Chain of Survival.

Healthcare providers should frequently review the anatomy and physiology of the respiratory, cardiovascular, and cerebro-vascular systems to help ensure long-term retention of knowledge and skills related to BLS.

Summary of Key Concepts

- Lung, heart, and brain function are interdependent.

- The function of the respiratory system is to bring oxygen from the air into the lungs and to eliminate carbon dioxide from the body.

- The function of the heart is to pump blood to the lungs, brain, and body.

- One function of the brain is to regulate body function, including the respiratory and cardiovascular systems (for example, the respiratory center in the brain must function for respiration to occur).

- The most common cause of airway obstruction is occlusion by upper airway structures, such as the tongue and epiglottis.

- Sudden blockage of blood supply to a specific area of the brain can result in a stroke, with a reduction or loss of function on the opposite side of the body.

Review Questions

1. A 55-year-old man suddenly experiences severe substernal chest pressure with shortness of breath, sweating, and nausea. The discomfort travels to his jaw and down his left arm. What is the most likely cause of his condition?

   a. a stroke

   b. a seizure

   c. a heart attack

   d. respiratory arrest

2. You find a victim who has been in cardiac arrest for 20 minutes. Despite vigorous resuscitative efforts, he does not regain spontaneous breathing. This is most likely caused by irreversible damage to the respiratory center in the brain. Where is the respiratory center located?

   a. the cerebrum

   b. the brain stem

   c. the spinal cord

   d. the peripheral nerves

3. A 68-year-old woman suddenly becomes dizzy and lightheaded, with weakness in her right arm and leg. She is having difficulty speaking. What is the most likely cause of her symptoms?

   a. a heart attack

   b. an upper airway obstruction

   c. a cardiac arrest

   d. a stroke in the left hemisphere

4. A 55-year-old male coworker suddenly collapses while on the job. You determine unresponsiveness, have someone call 911, and find that the victim is in cardiac arrest. When you attempt initial rescue breathing, you are unable to ventilate (move air into the victim's lungs). The most likely cause for this is

   a. a foreign-body airway obstruction

   b. lack of forceful expiration

   c. obstruction of the airway by the victim's tongue and epiglottis

   d. collapse of the victim's lungs

How did you do?

Answers: **1,** c; **2,** b; **3,** d; **4,** c.

References

1. Fingerhut LA, Cox CS, Warner M. Advance data from Vital and Health Statistics of the Centers for Disease Control and Prevention. International Comparative Analysis of Injury Mortality: Findings From the *International Collaborative Effort (ICE) on Injury Statistics*. Number 303. October 7, 1998.

2. National Center for Health Statistics and National Safety Council. *Data on odds of death due to choking*. May 7, 1998.

3. National Safety Council. *Accident Facts 1997*. Chicago, Ill: National Safety Council; 1997.

4. Canadian Hospitals Injury Reporting and Prevention Program. Summary statistics, CHIRPP database for 1997.

5. Tang W, Weil MH, Sun SJ, Kette D, Kette F, Gazmuri RJ, O'Connell F, Bisera J. Cardiopulmonary resuscitation by precordial compression but without mechanical ventilation. *Am J Resp Crit Care Med*. 1994;150:1709-1713.

6. Noc M, Weil MH, Sun SJ, Tang W, Bisera J. Spontaneous gasping during cardiopulmonary resuscitation without mechanical ventilation. *Am J Resp Crit Care Med*. 1994;150:861-864.

7. Clark JJ, Larsen MP, Culley LL, Graves JR, Eisenberg MS. Incidence of agonal respirations in sudden cardiac arrest. *Ann Emerg Med*. 1992;21:1464-1467.

8. Brouwer MA, Martin JS, Maynard C, Wirkus M, Litwin PE, Verheugt FW, Weaver WD. Influence of early prehospital thrombolysis on mortality and event-free survival (the Myocardial Infarction Triage and Intervention [MITI] Randomized Trial): MITI Project Investigators. *Am J Cardiol*. 1996;78:497-502.

9. Raitt MH, Maynard C, Wagner GS, Cerqueira MD, Selvester RH, Weaver WD. Relation between symptom duration before thrombolytic therapy and final myocardial infarct size. *Circulation*. 1996;93:48-53.

10. Wackers FJ, Terrin ML, Kayden DS, Knatterud G, Forman S, Braunwald E, Zaret BL. Quantitative radionuclide assessment of regional ventricular function after thrombolytic therapy for acute myocardial infarction: results of phase I Thrombolysis in Myocardial Infarction (TIMI) trial. *J Am Coll Cardiol*. 1989;13:998-1005.

11. Res JC, Simoons ML, van der Wall EE, van Eenige MJ, Vermeer F, Verheugt FW, Wijns W, Braat S, Remme WJ, Serruys PW, et al. Long term improvement in global left ventricular function after early thrombolytic treatment in acute myocardial infarction: report of a randomised multicentre trial of intracoronary streptokinase in acute myocardial infarction. *Br Heart J*. 1986;56:414-421.

12. Mathey DG, Sheehan FH, Schofer J, Dodge HT. Time from onset of symptoms to thrombolytic therapy: a major determinant of myocardial salvage in patients with acute transmural infarction. *J Am Coll Cardiol*. 1985;6:518-525.

13. Serruys PW, Simoons ML, Suryapranata H, Vermeer F, Wijns W, van den Brand M, Bar F, Zwaan C, Krauss XH, Remme WJ, et al. Preservation of global and regional left ventricular function after early thrombolysis in acute myocardial infarction. *J Am Coll Cardiol*. 1986;7:729-742.

14. Newby LK, Rutsch WR, Califf RM, Simoons ML, Aylward PE, Armstrong PW, Woodlief LH, Lee KH, Topol EJ, van de Werf F. Time from symptom onset to treatment and outcomes after thrombolytic therapy: GUSTO-1 Investigators. *J Am Coll Cardiol*. 1996;27: 1646-1655.

15. Anderson JL, Karagounis LA, Califf RM. Metaanalysis of five reported studies on the relation of early coronary patency grades with mortality and outcomes after acute myocardial infarction. *Am J Cardiol*. 1996;78:1-8.

16. Eisenberg MS, Cummins RO, Damon S, Larsen MP, Hearne TR. Survival rates from out-of-hospital cardiac arrest: recommendations for uniform definitions and data to report. *Ann Emerg Med*. 1990;19:1249-1259.

17. Eisenberg MS, Copass MK, Hallstrom A, Cobb LA, Bergner L. Management of out-of-hospital cardiac arrest: failure of basic emergency medical technician services. *JAMA*. 1980;243:1049-1051.

18. Eisenberg MS, Hallstrom AP, Copass MK, Bergner L, Short F, Pierce J. Treatment of ventricular fibrillation: emergency medical technician defibrillation and paramedic services. *JAMA*. 1984;251:1723-1726.

19. Weaver WD, Copass MK, Bufi D, Ray R, Hallstrom AP, Cobb LA. Improved neurologic recovery and survival after early defibrillation. *Circulation*. 1984;69:943-948.

20. Larsen MP, Eisenberg MS, Cummins RO, Hallstrom AP. Predicting survival from out-of-hospital cardiac arrest: a graphic model. *Ann Emerg Med*. 1993;22:1652-1658.

21. Eisenberg M, Bergner L, Hallstrom A. Paramedic programs and out-of-hospital cardiac arrest, II: impact on community mortality. *Am J Public Health*. 1979;69:39-42.

22. Fletcher GF, Cantwell JD. Ventricular fibrillation in a medically supervised cardiac exercise program: clinical, angiographic, and surgical correlations. *JAMA*. 1977;238:2627-2629.

23. Haskell WL. Cardiovascular complications during exercise training of cardiac patients. *Circulation*. 1978;57:920-924.

24. Hossack KF, Hartwig R. Cardiac arrest associated with supervised cardiac rehabilitation. *J Cardiac Rehabil*. 1982;2:402-408.

25. Van Camp SP, Peterson RA. Cardiovascular complications of outpatient cardiac rehabilitation programs. *JAMA*. 1986;256:1160-1163.

You are a BLS ambulance provider in a rural area. You are called to the home of a 65-year-old man who is experiencing "weakness." When you arrive the patient is sitting on the couch clutching his chest. He appears pale and sweaty and complains of chest discomfort radiating to his jaw and down his left arm for the past 30 minutes. He has no history of heart disease. According to the protocol, you provide oxygen at 4 L/min and administer sublingual nitroglycerin and aspirin while quickly performing a focused history and physical assessment.

When you prepare the patient for transport to the hospital, he refuses further medical attention. After several failed attempts to convince him to go to the hospital, you ask the EMS medical director — a physician — to talk with the patient. The doctor finally convinces the patient to come to the Emergency Department for evaluation.

At the hospital the patient is given fibrinolytic therapy and is discharged 5 days later with a very favorable prognosis. He calls to thank you for your persistent and thoughtful care.

Coronary Artery Disease and Acute Coronary Syndromes

Overview

This year approximately 7 to 8 million patients will be evaluated in a US Emergency Department (ED) for chest discomfort. Of these patients, more than 2 million (approximately 25%) will be diagnosed as having an acute coronary syndrome, including unstable angina and AMI. More than one half million of these patients will be hospitalized with a diagnosis of unstable angina,[1] and 1.5 million will experience an AMI.[2] Of the 1.5 million patients who experience AMI, approximately one half million will die, and 50% of those deaths will occur suddenly, within the first hour after the onset of symptoms.[3] When prehospital mortality is included, the first prolonged attack of ischemic chest pain has a 34% fatality rate, and in 17% of patients it is their first, last, and only symptom.[4]

Current management of ACS contrasts dramatically with the care given 2 decades ago. Fibrinolytic agents and percutaneous coronary interventions (PCIs) can reopen the blocked coronary vessels that cause myocardial ischemia. As a result, these treatments save lives and improve quality of life.[5-12] Early diagnosis and treatment of AMI significantly reduces mortality,[5] decreases the size of the infarction,[6] improves local[7] and overall left ventricular (LV) function,[8-10] and decreases incidence of heart failure.[11,12] To be most effective, however, these interventions must be administered within the first few hours of symptom onset.[5-12]

The time-limited treatments now available for ACS have highlighted the important role of lay rescuers, first responders,

Learning Objectives

1. Define the following terms:

   ▥ Coronary artery disease (CAD)

   ▥ Acute coronary syndromes (ACS)

   ▥ Angina/angina pectoris

   ▥ Acute myocardial infarction (AMI)

2. Describe the "classic" pattern of ischemic-type chest pain

3. List 4 signs and symptoms of AMI

4. Describe the appropriate "actions for survival" that a rescuer should take for a patient with signs of chest discomfort (ischemic-type chest pain) and known heart disease versus those appropriate for a patient with signs of chest discomfort and no history of heart disease

5. List 3 types of patients who are likely to have an atypical presentation of AMI

6. Explain how sudden cardiac death occurs secondary to CAD

and emergency medical services (EMS) personnel. Early recognition, early access, and early transport to the hospital of victims with suspected ACS substantially reduce morbidity and mortality by making early definitive hospital-based treatment possible.

Definition of Terms

Arteriosclerosis, commonly called "hardening of the arteries," includes a variety of conditions that cause the artery walls to thicken and lose elasticity.

Atherosclerosis is a form of arteriosclerosis in which the inner layers of artery walls become thick and irregular because of deposits of a fatty substance. As the interior artery walls become lined with layers of these deposits, the arteries become narrowed. This narrowing reduces the flow of blood through the arteries and decreases their ability to dilate when needed to supply more blood to the heart (eg, during exercise or stress).

Coronary artery disease is the presence of atherosclerosis in the coronary arteries.

The term **acute coronary syndromes** encompasses a spectrum of symptomatic clinical conditions representing acute closure of the coronary arteries with varying degrees of cholesterol plaque, clot, and spasm. These syndromes include unstable angina and AMI. Sudden death may occur with ACS.

Myocardial ischemia is inadequate delivery of oxygen to the heart muscle, which may produce chest discomfort, or angina pectoris.

Chest discomfort/ischemic-type chest pain/angina pectoris are symptoms caused by inadequate blood flow and oxygen delivery to the myocardium (myocardial ischemia). Typically the discomfort is described as crushing chest pressure that may radiate to the arms, shoulders, jaw, or back. This sensation may be "classic" or may be described as diffuse chest or back discomfort or ache.

Because many patients with angina/ischemic-type chest pain perceive the sensation as "pressure," they may deny that they are in pain. To avoid confusion and to aid in the prompt recognition of warning signs of myocardial infarction (MI), the term chest discomfort should be used when asking patients if they are experiencing symptoms of angina or ischemic-type chest pain.

Myocardial infarction is defined as the death of heart muscle (myocardium) as

the result of prolonged inadequate blood flow and oxygen delivery.

A **thrombus** is a clot formed by the blood's coagulation system in response to injury. Some components include platelets, clot-activating proteins (for example, thrombin), and strands that link and strengthen the clot (fibrin). When a thrombus forms in a coronary artery, it blocks some or all blood flow to an area of heart muscle. This can create myocardial ischemia, ischemic-type chest pain, and MI.

Pathology and Natural History of CAD: A Problem of Supply and Demand

Atherosclerosis is a slow, progressive disease that usually begins early in life — significant disease may be present before the age of 20. It is a generalized disease process that may involve arteries in different areas, such as the heart (leading to a heart attack), the brain (leading to a stroke), or the legs (leading to pain precipitated by walking or leg cramps during exercise, called *claudication*).

Atherosclerosis of the coronary arteries places the patient at risk for development of angina, AMI, or sudden cardiac death. Long before the function of the heart muscle is impaired, there is an asymptomatic period in which risk factor modification may halt the process. The inner portion of the arterial wall becomes thickened with deposits of fats (lipid, cholesterol) and eventually calcium. The result is a gradual narrowing of the arterial lumen.

Patients who develop ACS have varying degrees of coronary artery occlusion. The development of ACS typically is caused by rupture or erosion of a lipid-laden plaque (see Figure 1).[13,14] The plaque may be hemodynamically insignificant before rupture, but an inflammatory component is often present just under the surface of the lining of the wall, weakening the plaque and predisposing it to rupture.[15] Blood flow velocity, turbulence, and

FIGURE 1. The natural history of coronary artery disease: evolution to the major acute coronary syndromes.

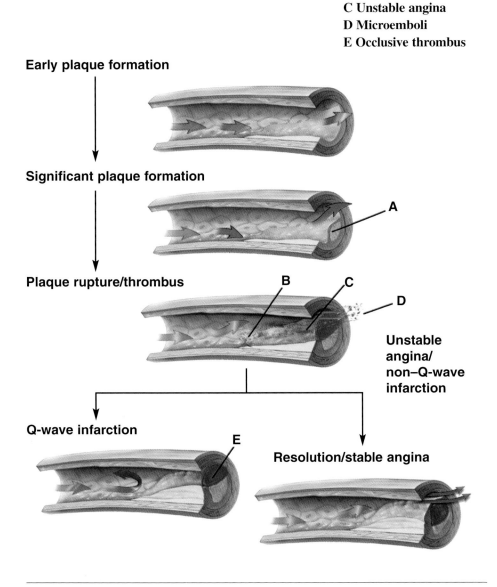

A Unstable plaque
B Plaque rupture
C Unstable angina
D Microemboli
E Occlusive thrombus

Early plaque formation

Significant plaque formation

Plaque rupture/thrombus

Q-wave infarction

Unstable angina/non–Q-wave infarction

Resolution/stable angina

vessel anatomy are important contributing factors to plaque disruption.

After the plaque ruptures or erodes, the body attempts to close this internal "cut" through activation of platelets and the body's coagulation system. Blood platelets cover the surface of the ruptured plaque, and other platelets are recruited to the site (see Figure 1, B). Administration of aspirin at this time can be effective because it reduces the ability of platelets to clump.

Activation of the coagulation system results in generation of thrombin, the body's most active clot-making substance. At this time a platelet-rich thrombus is present that *partially occludes* the coronary artery, compromising oxygen delivery to a portion of the myocardium, causing myocardial ischemia. This ischemia may cause prolonged chest discomfort or ischemic-type chest pain (see Figure 1, C).

Currently treatment with *antiplatelet* drugs, including aspirin and newer therapies (such as glycoprotein IIb/IIIa inhibitors), will be most effective. Fibrinolytic therapy is not effective and may worsen the occlusion.[16]

Patients with ACS may present with a variety of forms of MI or a risk of MI. The patient presentation is determined by the site of artery occlusion, the size of the occluded artery, the duration and severity of the occlusion, and the presence or absence of "helper arteries" called collaterals that have formed to help maintain blood flow to the myocardium (see Figure 1, C and D). Different presentations of MI are treated differently. The various types of MI may be identified by characteristic changes in the ECG and possibly by serum markers of myocardial injury, previously called cardiac enzymes.[16]

If the thrombus occludes the coronary artery for a prolonged period, the patient will develop a specific type of MI called *Q-wave infarction* (characterized by a Q wave visible on the ECG). This type of long-standing thrombus is rich in

platelets (see Figure 1, E) and will be most responsive to early treatment with fibrinolytics (so-called clotbusters) and direct percutaneous transluminal angioplasty (PTA).[16]

ACS and Myocardial Infarction

Clinical Presentation of CAD

CAD begins in the late teens or early 20s and progresses silently until either critical narrowing of the coronary artery is present or acute plaque rupture or erosion occurs. There are 2 symptomatic presentations of CAD. The patient may develop gradual narrowing of the coronary artery until the artery is narrowed by approximately 70% to 90%. Then the patient will develop chest discomfort (angina) with exertion. As narrowing of the coronary artery progresses, the patient will develop more severe angina with less exertion and may ultimately experience angina at rest.

At any time patients may develop ACS caused by plaque rupture or erosion. These patients can become acutely symptomatic as the result of underlying CAD and artery narrowing, compounded by the development of a thrombus after plaque rupture or erosion. Patients with ACS may then develop unstable angina (angina at rest, angina that wakes the patient at night — nocturnal angina,

angina that is triggered with minimal exertion) or MI. Sudden death may complicate either clinical presentation of CAD.

Angina Pectoris

Angina pectoris, a common symptom of CAD, is a transient discomfort (which may or may not be perceived as pain) caused by an inadequate blood flow and oxygen delivery to the heart muscle. The discomfort is frequently located in the center of the chest (called precordial or substernal) but may be more diffuse throughout the front of the chest.

Angina is a steady discomfort, often brought on by any factor that increases the heart rate, including exercise, unusual exertion, and emotional or psychological stress. It commonly lasts from 2 to 15 minutes. It is usually described as crushing, pressing, constricting, oppressive, or heavy (Figure 2). The discomfort may spread to one (more often the left) or both shoulders or arms or to the neck, jaw, back, or upper mid portion of the abdomen (epigastrium).

Some patients deny pain but freely admit to severe discomfort. For this reason the terms chest discomfort or ischemic-type chest pain or angina (or even anginal pain) are used instead of the simple but frequently misunderstood term chest pain.

Women, the elderly, and persons with diabetes often present with angina that

FIGURE 2. Typical locations of chest pain in persons having a heart attack.

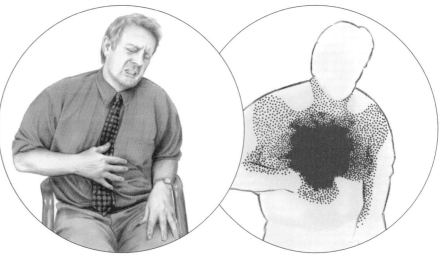

is more diffuse in location and vague in description than classic angina. These patients may describe shortness of breath, syncope, lightheadedness, weakness, or diffuse pain.[17-21]

The most frequent cause of angina is coronary atherosclerosis. As the severity of the coronary narrowing increases, the amount of exertion needed to bring on angina decreases.

Angina is usually promptly relieved by rest or nitroglycerin. If exertional angina is not relieved by rest or (in the case of the patient with known CAD) 3 nitroglycerin tablets over 10 minutes, emergency medical evaluation is required (phone 911).

Unstable angina is a term used by many different groups with many different definitions. It most often is used to describe angina that is continuing, prolonged, or occurring at rest (possibly awakening the patient at night). The patient with **angina that occurs at rest and is prolonged (lasting more than 20 minutes), angina that is of recent onset and progressive in nature, or nocturnal angina is at increased risk for AMI and sudden death. Phone 911 or other emergency response number** (see Tables 1 and 2).[22] In the patient with known heart disease, prolonged angina unrelieved by rest or nitroglycerin is an indication to phone 911 or other emergency response number.

Patients should seek medical advice if they have angina of new onset (onset more than 2 weeks ago but within 2 months); increased frequency, severity, or duration; or occurring at lower activity levels. These forms of angina are thought to have a relatively low risk of adverse cardiac events.[22]

AMI (Heart Attack)

A heart attack occurs when an area of the heart muscle is deprived of blood flow and oxygen for a prolonged period (usually more than 20 to 30 minutes) and the muscle begins to die. A heart attack is usually the result of severe narrowing or complete blockage of a diseased coronary artery or plaque rupture or erosion with secondary thrombus formation.

Rarely heart attack is caused by a spasm of the arteries, dissection of the coronary artery, or an embolism. Blood vessel spasm (either spontaneous or secondary to drugs such as cocaine) blocks blood flow to heart muscle, causing a heart attack.

When blood flow to the heart muscle is blocked for a sufficient period, the muscle becomes ischemic (damaged as a result of inadequate oxygenation). If blood flow through the artery is not quickly restored, the heart muscle cells supplied by that artery will begin to die (necrosis).

Ischemic heart muscle (muscle that does not receive sufficient oxygen) may develop abnormal electrical rhythms, including ventricular fibrillation (VF). The VF most often develops within the first hour of the onset of symptoms. For this reason it is extremely important to phone 911 when symptoms of new or prolonged angina (unrelieved by rest and nitroglycerin) or nocturnal angina develop.

"Red Flags" or Warning Signs of Heart Attack

■ Chest discomfort is the most important signal of a heart attack. The discomfort is similar to previous anginal episodes in character, location, and radiation but lasts considerably longer and is not relieved — or is only partially relieved — by rest or nitroglycerin.[22] Some patients describe intense pain, but this is not universal.

■ Other signs may include sweating, nausea, vomiting, or shortness of breath.

■ A feeling of weakness may accompany chest discomfort.

■ Be alert to the fact that

— The discomfort may not be severe and the patient may complain only of related symptoms, such as short-

Critical Concepts:
Atypical Presentations of AMI

The elderly,[23] patients with diabetes, and women[17-19] are more likely to present with unusual, atypical angina without classic symptoms or with only vague, nonspecific complaints. Diabetic patients may present only with weakness. Symptoms such as shortness of breath, syncope, or lightheadedness may be the only symptoms in diabetic patients. In a long-term follow-up of the Framingham study, one third of first infarctions in men and half of those in women were clinically unrecognized.[20] About one half of these were truly silent, but the other 50% had atypical presentations.[21]

The BLS provider must be aware of the many ways that patients may present with angina and be prepared to activate the EMS system even in the absence of typical signs and symptoms of AMI.

TABLE 1. Principal Presentations of Unstable Angina.

Rest angina	Angina occurring at rest and usually prolonged (>20 min), occurring within 1 week of presentation
New-onset angina	Angina of at least CCSC III (marked limitation of ordinary physical activity) severity, with onset within 2 mo of initial presentation
Increasing angina	Previously diagnosed angina that is distinctly more frequent, longer in duration, or lower in threshold (ie, increased by at least 1 CCSC within 2 mo of initial presentation to at least CCSC III severity)

Adapted from 1994 AHCPR guidelines. CCSC indicates Canadian Cardiovascular Society Classification.

ness of breath. However, you should suspect that these symptoms represent atypical angina if they are prolonged and not relieved by rest or nitroglycerin, particularly in an elderly, diabetic, or female patient.

— The person does not necessarily have to "look bad" or have all the symptoms for an MI to be present — if in doubt, phone 911 (or other emergency response number).

— Stabbing, momentary twinges of pain are usually not signals of a heart attack. Sharp or stabbing pain that can be localized by the tip of a finger and reproduced by pushing on the spot is rarely cardiac in origin.

— If the patient uses the term sharp to describe the pain, ask him or her to use another word to clarify the meaning. One-word descriptions of pain can be ambiguous, and some patients use the term sharp when they mean *intense,* whereas others use it to describe the quality of the pain. Intense pain may be angina, whereas stabbing pain often is not.

■ Signals of an MI can develop in either sex, even in young adults, at any time and in any place.

FYI: Precipitating Events of AMI

AMI can occur under a wide variety of circumstances. Most episodes of acute coronary syndromes occur at rest or with modest daily activity. Heavy physical exertion is a precipitating event in a minority of patients, perhaps 10% to 15%.[24,25] Emotional stress and life events with a powerful personal impact (for example, the death of a spouse or other loved one, divorce, or loss of job) are commonly observed before MI and may be correlated.[26,27] Illicit drugs such as cocaine have clearly been shown to cause heart attacks and ventricular arrhythmias.[28,29]

Actions for Survival From ACS
Critical Role of Early EMS Activation

Many deaths from heart attack occur before the victim reaches the hospital. A great number of these fatalities could be prevented by calling 911 or other emergency response number in the first few minutes after the onset of symptoms. The most common cause of prehospital death in heart attack victims is ventricular fibrillation. VF can often be successfully treated

with a defibrillator, but it will become fatal if it develops when the victim is alone, at home, or in another location away from a defibrillator and persons trained in its use.

Despite efforts to educate the public about risk factors and the early warning signals of heart attack, the rate of death from this major killer remains at an appallingly high level. More than half of all heart attack victims die outside the hospital, most within 1 hour of initial symptoms.[3] It is essential to know and be able to recognize the signals of heart attack.

The initial treatment should be to have the victim rest quietly. Because both angina pectoris and heart attack are caused by a lack of adequate blood supply to the heart, the appropriate treatment for both is to reduce activity. When heart rate or blood pressure increases, such as during activity, the heart requires more oxygen. Rest reduces heart rate and oxygen requirements of the heart and body. The victim should be allowed either to lie down or sit up, whichever allows the most comfort and the easiest breathing.

Appropriate Response to Symptoms of Possible AMI

If chest discomfort lasts for more than a few minutes, contact the local EMS system (or other emergency response number) unless the victim has known

TABLE 2. Short-Term Risk of Adverse Cardiac Events in Patients With Unstable Angina.

High risk	Intermediate risk	Low risk
Prolonged ongoing (>20 min) ischemic pain	Prolonged (>20 min) rest angina, now resolved, with moderate or high likelihood of CAD	Increased angina frequency, severity, or duration
Pulmonary edema, most likely related to ischemia	Rest angina (>20 min or relieved with rest or sublingual nitroglycerin)	Angina provoked at a lower threshold
Angina at rest with dynamic ST changes >1 mm	Nocturnal angina	New-onset angina with onset 2 wk to 2 mo before presentation
Angina with new or worsening MR murmur	Angina with dynamic T-wave changes	Normal or unchanged ECG
Angina with S_3 or new/worsening rales	New onset CCSC III or IV angina in the past 2 wk with moderate or high likelihood of CAD	
Angina with hypotension	Pathological Q waves or rest ST depression <1 mm in multiple-lead groups (anterior, inferior, lateral)	
Elevated serum troponin I or T level	Age >65 y	

In general, final assignment of risk is based on highest risk feature; however, the table should not be interpreted as an inflexible algorithm. Adapted from 1994 AHCPR Guidelines, with modifications reflecting 1998 ICF workshops.
CCSC indicates Canadian Cardiovascular Society Classification; MR, mitral regurgitation.

cardiovascular disease with physician's instructions to take nitroglycerin first. Nitroglycerin may be taken as a tablet or as a spray under the tongue. Use of the nitroglycerin patch or ointment is not recommended because their onset of action is too slow, and absorption of the drug through the skin is unpredictable in the presence of MI. If the victim is taking nitroglycerin tablets and 1 tablet of nitroglycerin does not relieve angina, the patient should take a second and a third tablet as needed at 3- to 5-minute intervals.

Nitroglycerin is a vasodilator that dilates coronary arteries and relieves the discomfort of ischemic-type chest pain/angina pectoris. Because nitroglycerin lowers blood pressure, the victim taking the drug should sit or lie down. Nitroglycerin may produce a stinging sensation under the tongue and may cause a headache. The absence of these symptoms, however, does not mean the tablets are old or ineffective. Nitroglycerin tablets

often work, but they may be ineffective if CAD is severe or if the patient develops ACS (with rupture and erosion of a plaque and thrombus formation).

Age and light may deactivate nitroglycerin tablets. It is best to keep a fresh supply in a dark place and carry only a few tablets in a small, dark bottle, changing to fresh tablets every month or so. If the patient is using "old" nitroglycerin tablets, ask where he keeps fresh tablets that have not been exposed to light. Some nitroglycerin sprays are effective for 2 years, and this form of nitroglycerin therapy may be delivered more reliably.

In general, if chest discomfort persists for 5 to 10 minutes despite rest, the EMS system (or other emergency response number) should be notified. In patients with known heart disease, this notification should occur if typical symptoms persist for 10 minutes despite rest and ingestion of 3 nitroglycerin tablets (see Figure 3).

If chest discomfort or other signs of ischemic-type chest pain/angina develop in a person with no known CAD, take the following actions:

1. Recognize the signals.

2. Have the victim stop activity and sit or lie down.

3. If discomfort persists for 5 minutes or more, phone 911 (or other emergency response number). If an EMS system is not available, take the victim immediately to the nearest hospital ED that provides 24-hour emergency care.

If chest discomfort or other signs of ischemic-type chest pain/angina develop in a person with known CAD who has recently been taking prescribed nitroglycerin, take the following actions:

1. Recognize the signals.

2. Have the victim stop activity and sit or lie down.

FIGURE 3. Emergency action plan for a person with signals of heart attack.

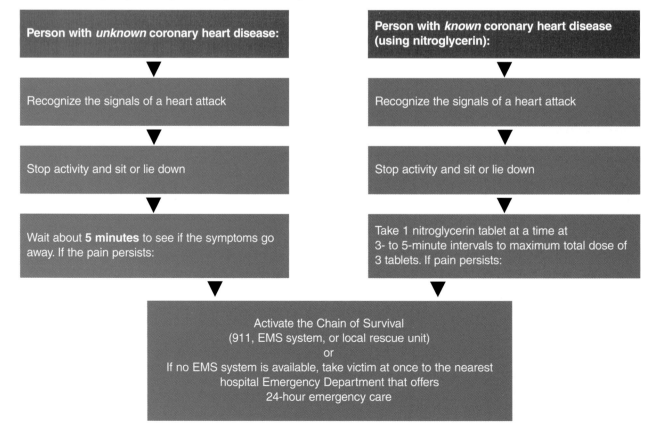

Person with *unknown* coronary heart disease:	Person with *known* coronary heart disease (using nitroglycerin):
▼	▼
Recognize the signals of a heart attack	Recognize the signals of a heart attack
▼	▼
Stop activity and sit or lie down	Stop activity and sit or lie down
▼	▼
Wait about **5 minutes** to see if the symptoms go away. If the pain persists:	Take 1 nitroglycerin tablet at a time at 3- to 5-minute intervals to maximum total dose of 3 tablets. If pain persists:

Activate the Chain of Survival
(911, EMS system, or local rescue unit)
or
If no EMS system is available, take victim at once to the nearest hospital Emergency Department that offers 24-hour emergency care

3. Place 1 nitroglycerin tablet under the victim's tongue or administer spray sublingually. Repeat at 3- to 5-minute intervals to a total dose of 3 tablets if discomfort is not relieved (a maximum of 10 minutes). If you are at the victim's home and the discomfort is unrelieved after the first nitroglycerin tablet, ask the victim to direct you to a fresh supply of nitroglycerin tablets and administer a fresh tablet for the second and third doses if possible.

Lay rescuers should be cautious, however, when administering nitroglycerin because the victim may already have taken some nitroglycerin and because tablet strengths may vary. Phone 911 if the discomfort persists after 10 minutes or after the victim has taken a total of 3 nitroglycerin tablets.

4. If signals persist, phone 911 (or other emergency response number). If an EMS system is not available, the victim should be taken immediately to the nearest hospital ED that provides 24-hour emergency care.

Everyone should have an emergency action plan at home and at work (see Critical Concepts: Emergency Action Plan).

Critical Concepts:
Emergency Action Plan

1. Know the appropriate emergency response telephone number (usually 911).

2. Know the location of the nearest hospital Emergency Department that provides 24-hour emergency care.

3. Before the need for emergency services arises, discuss with the family physician the hospital of choice, the distance to be traveled, and the emergency capabilities of hospitals under consideration

Because the victim may deny the possibility of a heart attack, it is essential that bystanders activate the emergency action plan. These bystanders must be prepared to render BLS if necessary.

If you observe someone experiencing symptoms of chest discomfort and possible heart attack that last 5 minutes or longer (10 minutes or longer in the patient with known heart disease), you should act quickly.

Expect denial on the part of the patient — but insist on taking prompt action. Do the following:

1. Phone first! Phone 911 or other emergency response number. If EMS is not available, take the victim to the nearest hospital ED that provides 24-hour emergency care.

2. Be prepared to provide CPR (rescue breathing and chest compressions) if necessary.

Monitor the victim's responsiveness and breathing continuously. It can be helpful to palpate the victim's pulse to evaluate heart rate and regularity. Electrocardiographic monitoring should be initiated as soon as possible. Without warning, the victim may develop a rhythm disturbance that may cause cardiac arrest. Rescue personnel should administer oxygen if available.

If the victim becomes unresponsive, begin the ABCs of CPR by opening the airway, assessing for breathing, and providing rescue breathing if needed. You will then attempt to palpate the carotid artery while looking for other signs of circulation (normal breathing, coughing, or movement in response to the rescue breaths). If there is no pulse and no signs of circulation are present, provide chest compressions.

Continue CPR until the arrival of another rescuer with an AED or other EMS personnel capable of providing advanced cardiovascular life support (see chapter 6, "Adult Cardiopulmonary Resuscitation").

Denial: The Deadly Response to a Heart Attack

Victims of heart attack frequently deny the possibility of a heart attack with rationalizations such as the following:

- *It's indigestion or something I ate.*

- *It can't happen to me. I'm too healthy.*

- *I don't want to bother my doctor.*

- *I don't want to frighten anyone.*

- *I'll use a home remedy.*

- *I'll feel ridiculous if it isn't a heart attack.*

When the victim starts looking for reasons why he or she can't be having a heart

Critical Concepts:
The Psychology of Denial of AMI

Denial is a common reaction to emergencies such as AMI. The victim's first tendency may be to deny the possibility of a heart attack. This denial is not limited to the victim — it may also persuade the rescuer. The tendency of people involved in an emergency to deny or downplay the serious nature of the presenting problem is a natural one that must be overcome to provide rapid intervention and maximize the victim's chance of survival. Denial of the serious nature of the symptoms delays treatment and increases the risk of death.[30,31]

The elderly, women, and persons with diabetes, hypertension, or known CAD are most likely to delay calling the EMS system.[11]

Because the victim may deny the possibility of a heart attack, rescuers must be prepared to activate the EMS system and provide BLS as necessary. Public education campaigns have been effective in increasing public awareness of this important issue.[32,33]

attack, it is a signal for positive action by a bystander or family member.

Prehospital death from MI is often preventable. If VF develops after EMS personnel arrive, they will be prepared to provide CPR and defibrillation. Paramedics are also capable of establishing intravenous (IV) access, administering drugs, and providing advanced support of ventilation. But none of these therapies will be available to the victim unless the EMS system is notified.

Sudden Cardiac Death (Cardiac Arrest)

Sudden death occurs when the heart stops beating and breathing ceases abruptly or unexpectedly. Sudden cardiac death, or cardiac arrest, may occur as the initial and only symptom of CAD. Sudden cardiac death may occur before any other symptoms develop. It may also occur in persons with known CAD and may complicate a heart attack. It most commonly occurs within the first hour after the onset of symptoms of a heart attack.

Within seconds after cardiac arrest the victim becomes unresponsive and stops breathing. The sooner circulation to the brain is restored, the greater the chance for full recovery of brain function. After 4 to 6 minutes of cardiac arrest, significant brain damage usually develops unless CPR is provided immediately. Occasionally persons exposed to extreme cold (for example, a small child submerged in icy water) or a barbiturate overdose may recover normal brain function after longer periods of cardiac arrest. Such a recovery or survival, however, is not the norm. Patients who develop cardiac arrest need immediate CPR and use of a defibrillator as soon as it is available.

Causes of Sudden Cardiac Arrest

CAD is the most common cause of cardiac arrest. Yet any condition that interferes with the delivery of oxygen or blood to the heart or that causes irritation of the

heart muscle itself may lead to cardiac arrest. These conditions include primary respiratory arrest, direct injury to the heart, use of drugs, or disturbances in heart rhythm. Several of the most common noncardiac causes of cardiac arrest are presented in Chapter 11.

Brain injury does not invariably lead to cardiac arrest, because the heart does not require normal brain function to continue beating. If the brain injury causes respiratory arrest, this can precipitate a cardiac arrest. Even when respiration ceases, however, the heart may continue to beat for several minutes until the oxygen level in the blood is so low that the heart stops beating.

In most episodes of sudden cardiac death the direct cause of the cardiac arrest is VF (an abnormal, chaotic, uncoordinated quivering of the heart muscle), which results in the lack of an effective heartbeat. VF develops in approximately 5% of patients with AMI, and this incidence has not changed over time.[34] VF is responsible for most prehospital deaths in patients with AMI and is linked to increased in-hospital mortality.[34]

Treatment of Sudden Cardiac Arrest

VF cannot be converted to an effective heartbeat without electrical defibrillation. Until defibrillation can be attempted, however, CPR may maintain vital organ perfusion for several minutes. Defibrillation is the key to resuscitation from VF. It consists of the application of electric shock to the heart through the chest wall. The electric shock depolarizes all myocardial cells at the same time, which may enable spontaneous coordinated electrical activity to return. Defibrillation should be performed as soon as possible at the scene.

If CPR is initiated promptly and defibrillation provided rapidly, the victim's chance of survival is high. Early defibrillation is a vital link in the Chain of Survival.[35] It has been shown to significantly improve outcome in victims of

out-of-hospital cardiac arrest.[36-41] It can be performed by minimally trained personnel using automated external defibrillators (AEDs)[42-44] (see Chapter 7, "Automated External Defibrillation"). BLS providers employed by healthcare systems that have AEDs should learn how to use them.

Out-of-Hospital Care for ACS

Rapid access of the EMS system after recognition of the signs and symptoms of ACS has many benefits. Emergency dispatchers can send the appropriate emergency team and provide patient care instructions for the patient before their arrival.[45] BLS-trained ambulance providers can administer oxygen, nitroglycerin, and aspirin out-of-hospital.[46,47] Nitroglycerin is effective for relief of symptoms,[48] and aspirin has been shown to reduce mortality in ACS.[49] Oxygen has been shown to reduce the degree of ECG changes associated with heart attack. Routine out-of-hospital administration of these medications by BLS ambulance providers is expected to reduce AMI morbidity and mortality.[50]

ACLS-trained ambulance providers monitor the heart rhythm continuously to immediately detect potentially lethal cardiac arrhythmias. In many systems ACLS ambulance providers are equipped and authorized to perform a 12-lead ECG and transmit it to the receiving facility. This enables diagnosis of a heart attack in progress and significantly reduces time to treatment, including fibrinolytic therapy, upon arrival at the hospital.[51-56] In the event of a complication (either at the scene or en route to the hospital), ACLS ambulance providers can administer lifesaving therapies, including rapid defibrillation, airway management, and IV medications.

Initial Assessment and Stabilization

BLS providers must assess responsiveness, airway, breathing, and circulation. If the victim is unresponsive, open the airway and assess breathing. When needed, provide ventilation with a bag mask or other device capable of delivering oxygen. All victims with suspected ACS should receive supplemental oxygen even if initial evidence of oxygenation is good. If the victim is unresponsive and has no breathing with no signs of circulation (including no pulse) after delivery of 2 rescue breaths, use of an AED is indicated.

History and Physical Assessment

The BLS ambulance provider obtains a focused history during preparation for transport, but obtaining the history should not delay transport of the ACS victim. The history should include questions about the quality, intensity, location, radiation, and duration of chest discomfort, initiating and relieving factors, and activity at onset of symptoms. The EMS provider should also obtain a significant past medical history and risk factors for ACS.

The physical assessment of the victim should not delay transport. It should focus on vital signs and assessment of signs of oxygenation and perfusion. The BLS ambulance provider should routinely evaluate skin color, temperature, and moisture. Typically victims with ACS will exhibit signs of a stress response, including cool, pale, and sweaty skin. The physical examination should include auscultation of breath sounds and evaluation for evidence of congestive heart failure (distended neck veins, shortness of breath, and peripheral edema).

Management

In the out-of-hospital setting provide supplemental oxygen at 4 L/min to all victims with suspected ACS and titrate as needed. If the victim is experiencing chest discomfort and has a recent prescription for nitroglycerin, the BLS ambulance provider can help administer it, provided that the victim's systolic blood pressure is greater than 90 mm Hg. The victim can take up to 3 nitroglycerin tablets at intervals of 3 to 5 minutes. Monitor blood pressure closely for signs of hypotension after administration of each nitroglycerin tablet. Place the victim in a position of comfort and transport to the hospital as soon as possible.

Aspirin (160 to 325 mg) can be administered en route according to local protocols. Prearrival notification of the receiving hospital is essential to shorten the time to definitive treatment after arrival at the hospital.

ACLS ambulance providers may provide additional therapies, including administration of IV morphine; medications to manage arrhythmias, shock, and pulmonary congestion; and transcutaneous pacing if needed. The mnemonic "MONA" (morphine, oxygen, nitroglycerin, and aspirin) is used as a reminder of the core out-of-hospital therapies for ACS. This mnemonic, however, does not indicate the appropriate order of these therapies: oxygen, nitroglycerin, and aspirin are often administered by BLS providers, whereas morphine is administered by ACLS providers.

Summary of CAD

Take time to review the prehospital BLS AMI algorithm (Figure 4).

Summary of Key Concepts

- Cardiovascular disease is the leading cause of death in the United States.

- The term *acute coronary syndromes* encompasses symptomatic conditions resulting in an inadequate blood supply to the heart, including unstable angina and AMI.

- Atypical symptoms of AMI are more likely to occur in patients with diabetes, women, and the elderly.

- Angina is a transient discomfort (usually less than 15 minutes) due to a temporary lack of adequate blood supply to the heart muscle.

- AMI is defined as death of heart tissue due to blockage of a coronary artery caused by atherosclerosis and thrombus formation.

- Chest discomfort associated with AMI is usually "pressure-like" and typically lasts longer than 15 to 20 minutes.

- Additional signs and symptoms associated with AMI include nausea; vomiting; sweating; radiation of discomfort to the neck, jaw, or arm; and difficulty breathing.

- Denial is a common reaction to emergencies such as AMI. When signs and symptoms are present, bystanders should be prepared to activate the EMS system and provide BLS as necessary.

- A patient with chest discomfort and known CAD should be encouraged to take up to 3 nitroglycerin tablets (1 tablet every 3 to 5 minutes) if needed for chest discomfort unrelieved by rest but should wait for no longer than 10 minutes before activating the EMS system.

- Patients with chest discomfort and no known history of CAD should wait only a few minutes (no more than 5 minutes) before activating the EMS system.

- The most common cause of sudden cardiac death associated with AMI and prolonged angina is VF (an abnormal, chaotic, uncoordinated quivering of the heart muscle), which results in the lack of an effective heartbeat.

- The only effective treatment for VF is defibrillation. Defibrillation must be attempted as soon as possible to maximize the victim's chance of survival. CPR buys time, maintaining minimal blood flow and oxygen delivery to vital organs until defibrillation can be attempted.

FIGURE 4. Algorithm for Prehospital BLS Management of Acute Myocardial Infarction.

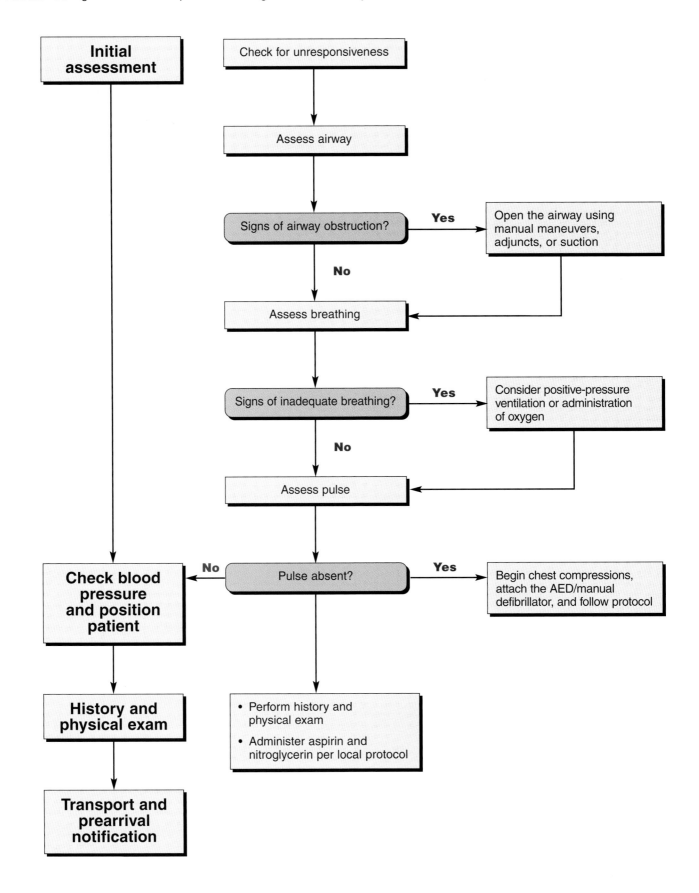

Review Questions

1. Mr. Jones developed his first episode of ischemic chest pain at the age of 43 and was diagnosed with angina pectoris. At the age of 50 he had an AMI that required bypass surgery. This gradual process of narrowing of the coronary arteries leading to the development of these diseases is called

   a. ischemia

   b. atherosclerosis

   c. angina

   d. thrombosis

2. The cardiovascular problems experienced by Mr. Jones fall into the general category of

   a. congestive heart failure

   b. acute coronary syndromes (ACS)

   c. cardiogenic shock

   d. valvular disease

3. Mrs. Anderson is an 83-year-old woman who suffered an AMI at home while vacuuming the floor. She has a history of high blood pressure, stroke, and diabetes. She did not experience chest pain but instead had a combination of less-dramatic symptoms, including mild shortness of breath, sweating, and dizziness. What factors in Mrs. Anderson's profile made her prone to an atypical presentation of AMI?

   a. age, gender, and a history of diabetes

   b. history of high blood pressure and activity at onset of event

   c. history of stroke and history of high blood pressure

   d. activity at the onset of illness and history of stroke

4. Your uncle, who has a history of angina, has been experiencing chest discomfort for 2 minutes. He routinely takes nitroglycerin for chronic angina. You should

   a. allow him to take up to 3 nitroglycerin tablets before activating EMS

   b. activate EMS and then help administer nitroglycerin

   c. not allow him to take the nitroglycerin because the pain has lasted too long

   d. allow him to take only 1 nitroglycerin tablet

5. A 55-year-old woman suddenly experiences crushing, substernal/central chest pain while at work. She has no known history of CAD. When should you activate EMS?

   a. if the pain is not relieved within a few hours

   b. if the pain is not relieved within a few minutes of rest

   c. after administering nitroglycerin obtained from a coworker

   d. the minute chest pain begins

6. A 62-year-old man suddenly collapses while walking on a treadmill at the health club. He is unresponsive, and you immediately ask someone to activate the EMS system while you begin CPR. The man is not breathing and has no signs of circulation. What abnormal heart rhythm is the most likely cause of this event?

   a. asystole

   b. bradycardia

   c. ventricular fibrillation

   d. pulseless electrical activity

7. What definitive treatment will be needed to convert this 62-year-old man back to a normal heart rhythm?

   a. CPR

   b. rescue breathing

   c. sublingual nitroglycerin

   d. defibrillation

How did you do?
Answers: **1,** b; **2,** b; **3,** a; **4,** a; **5,** b; **6,** c; **7,** d.

References

1. Graves EJ. National hospital discharge survey: annual summary, 1991. *Vital Health Statistics.* 1993;13:1-62.

2. *2000 Heart and Stroke Statistical Supplement.* Dallas, Tex: American Heart Association; 1999.

3. Gillum RF. Trends in acute myocardial infarction and coronary heart disease death in the United States. *J Am Coll Cardiol.* 1994;23: 1273-1277.

4. Kannel WB, Schatzkin A. Sudden death: lessons from subsets in population studies. *J Am Coll Cardiol.* 1985;5(suppl 6):141B-149B.

5. Brouwer MA, Martin JS, Maynard C, et al. Influence of early prehospital thrombolysis on mortality and event-free survival (the Myocardial Infarction Triage and Intervention [MITI] Randomized Trial): MITI Project Investigators. *Am J Cardiol.* 1996;78:497-502.

6. Raitt MH, Maynard C, Wagner GS, et al. Relation between symptom duration before thrombolytic therapy and final myocardial infarct size. *Circulation.* 1996;93:48-53.

7. Wackers FJ, Terrin ML, Kayden DS, et al. Quantitative radionuclide assessment of regional ventricular function after thrombolytic therapy for acute myocardial infarction: results of phase I Thrombolysis in Myocardial Infarction (TIMI) trial. *J Am Coll Cardiol.* 1989;13:998-1005.

8. Res JC, Simoons ML, van der Wall EE, et al. Long term improvement in global left ventricular function after early thrombolytic treatment in acute myocardial infarction: report of a randomised multicentre trial of intracoronary streptokinase in acute myocardial infarction. *Br Heart J.* 1986;56:414-421.

9. Mathey DG, Sheehan FH, Schofer J, Dodge HT. Time from onset of symptoms to thrombolytic therapy: a major determinant of myocardial salvage in patients with acute transmural infarction. *J Am Coll Cardiol.* 1985;6:518-525.

10. Serruys PW, Simoons ML, Suryapranata H, et al. Preservation of global and regional left ventricular function after early thrombolysis in acute myocardial infarction. *J Am Coll Cardiol.* 1986;7:729-742.

11. Newby LK, Rutsch WR, Califf RM, et al. Time from symptom onset to treatment and outcomes after thrombolytic therapy: GUSTO-1 Investigators. *J Am Coll Cardiol.* 1996;27: 1646-1655.

12. Anderson JL, Karagounis LA, Califf RM. Metaanalysis of five reported studies on the relation of early coronary patency grades with mortality and outcomes after acute myocardial infarction. *Am J Cardiol.* 1996;78:1-8.

13. Chesebro JH, Rauch U, Fuster V, Badimon JJ. Pathogenesis of thrombosis in coronary artery disease. *Haemostasis.* 1997;27(suppl 1):12-18.

14. Fuster V, Fallon JT, Badimon JJ, Nemerson Y. The unstable atherosclerotic plaque: clinical significance and therapeutic intervention. *Thromb Haemost.* 1997;78:247-255.

15. Azar RWD. The inflammatory etiology of unstable angina. *Am Heart J.* 1996;132: 1101-1106.

16. American College of Cardiology/American Heart Association Task Force on Practice Guidelines, Committee on Management of Acute Myocardial Infarction. 1999 update: ACC/AHA guidelines for the management of patients with myocardial infarction. *J Am Coll Cardiol.* 1999;34:890-911.

17. Peberdy MA, Ornato JP. Coronary artery disease in women. *Heart Dis Stroke.* 1992;1: 315-319.

18. Douglas PS, Ginsburg GS. The evaluation of chest pain in women. *N Engl J Med.* 1996;334: 1311-1315.

19. Sullivan AK, Holdright DR, Wright CA, et al. Chest pain in women: clinical, investigative, and prognostic features. *Br Med J.* 1994;308: 883-886.

20. Brand FN, Larson M, Friedman LM, Kannel WB, Castelli WP. Epidemiologic assessment of angina before and after myocardial infarction: the Framingham study. *Am Heart J.* 1996;132(pt 1):174-178.

21. Sigurdsson E, Thorgeirsson G, Sigvaldason H, Sigfusson N. Unrecognized myocardial infarction: epidemiology, clinical characteristics, and the prognostic role of angina pectoris: the Reykjavik Study. *Ann Intern Med.* 1995;122: 96-102.

22. Antman EM, Fox KM, for the International Cardiology Forum. Guidelines for the diagnosis and management of unstable angina and non–Q-wave myocardial infarction: proposed revisions. *Am Heart J.* 2000;139:461-475.

23. Solomon CG, Lee TH, Cook EF, et al. Comparison of clinical presentation of acute myocardial infarction in patients older than 65 years of age to younger patients: the Multicenter Chest Pain Study experience. *Am J Cardiol.* 1989;63:772-776.

24. Behar S, Halabi M, Reicher-Reiss H, et al. Circadian variation and possible external triggers of onset of myocardial infarction: SPRINT Study Group. *Am J Med.* 1993;94:395-400.

25. Smith M, Little WC. Potential precipitating factors of the onset of myocardial infarction. *Am J Med Sci.* 1992;303:141-144.

26. Jenkins CD. Recent evidence supporting psychologic and social risk factors for coronary disease. *N Engl J Med.* 1976;294:1033-1038.

27. Rahe RH, Romo M, Bennett L, Siltanen P. Recent life changes, myocardial infarction, and abrupt coronary death: studies in Helsinki. *Arch Intern Med.* 1974;133:221-228.

28. Castro VJ, Nacht R. Cocaine-induced brady-arrhythmia: an unsuspected cause of syncope. *Chest.* 2000;117:275-277.

29. Mittleman MA, Mintzer D, Maclure M, Tofler GH, Sherwood JB, Muller JE. Triggering of myocardial infarction by cocaine. *Circulation.* 1999;2737-2741.

30. Kereiakes DJ, Weaver WD, Anderson JL, Feldman T, Gibler B, Aufderheide T, Williams DO, Martin LH, Anderson LC, Martin JS, et al. Time delays in the diagnosis and treatment of acute myocardial infarction: a tale of eight cities: report from the Pre-hospital Study Group and the Cincinnati Heart Project. *Am Heart J.* 1990;120:773-780.

31. Weaver WD. Time to thrombolytic treatment: factors affecting delay and their influence on outcome. *J Am Coll Cardiol.* 1995;25(suppl 7): 3S-9S.

32. Blohm M, Herlitz J, Schroder U, et al. Reaction to a media campaign focusing on delay in acute myocardial infarction. *Heart Lung.* 1991;20:661-666.

33. Blohm MB, Hartford M, Karlson BW, Luepker RV, Herlitz J. An evaluation of the results of media and educational campaigns designed to shorten the time taken by patients with acute myocardial infarction to decide to go to hospital. *Heart.* 1996;76:430-434.

34. Thompson CA, Yarzebski J, Goldberg RJ, Lessard D, et al. Changes over time in the incidence and case-fatality rates of primary ventricular fibrillation complicating acute myocardial infarction: perspectives from the Worcester Heart Attack Study. *Am Heart J.* 2000;139:1014-1021.

35. Cummins RO, Ornato JP, Thies WH, Pepe PE. Improving survival from sudden cardiac arrest: the "chain of survival" concept: a statement for health professionals from the Advanced Cardiac Life Support Subcommittee and the Emergency Cardiac Care Committee, American Heart Association. *Circulation.* 1991;83:1832-1847.

36. Larsen MP, Eisenberg MS, Cummins RO, Hallstrom AP. Predicting survival from out-of-hospital cardiac arrest: a graphic model. *Ann Emerg Med.* 1993;22:1652-1658.

37. Auble TE, Menegazzi JJ, Paris PM. Effect of out-of-hospital defibrillation by basic life support providers on cardiac arrest mortality: a metaanalysis. *Ann Emerg Med.* 1995;25: 642-648.

38. Holmberg M, Holmberg S, Herlitz J, Gardelov B. Survival after cardiac arrest outside hospital in Sweden. Swedish Cardiac Arrest Registry. *Resuscitation.* 1998;36:29-36.

39. White RD, Asplin BR, Bugliosi TF, Hankins DG. High discharge survival rate after out-of-hospital ventricular fibrillation with rapid defibrillation by police and paramedics. *Ann Emerg Med*. 1996;28:480-485.

40. White RD, Hankins DG, Bugliosi TF. Seven years' experience with early defibrillation by police and paramedics in an emergency medical services system. *Resuscitation*. 1998;39:145-151.

41. Nichol G, Hallstrom AP, Ornato JP, Riegel B, Stiell IG, Valenzuela T, Wells GA, White RD, Weisfeldt ML. Potential cost-effectiveness of public access defibrillation in the United States. *Circulation*. 1998;97:1315-1320.

42. White RD, Vukov LF, Bugliosi TF. Early defibrillation by police: initial experience with measurement of critical time intervals and patient outcome. Ann Emerg Med. 1994;23:1009-1013.

43. O'Rourke MF, Donaldson E, Geddes JS. An airline cardiac arrest program. *Circulation*. 1997;96:2849-2853.

44. Page RL, Hamdan MH, McKenas DK. Defibrillation aboard a commercial aircraft. *Circulation*. 1998;97:1429-1430.

45. Rossi R. The role of the dispatch centre in preclinical emergency medicine. *Eur J Emerg Med*. 1994;1:27-30.

46. Haynes BE, Pritting J. A rural emergency medical technician with selected advanced skills. *Prehosp Emerg Care*. 1999;3:343-346.

47. Funk D, Groat C, Verdile VP. Education of paramedics regarding aspirin use. *Prehosp Emerg Care*. 2000;4:62-64.

48. Held P. Effects of nitrates on mortality in acute myocardial infarction and in heart failure. *Br J Clin Pharmacol*. 1992;34(suppl 1):25S-28S.

49. Verheugt FW, van der Laarse A, Funke-Kupper AJ, Sterkman LG, Galema TW, Roos JP. Effects of early intervention with low-dose aspirin (100 mg) on infarct size, reinfarction and mortality in anterior wall acute myocardial infarction. *Am J Cardiol*. 1990;66:267-277.

50. Tan WA, Moliterno DJ. Aspirin, ticlopidine, and clopidogrel in acute coronary syndromes: underused treatments could save thousands of lives. *Cleve Clin J Med*. 1999;66:615-618, 621-624,627-628.

51. Aufderheide TP, Hendley GE, Woo J, et al. A prospective evaluation of prehospital 12-lead ECG application in chest pain patients. *J Electrocardiol*. 1992;24(suppl):8-13.

52. Aufderheide TP, Keelan MH, Hendley GE, et al. Milwaukee Prehospital Chest Pain Project, phase 1: feasibility and accuracy of prehospital thrombolytic candidate selection. *Am J Cardiol*. 1992;69:991-996.

53. Selker HP, Zalenski RJ, Antman EM, Aufderheide TP, et al. An evaluation of technologies for identifying acute cardiac ischemia in the emergency department: a report from a National Heart Attack Alert Program Working Group. *Ann Emerg Med*. 1997;29:13-87.

54. Aufderheide TP, Kereiakes DJ, Weaver WD, et al. Planning, implementation, and process monitoring for prehospital 12-lead ECG diagnostic programs. *Prehosp Disaster Med*. 1996;11:162-171.

55. National Heart Attack Alert Program Coordinating Committee, 60 Minutes to Treatment Working Group. Emergency department: rapid identification and treatment of patients with acute myocardial infarction. *Ann Emerg Med*. 1994;23:311-329.

56. Canto JG, Rogers WJ, Bowlby LJ, et al. The prehospital electrocardiogram in acute myocardial infarction: is its full potential being realized? *J Am Coll Cardiol*. 1997;29:498-505.

You are an EMT called to the home of an elderly woman. Upon your arrival the woman's husband tells you that 20 minutes ago, while sitting in a chair watching television, his wife began slurring her words. She has been unable to get up because of weakness in her right leg.

Initial assessment reveals no problems with airway, breathing, or circulation. You quickly perform the Cincinnati Prehospital Stroke Scale and identify left facial droop, right arm weakness, and slurring of speech. You assess her level of consciousness and determine that her Glasgow Coma Scale score is 14. You strongly suspect a stroke, with a time of onset at 2:50 PM (27 minutes ago), based on the husband's history.

Both the wife and husband ask that you take her to the community hospital nearby. You realize, however, that she may be a candidate for fibrinolytic therapy, and you know that the community hospital does not have computed tomography (CT). You think the woman may benefit from treatment at another hospital that you know is capable of managing acute stroke. After explaining your concern to the couple, they agree to your recommendation.

You expedite transport, notifying the receiving hospital of the time of symptom onset and the results of the Cincinnati Prehospital Stroke Scale and Glasgow Coma Scale. A stroke team is waiting for you when you arrive at the hospital at 3:30 PM.

You get a call from the husband 2 days later. He thanks you profusely and says that his wife received fibrinolytic therapy shortly after arrival at the hospital and that all her symptoms have resolved.

Acute Stroke

Overview

Stroke is the third leading cause of death in the United States and the leading cause of brain injury in adults. Each year approximately 500 000 Americans suffer a new or recurrent stroke and nearly a quarter of those die (Figure 1).[1] Until recently care of the stroke patient was largely supportive, with therapy focusing on treatment of complications.[2] Because no treatment was available to alter the course of the stroke itself, little emphasis was placed on rapid transport or intervention.[2]

Now fibrinolytic therapy offers the opportunity to limit neurologic insult and improve outcome in ischemic stroke patients.[3-10] Fibrinolytic therapy reduces disability from stroke in eligible patients.[3-10] Patients treated with fibrinolytics are more likely to be discharged home and less likely to be discharged to a nursing home.[7,11] This therapy is cost-effective and results in sustained improvement in quality of life.[7,11]

For these reasons all patients presenting to the hospital within 3 hours of the onset of signs and symptoms consistent with acute ischemic stroke should be considered for intravenous fibrinolytic therapy.[3,6,7,10] Use of intra-arterial fibrinolytic agents within 3 to 6 hours of symptom onset may also be beneficial in patients with stroke caused by middle cerebral artery occlusions. They should be administered in hospitals experienced with this therapy.[4,8,9]

Learning Objectives

1. Recognize that new therapy for acute stroke limits disability if provided within 3 hours of stroke onset.

2. Define transient ischemic attack (TIA), acute stroke, ischemic stroke, and hemorrhagic stroke.

3. Describe the key points in stroke care (the 7 "D's" of stroke) and the importance of avoiding delays at each point.

4. Recognize the time-critical nature of treatment for acute stroke, including the importance of rapid identification and transport to a hospital capable of caring for patients with acute stroke.

5. Recognize the importance of educating at-risk patients and their families to phone 911 (or other emergency response number) immediately if symptoms of a possible stroke appear.

6. List the goals of prehospital assessment and management of patients with suspected stroke.

7. Describe the Cincinnati Prehospital Stroke Scale and the Los Angeles Prehospital Stroke Screen.

8. Describe the Glasgow Coma Scale.

9. Recognize the need for BLS ambulance providers to obtain the following information and communicate it to the receiving hospital before arrival:

   a. The time of suspected stroke onset

   b. The results of a prehospital stroke scale or stroke screen

   c. Results of the Glasgow Coma Scale

The time available to provide this beneficial therapy is brief. For most stroke victims, definitive hospital-based intervention must occur within 3 hours of symptom onset. These time-limited treatments now available for stroke highlight the important role of lay rescuers, first responders, and emergency medical services (EMS) personnel. Early recognition, early intervention, and early transport of victims with suspected stroke from the scene to a *hospital capable of managing acute stroke patients* can substantially reduce morbidity and mortality.

FIGURE 1. Estimated prevalence of stroke by age and sex, United States, 1988-1994.

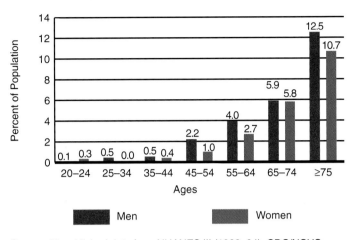

Source: Unpublished data from NHANES III (1988–94), CDC/NCHS.

Pathophysiology and Classification of Cerebrovascular Disease

The pathophysiology of an ischemic stroke is similar to that of a myocardial infarction.[12] In both cases there is inadequate blood supply and oxygen delivery, usually as the result of an obstructing blood clot. This blood clot often obstructs flow in an artery that is already narrowed by atherosclerosis. Rapid intervention with fibrinolytic therapy can improve the outcome of stroke, just as fibrinolytic therapy can improve the outcome of acute myocardial infarction (AMI).[3] The pathophysiology of hemorrhagic stroke is somewhat different; this type of stroke occurs when a vessel ruptures.

A *transient ischemic attack, or TIA,* is a reversible episode of focal neurologic dysfunction that typically lasts a few minutes to a few hours. It is impossible to distinguish between a TIA and a stroke at the time of onset. If the neurologic symptoms completely resolve within 24 hours, the event is then classified as a TIA. In fact, most TIAs are less than 60 minutes in duration.[13] TIAs are a significant indicator of stroke risk. Approximately 5% of patients with a

TIA will develop a stroke within 1 month if untreated.[2,14] Approximately one fourth of patients presenting with stroke have had a previous TIA.[15] Patients who experience a TIA should be evaluated by a physician to identify therapies that may reduce the risk of stroke. Antiplatelet agents such as aspirin can reduce the risk of subsequent stroke in patients with TIA.

A stroke is a disruption in blood supply to a region of the brain that causes sudden neurologic impairment. Approximately 85% of strokes are *ischemic,* resulting from complete occlusion of a cerebral artery caused by cerebral thrombosis (blood clot) or embolism (blockage of a vessel by a clot that has traveled from another location). Hemorrhagic strokes are caused by cerebral artery rupture with bleeding into the surface of the brain (subarachnoid hemorrhage) or bleeding into the tissue of the brain (intracerebral hemorrhage). The most common cause of a subarachnoid hemorrhage is an aneurysm.[16,17] The most common cause of intracerebral hemorrhage is hypertension.[18,19]

Although both ischemic and hemorrhagic stroke can be life-threatening, ischemic stroke rarely leads to death within the first hour. By comparison, hemorrhagic stroke can be fatal at onset. Patients with

ischemic stroke can often be treated with fibrinolytic therapy if they arrive within 2 hours at a hospital capable of treating acute stroke (with protocols for providing fibrinolytic therapy) and receive the drug within 3 hours of symptom onset. Fibrinolytic therapy *cannot* be administered to patients with hemorrhagic stroke because it would worsen intracerebral bleeding. Some patients with hemorrhagic stroke can benefit from operative intervention.[20,21]

The AHA ECC Chain of Survival for the Stroke Victim

The metaphor of a Chain of Survival has been used to describe the sequence of events needed to survive sudden cardiac death[22]:

- Early access to EMS

- Early CPR

- Early defibrillation

- Early advanced care

The AHA and the American Stroke Association have also developed a community-oriented "stroke chain of survival" that links specific actions to be taken by patients and family members with recommended actions by out-of-hospital healthcare responders, emergency department personnel, and in-hospital specialty services:

- Rapid recognition and reaction to stroke warning signs

- Rapid start of prehospital care

- Rapid EMS system transport and hospital pre-notification

- Rapid diagnosis and treatment in the hospital

Stroke victims will rarely require defibrillation, although arrhythmias are common during the first 24 hours after a stroke.[23] Stroke victims do require early advanced care with rapid transport and prearrival notification to a hospital capable of treating acute stroke.

The Key Points in Stroke Management: The 7 "D's" of Stroke Care

Key points in the management of the stroke patient can be remembered using the 7 "D's" mnemonic[24]: **D**etection, **D**ispatch, **D**elivery, **D**oor, **D**ata, **D**ecision, and **D**rug.[24] Delay may occur at any of these points of management, so at each point, response to and management of the stroke victim must be skilled and efficient.

The first 3 D's (**d**etection, **d**ispatch, and **d**elivery) are the responsibility of BLS providers in the community, including the lay public and EMS responders. **D**etection occurs when a patient, family member, or bystander recognizes the signs and symptoms of a stroke or TIA and phones 911 (or activates the EMS system). EMS dispatchers must then prioritize the call for a suspected stroke patient as they would a victim of AMI or serious trauma and dispatch the appropriate EMS team with high transport priority. EMS providers must respond quickly, confirm the signs and symptoms of a suspected stroke, transport (**deliv**ery) the patient to a hospital capable of caring for patients with acute stroke (this includes provision of fibrinolytic therapy within 1 hour after arrival at the Emergency Department). These 3 points are discussed in greater detail below.

The remaining 4 D's are initiated in-hospital: **d**oor (initial Emergency Department triage and evaluation), **d**ata (acquiring a CT scan to diagnose the type of stroke), **d**ecision (identifying candidates eligible for fibrinolytic therapy), and **d**rug (treating with fibrinolytic therapy).

Detection of Warning Signs of Stroke

Recognition of the signs and symptoms of stroke is critical to early intervention and treatment. The presentation of stroke may be subtle. Signs and symptoms of stroke may include only mild facial paralysis or difficulty with speaking that may go unnoticed or be denied by the patient or family member.[25] Other signs and symptoms include alteration in responsiveness (confusion, stupor, or coma); sudden weakness or numbness of the face, arm, or leg on one side of the body; slurred or incoherent speech; unexplained dizziness; unsteadiness; sudden falls; and dimness or loss of vision, particularly in one eye.

Patients at high risk for stroke and their families should be taught the warning signs of stroke and should be instructed to phone 911 whenever signs of stroke are suspected. In one recent study of stroke patients, only 8% had been educated about the signs of stroke, yet nearly half had experienced a prior TIA or stroke.[26] The education of at-risk patients and their families is the responsibility of healthcare providers, and the information should be reinforced in every contact with the patient and family.

Dispatch: Early EMS Activation and Dispatch Instructions

As soon as signs or symptoms of a stroke are suspected, family members or other bystanders should immediately activate the EMS system (phone 911 or other emergency response number). This is the first critical link in the Chain of Survival. Activation of the EMS system begins to link the stroke victim to medical care; this first link will make possible therapies such as fibrinolytics, which can improve survival and function after stroke.

Rapid access of the EMS system after recognition of stroke is beneficial for several reasons. Most important, stroke patients who are transported by the EMS system arrive at the hospital faster than those who are not. Studies have documented that contacting the family physician or having a family member drive the victim to the hospital actually delays the stroke victim's arrival at the hospital, and the delay is often sufficient to make the patient ineligible for treatment.[25,27-29] Arrival at a hospital capable of caring for patients with acute stroke within 1 to 2 hours of the onset of stroke symptoms increases the likelihood that the stroke victim will be eligible for time-critical therapy, such as fibrinolytics.[25,27,30-36]

When the EMS system is accessed, emergency dispatchers can send the appropriate emergency team and provide patient care instructions before their arrival.[28,37,38] EMS responders can then transport the victim to a hospital capable of caring for patients with acute stroke and notify that facility before arrival to ensure rapid hospital-based evaluation and treatment.

EMS dispatchers play a critical role in the timely treatment of potential stroke victims. They are responsible for suspecting a stroke when they receive a call for help, and they must prioritize the call appropriately to ensure a rapid response by the EMS system.

Although highly skilled dispatchers can be effective in triaging emergencies over the telephone, the available evidence suggests that dispatchers require additional education about stroke. In a recent study just over half of the EMS dispatchers correctly diagnosed stroke from the initial EMS call.[28]

Currently only half of stroke victims in the United States are transported to the hospital by the EMS system.[25,39] Strokes that occur when the victim is alone or sleeping may further delay prompt recognition and action.[40] Eighty-five percent of strokes occur at home.[39] As a result, public education programs have focused their efforts on persons at risk for stroke and their friends and family members.[39] Public education has been successful in reducing time to arrival at the Emergency Department.[30,41]

After telephoning 911 (or appropriate emergency response number), the lay BLS rescuer should provide supportive care, including reassurance, use of the recovery position, rescue breathing, and CPR if needed.

Dealing With Denial

Stroke victims may either be unable to understand that they are having a stroke or, like AMI victims, may deny their symptoms with rationalizations.[42] Most stroke victims delay access to care for hours after symptom onset.[12,25,26,30,39,41-46] Tragically this delay often eliminates any possibility of provision of fibrinolytic therapy. Because victims may deny that they have the symptoms of a stroke or are unable to understand, lay rescuers should activate the EMS system, providing additional BLS as necessary.

Delivery: Prehospital Management and Rapid Transport

The goals of prehospital management of patients with suspected stroke include rapid identification of the stroke, support of vital functions, rapid transport of the victim to the receiving facility, and prearrival notification of the receiving facility. This care is presented in more detail below.

Prehospital Management of Stroke

The EMS System and BLS Care

In the past BLS ambulance providers received minimal training in stroke assessment and care.[28,37,38,47,48] Effective programs are needed to train EMS personnel to accurately recognize and prioritize stroke.[49,50] BLS ambulance providers now play a critical role in the recognition and stabilization of the stroke victim, selection of a receiving hospital capable of administering fibrinolytic therapy, and rapid transport.

Emergency ambulance service policies should give the same high dispatch, treatment, and transport priorities to patients with signs and symptoms of an acute ischemic stroke as those given to patients with signs and symptoms of AMI or major trauma. Patients with suspected stroke with airway compromise or altered level of consciousness should be given the same high dispatch, treatment, and transport priorities as similar patients without stroke symptoms.

The goals of out-of-hospital management by BLS ambulance providers for patients with suspected stroke include

1. Priority dispatch and response

2. Initial assessment and management

3. Rapid identification of stroke (using a standardized stroke scale)

4. Rapid transport of the victim to a hospital capable of caring for patients with acute stroke (capable of delivering fibrinolytics within 1 hour of arrival)

5. Prearrival notification of the hospital

Initial Prehospital Assessment of ABCs

The initial assessment of the stroke victim should be accomplished as quickly as possible by addressing the ABCs (airway, breathing, and circulation). Airway obstruction (most commonly caused by the tongue and epiglottis) may develop if the patient is unresponsive or obtunded. In an unresponsive patient, an airway obstructed by the tongue is opened with a head tilt–chin lift or jaw thrust.

Inadequate ventilation may occur for similar reasons, and rescue breathing may be required. Because the patient may vomit, suction or manual techniques may be needed to clear and maintain a patent airway. Use of an oropharyngeal or nasopharyngeal airway as well as administration of oxygen may be appropriate. Hypotension, if present, is rarely due to stroke, so other causes should be considered.

History and Physical Assessment

Stroke should be suspected in any patient with sudden loss of neurologic function on one side of the body or sudden alteration in consciousness. For BLS ambulance providers, a comprehensive list of stroke symptoms is presented in Table 1. Symptoms occasionally occur alone, or they can occur in any combination. The findings can be most severe at the beginning, wax and wane, or worsen progressively. The clinical presentations of ischemic and hemorrhagic stroke often overlap. Both types of stroke are likely to cause facial droop, unilateral motor weakness or paralysis, and difficulties in speech, But some symptoms are useful for initially distinguishing ischemic from hemorrhagic stroke.

TABLE 1. Clinical Presentations of Acute Stroke

- Alteration in consciousness (coma, stupor, confusion, seizures, delirium)

- Intense or unusually severe headache of sudden onset or any headache associated with decreased level of consciousness or neurologic deficit; unusual and severe neck or facial pain

- Aphasia (incoherent speech or difficulty understanding speech)

- Facial weakness or asymmetry (paralysis of the facial muscles, usually noted when the patient speaks or smiles); may be on the same side as limb paralysis or on the opposite side

- Incoordination, weakness, paralysis, or sensory loss of one or more limbs; usually involves one half of the body, particularly the hand

- Ataxia (poor balance, clumsiness, or difficulty walking)

- Visual loss (monocular or binocular); may be a partial loss of visual field

- Dysarthria (slurred or indistinct speech)

- Intense vertigo, double vision, unilateral hearing loss, nausea, vomiting, photophobia, or phonophobia

In general, patients with hemorrhagic stroke appear to be more seriously ill and have a more rapid course of deterioration than patients with ischemic stroke. Headaches (often described by the victim as a sudden onset of "the worst headache of my life"), disturbances in consciousness, nausea, and vomiting are more prominent with hemorrhagic stroke than with ischemic stroke. Loss of consciousness may be transient, with resolution by the time the patient receives medical attention. Patients with subarachnoid hemorrhage may have an intense headache without focal neurologic signs.

It is important to note that clinical presentation alone cannot distinguish between ischemic and hemorrhagic stroke. A CT scan will be required to rule out hemorrhagic stroke before fibrinolytics can be administered.

The patient with an *ischemic* stroke may be eligible for in-hospital treatment with fibrinolytic therapy. However, the drug must be administered within 3 hours of onset of symptoms. This requires that a treatment team be mobilized at the receiving hospital, eligibility determined (with a CT scan obtained and interpreted), and then therapy administered, all within the 3-hour time limit. Awareness of these time-critical factors should be incorporated into out-of-hospital assessment and management.

History

After a stroke the patient may be able to communicate well. If at all possible, establish the chief complaint and symptoms such as headache, dizziness, nausea, vomiting, weakness, seizure, or difficulty speaking. BLS ambulance providers should establish the time of onset of signs and symptoms of stroke: this timing has important implications for potential therapy. The onset of symptoms is viewed as the beginning of the stroke, and eligibility for fibrinolytic therapy ends 3 hours from that time. Ask family members or friends at the scene when the patient *last appeared to be normal* (eg, when the

patient went to bed or other information that will give the receiving hospital some estimate of the time of onset of symptoms).

The differential diagnosis of stroke is not extensive. Few neurologic illnesses have a similar sudden course. The number of alternative diagnoses is larger when the patient is comatose or no history of the current illness is available.

Hypoglycemia (low blood sugar) can cause confusion and focal neurologic deficits without a major alteration in consciousness and is an important consideration in a diabetic patient with stroke. Seizures can be unwitnessed, and the patient may be found with only focal neurologic signs after the seizure (postictal paralysis) that can last several hours. Patients with stroke may fall, which may also cause a head injury.

Physical Exam

The physical exam consists of a brief general medical assessment, rapid identification of the suspected stroke, and evaluation of the victim's level of consciousness.

After ensuring an adequate airway and obtaining vital signs, conduct a brief general medical assessment. Look for trauma to the head or neck, cardiovascular compromise, ocular signs, or other abnormalities.

It is impractical to perform an extensive neurologic exam out-of-hospital because it will delay transporting the patient to a hospital capable of caring for patients with acute stroke. The abbreviated out-of-hospital neurologic exam should use a validated tool such as the Cincinnati Prehospital Stroke Scale[29] (Table 2) or the Los Angeles Prehospital Stroke Screen (LAPSS)[35,36] (Table 3).

The Cincinnati Prehospital Stroke Scale evaluates 3 major physical findings: facial droop (Figure 2), arm drift (Figure 3), and speech.[30] Unilateral abnormality in any of the 3 areas is strongly suggestive of a stroke.

The Los Angeles Prehospital Stroke Screen (LAPSS) is used for evaluation

TABLE 2. Cincinnati Prehospital Stroke Scale

Try to elicit one of the following signs (abnormality in any one is strongly suggestive of stroke):

Facial droop (have patient show teeth or smile):

- Normal: both sides of face move equally well
- Abnormal: one side of face does not move as well as the other side

Arm drift (have patient close eyes and hold both arms straight out for 10 seconds):

- Normal: both arms move the same or both arms do not move at all (other findings, such as pronator drift, may be helpful)
- Abnormal: one arm does not move or one arm drifts down

Abnormal speech (have the patient say "you can't teach an old dog new tricks"):

- Normal: patient uses correct words with no slurring
- Abnormal: patient slurs words, uses the wrong words, or is unable to speak

From Reference 29.

of an acute, noncomatose, nontraumatic neurologic complaint. It requires that the provider give positive answers to a series of questions to rule out other causes of altered level of consciousness (eg, abnormal blood glucose). Then the provider must attempt to identify obvious right versus left asymmetry in facial smile or grimace, grip, and arm strength (Table 3).[35,36] Both have been proved sensitive and specific in identifying stroke patients.[29,36]

Either the Cincinnati Prehospital Stroke Scale or the LAPSS should be quickly accomplished. Note that the LAPSS will require determination of the patient's blood glucose level.

The patient's level of consciousness should then be assessed. The Glasgow Coma Scale (Table 4) is used to score the patient's response (eye opening, best motor response, and best verbal response) to simple stimuli such as voice and pain. The Glasgow Coma Scale is a well-known, reproducible scoring system that is reliable when used for stroke patients.[51]

Studies have shown an acceptable sensitivity and specificity of EMS identification of stroke patients.[52-58] *Once the diagnosis of stroke is suspected, time in the field should be kept to a minimum and the patient prepared for immediate transport to a hospital capable of caring for patients with acute stroke.*

Out-of-Hospital Management

Assessment and support of airway, breathing, and circulation must always be the first priority. Cardiac arrest in stroke patients is uncommon, but because many stroke victims have an altered level of consciousness, airway and breathing problems are frequent. BLS procedures include the head tilt–chin lift, jaw thrust, clearing of airway secretions, and rescue breathing as appropriate.

Seizures may complicate stroke. BLS treatment of a seizure requires

■ Protecting the victim's head (cradle the head or place something soft underneath it, such as a towel or your hands, to prevent injury)

■ Observing the victim during and after the seizure

■ At the end of the seizure assessing airway and breathing

If breathing is adequate, place the victim in a recovery position to allow pooled secretions to clear. *Do not place objects or fingers in the victim's mouth, and do not restrain the victim's movements.* Aspiration of food may occur as a complication of any seizure.

Many stroke victims demonstrate arrhythmias, including ventricular tachyarrhythmias and atrial fibrillation.[59-61] These

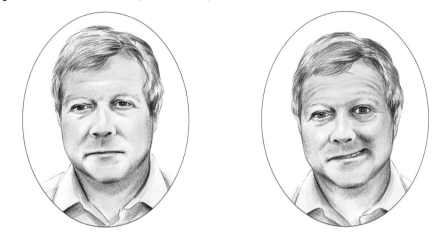

FIGURE 2. Facial droop in patient with stroke. A. Normal, B. Droop apparent on the right side of the face when patient attempts to smile.

TABLE 3. Los Angeles Prehospital Stroke Screen (LAPSS)

For evaluation of acute, noncomatose, nontraumatic neurologic complaint. If items 1 through 6 are **ALL checked "yes"** (or "unknown"), notify the receiving hospital before arrival of the potential stroke patient. If any are checked **"no,"** follow appropriate treatment protocol.

Interpretation: Ninety-three percent of patients with stroke will have positive findings (all items checked "yes" or "unknown") on the LAPSS (sensitivity = 93%), and 97% of those with positive findings will have a stroke (specificity = 97%). The patient may still be having a stroke if LAPSS criteria are not met.

Criteria	Yes	Unknown	No
1. Age >45 years	❏	❏	❏
2. History of seizures or epilepsy absent	❏	❏	❏
3. Symptom duration <24 hours	❏	❏	❏
4. At baseline, patient is not wheelchair bound or bedridden	❏	❏	❏
5. Blood glucose between 60 and 400	❏	❏	❏
6. *Obvious asymmetry* (right vs left) in *any* of the following 3 categories (must be unilateral)	❏	❏	❏

	Equal	R Weak	L Weak
Smile/grimace	❏	❏ Droop	❏ Droop
Grip	❏	❏ Weak grip	❏ Weak grip
	❏	❏ No grip	❏ No grip
Arm strength	❏	❏ Drifts down	❏ Drifts down
	❏	❏ Falls rapidly	❏ Falls rapidly

Adapted from Kidwell CS, Saver JL, Schubert GB, Eckstein M, Starkman S. Design and retrospective analysis of the Los Angeles Prehospital Stroke Screen (LAPSS). *Prehosp Emerg Care.* 1998;2: 267-273, and Kidwell CS, Starkman S, Eckstein M, Weems K, Saver JL: Identifying stroke in the field: prospective validation of the Los Angeles Prehospital Stroke Screen (LAPSS). *Stroke.* 2000;31:71-76.

FIGURE 3. Arm drift. When you ask the patient to close both eyes and hold both arms straight out, weakness on one side of the body may become more apparent.

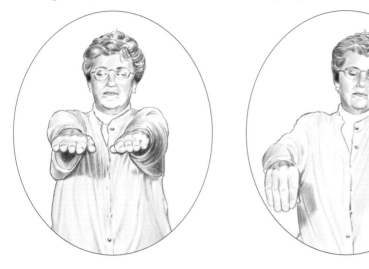

arrhythmias may point to an underlying cause of the stroke (eg, atrial fibrillation with embolism) or may be a consequence of the stroke. Bradycardia may indicate hypoxia or elevation in intracranial pressure.

Unless the patient requires stabilization, rapid patient transport should be the highest priority. Emergency ambulance services should transport a patient with stroke symptoms to an emergency receiving facility that has a proven capability of initiating fibrinolytic therapy for appropriate stroke patients within 1 hour of arrival unless such an emergency facility is more than 30 minutes away by ground ambulance.

A North American study has revealed that the vast majority of residents live within a 30-minute drive of a hospital with 24-hour CT scanning capability.[55] EMS physicians should work with neurologists and local hospitals to establish clear destination protocols for patients suspected of having an acute stroke.

Prearrival notification shortens the time to definitive hospital-based evaluation and intervention for patients with stroke.[3,47,48] In addition to standard information, *EMS systems should communicate the results of the Cincinnati Prehospital Stroke Scale, the LAPSS, the*

Glasgow Coma Scale, and the estimated time of symptom onset to the receiving hospital before arrival. This allows the receiving hospital time to prepare and coordinate the patient's time-critical care. The receiving facility should have a written plan to initiate therapy as quickly as possible.

The essential elements of out-of-hospital assessment of a patient with possible stroke are summarized in Figure 4.

TABLE 4. Glasgow Coma Scale

Eye opening	
Spontaneous	4
To speech	3
To pain	2
None	1
Best motor response	
Obeys	6
Localizes	5
Withdraws	4
Abnormal flexion	3
Abnormal extension	2
None	1
Best verbal response	
Oriented conversation	5
Confused conversation	4
Inappropriate words	3
Incomprehensible sounds	2
None	1

Summary of Key Concepts

✔ Fibrinolytic therapy is a new and effective treatment for acute ischemic stroke and limits disability if given within 3 hours of symptom onset.

✔ Treatment for acute ischemic stoke is time critical. Education of at-risk patients, early prehospital recognition, rapid assessment, and prompt transport with prearrival notification to a hospital capable of caring for patients with acute stroke are of key importance.

✔ Acute neurologic disability is a symptom of both TIA and stroke. If symptoms completely resolve within 24 hours, the event is classified as a TIA. TIAs are a risk factor for stroke.

✔ About 85% of strokes are ischemic, making the patient possibly eligible for treatment with fibrinolytics.

✔ Patients with hemorrhagic stroke are not eligible to receive fibrinolytic therapy. Generally they appear to be more seriously ill than those with ischemic stroke, and they have a more rapid course of deterioration.

✔ Laypersons should be educated to phone 911 immediately when experiencing or recognizing symptoms of a stroke to ensure rapid assessment and transport to a hospital capable of caring for patients with acute stroke.

✔ The goals of prehospital (EMS) management of suspected stroke are

1. Priority dispatch and response
2. Initial assessment and management
3. Rapid identification of stroke (using a standardized stroke scale)
4. Rapid transport of the victim to a hospital capable of acute stroke care (including delivery of fibrinolytics within 1 hour of the patient's arrival)
5. Prearrival notification of the receiving hospital.

✔ Prehospital notification should include the best estimate of the time of symptom onset, results of a stroke scale, and the Glasgow Coma Scale score.

FIGURE 4. Algorithm for Prehospital Management of Stroke.

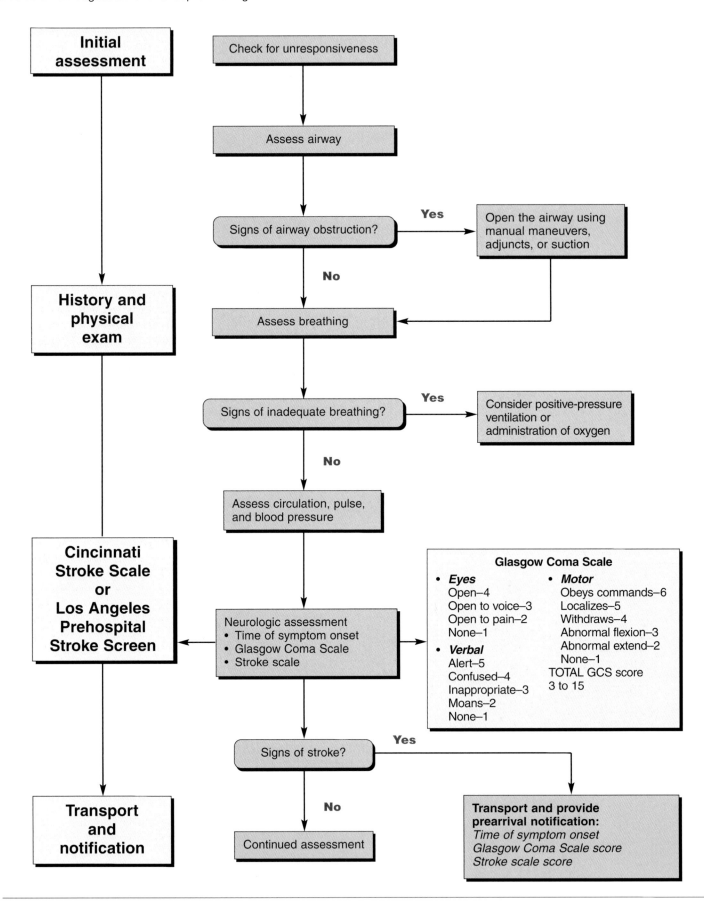

Review Questions

1. You are an EMT called to the side of an unresponsive 55-year-old woman. Family members state that she was complaining of being dizzy, feeling nauseated, and having difficulty speaking and moving her left arm and leg before she collapsed and became unresponsive. She is supine on the living room floor and cyanotic with snoring respirations. The most likely cause of the snoring respirations and cyanosis is

   a. respiratory arrest

   b. obstruction of the airway by the tongue and epiglottis

   c. cardiac arrest

   d. swelling of the vocal cords

2. A 19-year-old woman suddenly complains of the worst headache of her life, with nausea and vomiting. The most likely cause of her symptoms is

   a. hemorrhagic stroke

   b. ischemic stroke

   c. transient ischemic attack (TIA)

   d. hypoglycemia

3. You are a BLS ambulance provider. You respond to a call about a 78-year-old man who has difficulty speaking, right arm drift when he closes his eyes, and facial droop. Which 1 of these 3 scales evaluates the 3 abnormalities that this patient is demonstrating?

   a. Glasgow Coma Scale

   b. Cincinnati Prehospital Stroke Scale

   c. Stapleton Emergency Scale

   d. Kothari Stroke Screen

4. The family of an 86-year-old man notice that he is slurring his words and having difficulty walking, with weakness in the right arm and leg. He has a history of 2 TIAs 1 month ago. The most likely cause of his symptoms is

   a. hemorrhagic stroke

   b. ischemic stroke

   c. subarachnoid hemorrhage

   d. cerebral hemorrhage

5. You assess a patient who opens his eyes only in response to pain, moans incomprehensibly, and flexes in response to pain. The Glasgow Coma Scale score for this patient is

   a. 4

   b. 5

   c. 6

   d. 7

6. When transporting a patient with suspected stroke to the hospital, you contact the hospital, providing the estimated time of symptom onset, the results of a stroke scale evaluation, and the Glasgow Coma Scale score. The benefit of this communication is to allow the receiving hospital to

   a. calculate the patient's risk of dying

   b. assess bed availability

   c. estimate the chances of full recovery

   d. mobilize the stroke team and reduce time to treatment

How did you do?

Answers: **1,** b; **2,** a; **3,** b; **4,** b; **5,** d; **6,** d.

References

1. 2000 Heart and Stroke Statistical Update. Dallas, Tex: American Heart Association; 1999.

2. Easton JD, Hart RG, Sherman DG, Kaste M. Diagnosis and management of ischemic stroke, part I: threatened stroke and its management. Curr Probl Cardiol. 1983;8:1-76.

3. The National Institute of Neurological Disorders and Stroke rt-PA Stroke Study Group. Tissue plasminogen activator for acute ischemic stroke. N Engl J Med. 1995;333: 1581-1587.

4. Del Zoppo GJ, Higashida RT, Furlan AJ, Pessin MS, Rowley HA, Gent M, and the ProAct Investigators. ProAct: a phase II randomization trial of recombinant pro-urokinase by direct arterial delivery in acute middle cerebral artery stroke. Stroke. 1998;29:4-11.

5. Bendzus M, Urbach H, Ries F, Solymosi L. Outcome after local intra-arterial fibrinolysis compared with the natural course of patients with a dense middle cerebral artery on early CT. Neuroradiology. 1998;40:54-58.

6. Wardlaw JM, del Zoppo G, Yamaguchi T. Thrombolysis for acute ischaemic stroke. Cochrane Database of Systematic Reviews. 4th issue. 1999.

7. Kwiatkowski TG, Libman RB, Frankel M, Tilley BC, Morgenstern LB, Lu M, Broderick JP, Lewandowski CA, Marler JR, Levine SR, Brott T, for the NINDS r-tPA Stroke Study Group. Effects of tissue plasminogen activator for acute ischemic stroke at one year. N Engl J Med. 1999;340:1781-1787.

8. Furlan A, Higashida R, Wechsler L, Gent M, Rowley H, Kase C, Pessin M, Ahuja A, Callahan F, Clark WM, Silver F, Rivera F, for the PROACT investigators. Intra-arterial prourokinase for acute ischemic stroke: the PROACT II Study: a randomized controlled trial. JAMA. 1999;282:2003-2011.

9. Lewandowski CA, Frankel M, Tomsick TA, Broderick J, Frey J, Clark W, Starkman S, Grotta J, Spilker J, Khoury J, Brott T, and the EMS Bridging Trial Investigators. Combined intravenous and intra-arterial r-TPA versus intra-arterial therapy of acute ischemic stroke: Emergency Management of Stroke (EMS) Bridging Trial. Stroke. 1999;30:2598-2605.

10. Albers GW, Bates VE, Clark WM, Bell R, Verro P, Hamilton SA. Intravenous tissue-type plasminogen activator for treatment of acute stroke: the Standard Treatment with Alteplase to Reverse Stroke (STARS) Study. JAMA. 2000;283:1145-1150.

11. Fagan SC, Morgenstern LB, Petitta A, Ward RE, Tilley BC, Marler JR, Levine SR, Broderick JP, Kwiatkowski TG, Frankel M, Brott TG, Walker MD, and the NINDS rt-PA Study Group. Cost-effectiveness of tissue plasminogen activator for acute ischemic stroke. Neurology. 1998;50:883-890.

12. Pepe PE. The chain of recovery from brain attack: access, pre-hospital care, and treatment. In: Proceedings of the National Symposium on Rapid Identification and Treatment of Acute Stroke. Bethesda, Md: The National Institute of Neurological Disorders and Stroke; 1996; 20-42.

13. Kimura K, Minematsu K, Yasaka M, Wada K, Yamaguchi T. The duration of symptoms in transient ischemic attack. Neurology. 1999; 52:976-980.

14. Viitanen M, Eriksson S, Asplund K. Risk of recurrent stroke, myocardial infarction and epilepsy during long-term follow-up after stroke. Eur Neurol. 1988;28:227-231.

15. Antiplatelet Trialists' Collaboration. Collaborative overview of randomized trials of antiplatelet therapy, I: prevention of death, myocardial infarction, and stroke by prolonged antiplatelet therapy in various categories of patients. BMJ. 1994;308:81-106.

16. Weir B, ed. Aneurysms Affecting the Nervous System. Baltimore, Md: Williams & Wilkins; 1987.

17. Broderick JP, Brott T, Tomsick T, Huster G, Miller R. The risk of subarachnoid and intra-cerebral hemorrhages in blacks as compared with whites. N Engl J Med. 1992;326:733-736.

18. Brott T, Thalinger K, Hertzberg V. Hypertension as a risk factor for spontaneous intracerebral hemorrhage. Stroke. 1986;17:1078-1083.

19. Furlan AJ, Whisnant JP, Elveback LR. The decreasing incidence of primary intracerebral hemorrhage: a population study. Ann Neurol. 1979;5:365-373.

20. Kassell NF, Torner JC, Haley EC Jr, Jane JA, Adams HP, Kongable GL. The International Cooperative Study on the Timing of Aneurysm Surgery, part 1: overall management results. J Neurosurg. 1990;73:18-36.

21. Kassell NF, Torner JC, Jane JA, Haley EC Jr, Adams HP. The International Cooperative Study on the Timing of Aneurysm Surgery, part 2: surgical results. J Neurosurg. 1990;73: 37-47.

22. Cummins RO, Ornato JP, Thies WH, Pepe PE. Improving survival from sudden cardiac arrest: the 'chain of survival' concept. A statement for healthcare professionals from the Advanced Cardiac Life Support Subcommittee and the Emergency Cardiac Care Committee, American Heart Association. Circulation. 1991;83:1832-1847.

23. Korpelainen JT, Sotaniemi KA, Makikallio A. Dynamic behavior of heart rate in ischemic stroke. Stroke. 1999;30:1008-1013.

24. Hazinski MF. Demystifying recognition and management of stroke. Curr Emerg Cardiac Care. Winter 1996;7:8.

25. Barsan WG, Brott TG, Broderick JP, et al. Time of hospital presentation in patients with acute stroke. Arch Intern Med. 1993;153: 2558-2561.

26. Feldmann E, Gordon N, Brooks JM, et al. Factors associated with early presentation of acute stroke. Stroke. 1993;24:1805-1810.

27. Ferro JM, Melo TP, Oliveira V, Crespo M, Canhao P, Pinto AN. An analysis of the admission delay of acute strokes. Cerebrovasc Dis. 1994;4:72-75.

28. Kothari R, Barsan W, Brott T, Broderick J, Ashbrock S. Frequency and accuracy of pre-hospital diagnosis of acute stroke. Stroke. 1993;26:937-941.

29. Kothari R, Pancioli A, Liu T, Brott T, Broderick J. Cincinnati Prehospital Stroke Scale: reproducibility and validity [see comments]. Ann Emerg Med. 1999;33:373-378.

30. Alberts MJ, Perry A, Dawson DV, Bertels C. Effects of professional and public education on reducing the delay in presentation and referral of stroke patients. Stroke. 1992;23:352-356.

31. The National Institute of Neurological Disorders and Stroke (NINDS) rt-PA Stroke Study Group. A systems approach to immediate evaluation and management of hyperacute stroke: experience at eight centers and implications for community practice and patient care. Stroke. 1997;28:1530-1540.

32. Crocco TJ, Kothari RU, Sayre MR, Liu T. A nationwide prehospital stroke survey. Prehosp Emerg Care. 1999;3:201-206.

33. Kothari R, Jauch E, Broderick J, Brott T, Sauerbeck L, Khoury J, Liu T. Acute stroke: delays to presentation and emergency department evaluation. Ann Emerg Med. 1999; 33:3-8.

34. Morris DL, Rosamond WD, Hinn AR, Gorton RA. Time delays in accessing stroke care in the emergency department. Acad Emerg Med. 1999;6:218-223.

35. Kidwell CS, Saver JL, Schubert GB, Eckstein M, Starkman S. Design and retrospective analysis of the Los Angeles Prehospital Stroke Screen (LAPSS). Prehosp Emerg Care. 1998; 2:267-273.

36. Kidwell CS, Starkman S, Eckstein M, Weems K, Saver JL. Identifying stroke in the field: prospective validation of the Los Angeles Prehospital Stroke Screen (LAPSS). Stroke. 2000;31:71-76.

37. Zachariah B, Dunford J, Van Cott CC. Dispatch life support and the acute stroke patient: making the right call. In: Proceedings of the National Symposium on Rapid Identification and Treatment of Acute Stroke. Bethesda, Md: The National Institute of Neurological Disorders and Stroke; 1991:88-96.

38. Dávalos A, Castillo J, Martinez-Villa E. Delay in neurological attention and stroke outcome: Cerebrovascular Disease Study Group of the Spanish Society of Neurology. Stroke. 1995; 26:2233-2237.

39. Lyden PD, Rapp K, Babcock T, Rothrock J. Ultra-rapid identification, triage, and enrollment of stroke patients into clinical trials. J Stroke Cerebrovasc Dis. 1994;4:106-107.

40. Bornstein NM, Gur AY, Fainshtein P, Korczyn AD. Stroke during sleep: epidemiological and clinical features. Cerebrovasc Dis. 1999;9: 320-322.

41. Spilker JA. The importance of patient and public education in acute ischemic stroke. In: Proceedings of the National Symposium on Rapid Identification and Treatment of Acute Stroke. Bethesda, Md: The National Institute of Neurological Disorders and Stroke; 1996:119-125.

42. Grotta JC. The importance of time. In: Proceedings of the National Symposium on Rapid Identification and Treatment of Acute Stroke. Bethesda, Md: The National Institute of Neurological Disorders and Stroke; 1996;5-9.

43. Kwiatkowski T, Silverman R, Paiano R, et al. Delayed hospital arrival in patients with acute stroke. Acad Emerg Med. 1996;3:538.

44. Morris DL, Fordon RA, Hinn AR, et al. Delay in seeking care for stroke: demographic determinants: the delay in accessing stroke health-care study. Acad Emerg Med. 1996;3:539.

45. Kay R, Woo J, Poon WS. Hospital arrival time after onset of stroke. J Neurol Neurosurg Psychiatry. 1992;55:973-974.

46. Biller J, Shephard A. Delay beween onset of ischemic stroke and hospital arrival. Neurology. 1992;42(suppl I):390P.

47. Zachariah BS, Pepe PE. The development of emergency medical dispatch in the USA: a historical perspective. Eur J Emerg Med. 1995;2:109-112.

48. Sayre MR, Swor RA, Honeykutt KL. Prehospital identification and treatment. In: Proceedings of the National Symposium on Rapid Identification and Treatment of Acute Stroke. Bethesda, Md: The National Institute of Neurological Disorders and Stroke; 1996:97-119.

49. Pepe PE, Zachariah BS, Sayre MR, Floccare D. Ensuring the chain of recovery for stroke in your community: Chain of Recovery Writing Group. Prehosp Emerg Care. 1998;2:89-95.

50. Porteous GH, Corry MD, Smith WS. Emergency medical services dispatcher identification of stroke and transient ischemic attack. Prehosp Emerg Care. 1999;3:211-216.

51. Prasad K, Menon GR. Comparison of the 3 strategies of verbal scoring of the Glasgow Coma Scale in patients with stroke. Cerebrovasc Dis. 1998;8:79-85.

52. Kothari R, Hall K, Brott T, Broderick J. Early stroke recognition: developing an out-of-hospital NIH Stroke Scale. Acad Emerg Med. 1997;4:986-990.

53. Kothari R, Pio BJ, Sayre MR, Liu T. A prospective evaluation of the accuracy of prehospital diagnosis of acute stroke [abstract]. Prehosp Emerg Care. 1999;3:82.

54. Kothari R, Sauerbeck L, Jauch E, Broderick J, Brott T, Khoury J, Liu T. Patients' awareness of stroke signs, symptoms, and risk factors. Stroke. 1997;28:1871-1875.

55. Scott PA, Temovsky CJ, Lawrence K, Gudaitis E, Lowell MJ. Analysis of Canadian population with potential geographic access to intravenous thrombolysis for acute ischemic stroke. Stroke. 1998;29:2304-2310.

56. Zweifler RM, Drinkard R, Cunningham S, Brody ML, Rothrock JF. Implementation of a stroke code system in Mobile, Alabama: diagnostic and therapeutic yield. Stroke. 1997;28: 981-983.

57. Smith WS, Isaacs M, Corry MD. Accuracy of paramedic identification of stroke and transient ischemic attack in the field. Prehosp Emerg Care. 1998;2:170-175.

58. Williams LS, Bruno A, Rouch D, Marriott DJ. Stroke patients' knowledge of stroke: influence on time to presentation. Stroke. 1997;28: 912-915.

59. Oppenheimer SM, Hachinski VC. The cardiac consequences of stroke. Neurol Clin. 1992; 10:167-176.

60. Goldstein DS. The electrocardiogram in stroke: relationship to pathophysiological type and comparison with prior tracings. Stroke. 1979;10:253-259.

61. European Ad Hoc Consensus Group, Hacke W, chair. Optimizing intensive care in stroke: a European perspective. Cerebrovasc Dis. 1997;7:113-128.

You are a healthcare provider at a community hospital. You are talking with one of your patients, a 47-year-old man who has just been diagnosed with angina. He tells you that he smokes and will continue to smoke because his father was a smoker and lived to the age of 90.

You explain that controlling risk factors such as smoking will certainly reduce the risk of death from heart disease and stroke and many other diseases. You explain that because he has been diagnosed with angina, he already has evidence of coronary artery disease and is at high risk for heart attack and sudden death if he does not change his behavior.

You offer to help him find a method for quitting smoking that will work best for him, and you monitor his progress during subsequent visits. Three months later your diligent efforts have succeeded, and he quits smoking.

Risk Factors for Heart Disease and Stroke

Overview

Research in the causes of the "epidemic" of blood vessel diseases has identified a consistent association between specific attributes, conditions, and behaviors and the development of blood vessel disease.[1] The concept of risk factors developed from an awareness of these associations.

As healthcare providers and BLS educators, we have a responsibility to be familiar with the risk factors of heart disease and stroke and related information on prudent heart and brain living. Having this knowledge allows us to

1. Evaluate our own risk and do our best to live a healthy lifestyle

2. Educate our families and patients about such a lifestyle

3. Collect a medical history related to risk factors to appropriately diagnose and treat heart disease and stroke

It is now well known that heart attack and stroke occur much more frequently in persons who smoke and have elevated blood pressure. Other things being equal, the person who smokes 1 pack of cigarettes a day has a greater chance of heart attack, stroke, and sudden death than a person who does not smoke.

Persons who have more than 1 risk factor may have many more times the chance of developing vascular disease than persons who have none.[2,3] For example, the person who has an abnormal (high) serum

cholesterol level and smokes 2 packs of cigarettes a day may have as much as 10 times the chance of having a heart attack as the person who has a normal blood cholesterol level and does not smoke. But heart attacks also occur in the absence of risk factors.

Risk Factors: Heart Attack and Stroke

Heart attack and stroke are vascular diseases caused primarily by the effects of atherosclerosis. Atherosclerosis is a gradual process. It develops over the course of a lifetime and is affected by several factors, including age, gender, heredity, and lifestyle. Heart disease and stroke share many of the same risk factors. Some risk

factors are more significant for one disease than for the other. For example, high blood cholesterol is considered a major risk factor for heart disease and a secondary risk factor for stroke. High blood pressure is by far the major risk factor for hemorrhagic stroke. Heart disease itself is a risk factor for stroke.

Risk factors fall into 2 basic categories: those that can be changed or modified through heart-healthy living and those that cannot be changed. Healthcare providers should be aware of this distinction and educate their patients accordingly. Risk factors that cannot be changed can be used to identify patients at risk for heart attack and stroke. These patients and their families should be taught to identify warning signs of heart attack and stroke and what to do if these warning signs appear. Patients should also be taught how to modify those risk factors that can be changed.

Risk Factors That Cannot Be Changed

The Most Important: Age

The death rate from CAD increases with age. Nearly 1 in 4 deaths, however, occurs in persons younger than 65 years.[1] Coronary heart disease is the single largest killer of both men and women. This year approximately 1 100 000 persons will have a new or recurrent MI or fatal episode of coronary heart disease.[1] Approximately 1 300 000 patients will be discharged from

Emergency Departments with a diagnosis of CAD after evaluation for chest pain.

Age is the single most important risk factor for stroke worldwide; the incidence of stroke increases in both men and women after age 55. In fact, for persons 55 years of age and older, the incidence of stroke more than doubles with each successive decade. Although age is not modifiable, it must be considered when evaluating other risk factors such as high blood pressure or transient ischemic attacks (TIAs), because increasing age in combination with these modifiable risk factors results in a higher risk of stroke than any one risk factor alone. A common misconception is that only elderly people suffer strokes. In any given year about 28% of stroke victims are younger than 65.[1]

Heredity

A history of premature CAD in siblings or parents suggests an increased susceptibility that may be genetic.[4] Risk of stroke is greater for people who have a family history of stroke, but this risk is probably complicated by the presence of multiple common risk factors in families (eg, smoking, high blood pressure).

Gender

Before menopause women have a lower incidence of coronary atherosclerosis than men. Incidence increases significantly in postmenopausal women, who also have a worse clinical course compared with men. If hormone replacement therapy proves to be beneficial, this gender-associated risk may be modifiable.

Risk of stroke is higher in men than in women. Overall men have about a 19% greater chance of a stroke than women do. Among people under the age of 65, risk for men is even greater when compared with that of women.

Race

The risk of disability and death from stroke in African Americans is more than twice that of whites. Much of this risk can be explained by the greater number of risk factors (eg, smoking, high blood pressure, high blood cholesterol, and diabetes) present in African Americans.[1]

Risk Factors That Can Be Changed

Cigarette Smoking

The death rate from heart attack among people who do not smoke is considerably lower than that of people who do.[5] In those who quit smoking, the death rate eventually declines almost to that of people who have never smoked.[6-10]

Passive smoking (inhalation of environmental tobacco smoke) has also been shown to be associated with an increased risk of smoking-related disease.[11-15] Hence all people — and especially those with other risk factors — should try to avoid being exposed to passive smoke.

Cigarette smoking is also an important risk factor for stroke. Smoking can contribute to accelerated atherosclerosis and transient elevations in blood pressure that contribute to stroke. Smoking may also contribute to enzyme release, which has been linked to formation of aneurysms.[16] Carbon monoxide generated during smoking reduces the amount of oxygen carried in the blood. Cigarette smoking causes blood platelets to cluster, shortens platelet survival, decreases clotting time, and increases blood thickness. Cessation of cigarette smoking reduces risk of stroke.[16]

Cigarette smoking is a major independent risk factor that acts together with other risk factors (most notably elevated cholesterol and hypertension) to greatly increase the risk of CAD. Overall cigarette smokers experience a 70% greater rate of death from CAD than do nonsmokers. Heavy smokers (2 or more packs per day) have death rates from CAD 2 to 3 times those of nonsmokers.

FYI: Smoking and Sudden Death

Cigarette smoking has been found to elevate the risk of sudden death significantly. About 1 in 5 deaths from cardiovascular disease is attributed to smoking.[1] The risk appears to increase with the number of cigarettes smoked per day. With cessation of smoking, it diminishes to almost normal.

In 1997 an estimated 430 000 Americans died of smoking-related illnesses.[18] Nearly 30% of deaths from cardiovascular disease are attributable to smoking.[19]

Unless smoking habits change, perhaps 10% of all persons now alive may die prematurely of heart disease attributable to their smoking behavior.[20] The total number of such premature deaths may exceed 24 million.

"Warning: The Surgeon General Has Determined That Cigarette Smoking Is Dangerous to Your Health" — Many studies have shown (and the Surgeon General has verified) that cigarette smokers have a greater risk than nonsmokers of dying from a variety of diseases. If a smoker and a nonsmoker have the same disease, the disease is more likely to be fatal to the smoker. The same studies indicate that people who give up smoking have a lower death rate from heart attack than do persistent smokers. After a period of years the death rate of those who stop smoking is nearly as low as that of people who have never smoked. Some of the abnormal changes in lung tissue of heavy smokers have also been shown to gradually improve.[3,4]

Before menopause women have lower rates for CAD than men do. Part of this difference is due to the fact that fewer women smoke, and those who do tend to smoke fewer cigarettes per day and to inhale less deeply. However, among women whose smoking patterns are comparable to those of men, death rates from CAD are higher.

Cigarette smoking remains the leading preventable cause of coronary heart disease in women, with more than 50% of heart attacks among middle-aged women attributable to tobacco.

In recent years smoking rates have declined more slowly in women than in men. (Every year a smaller percentage of female smokers than male smokers quit.) Women who use oral contraceptives and smoke cigarettes increase their risk of MI approximately 10 times compared with women who neither use oral contraceptives nor smoke.[17]

The earlier a person begins to smoke, the greater the risk to the person's future health. There is considerable pressure on teenagers to smoke, and whether they resist may depend on the example set by their parents. In the majority of families in which the parents do not smoke, neither do the children.

Inhalation of environmental tobacco smoke, or "passive smoking," has been associated with an increased risk of smoking-related disease. Public buildings, hospitals, and many restaurants and businesses have implemented strong non-smoking policies. These efforts encourage patrons and employees to recognize the risks for both active and passive smokers. Ongoing efforts in this public health area should lead to a decrease in the incidence of disability and death from cigarette smoking.

Making the Decision to Quit

Despite all the data that exists about smoking, a large portion of the population continues to smoke. Quitting smoking is not easy. Nicotine is highly addictive, and the effects of withdrawal can be extremely uncomfortable for many people. Commercial advertising has been very effective in encouraging people to smoke. People must break the *habit* of smoking.

Healthcare providers can play an important role in a patient's decision to quit. A number of studies have documented that physician-delivered counseling interventions for smoking cessation can be effective. These studies have documented that 2 factors are especially important: the physician (or other healthcare professional) should receive training in counseling methods, and an office system that facilitates the delivery of such counseling and enhances its effect must be in place.[20-22] Healthcare financial incentives will also need to be changed to focus on primary and secondary prevention of smoking rather than tertiary care only. Take a moment to review *FYI: Smoking Intervention Guidelines*, which outlines the role of physicians and other healthcare providers in counseling patients during office visits.

Many programs are available today to help smokers who decide to quit. Smoking cessation programs sponsored by the American Heart Association and the American Lung Association are available nationwide. Nicotine patches, gums, pills, and inhalers can help persons who suffer from severe withdrawal symptoms. A change in lifestyle is also helpful during attempts to quit smoking.[23,24] Exercising to reduce stress, eating a balanced diet, and drinking plenty of water can be helpful in overcoming the stresses of smoking cessation.[25]

The most important variable is the motivation of the individual. Motivation can be provided by the onset of health problems, concern for the effects of second-hand smoke on a spouse or child, or even the death of a loved one from the effects of smoking. Healthcare providers and family members must provide a helpful, nonjudgmental atmosphere to help the smoker achieve his or her goal. It may take time to overcome the habit of smoking. Most smokers quit several times before they succeed.[18,22]

The American Heart Association and the American Lung Association offer support to anyone who wants to quit smoking. Visit their offices or websites for information.

High Blood Pressure

A major risk factor for heart attack, hypertension (high blood pressure) usually has no specific symptoms but can be detected by a simple, painless test.

As many as 50 million adults and children in the United States have high blood pressure.[1] It affects 1 in 4 American adults. Primary, or essential, hypertension is the most common type of hypertension. Its cause is unknown. Secondary hypertension is caused by another condition, such as kidney disease.

Experts who have studied high blood pressure report that a tendency toward hypertension is often found in families. People whose parents had high blood pressure are more likely to develop it than people whose parents did not. If there is a family history of stroke or heart attack at an early age or if parents have high blood pressure, all family members should have regular blood pressure checks.

High blood pressure increases the workload of the heart, causing it to enlarge and weaken over time. It also increases the risk of stroke, heart attack, kidney failure, and congestive heart failure. When high blood pressure is combined with older age, obesity, smoking, high blood cholesterol levels, or diabetes, the risk of heart attack or stroke increases several times.

Hypertension is one of the most powerful modifiable risk factors for both ischemic and spontaneous hemorrhagic stroke.[26,27] Risk of hemorrhagic stroke rises markedly with increases in systolic blood pressure.[26] Hypertension is relatively common, affecting more than 1 in 3 American adults by the age of 60 and more than half the population over the age of 80.[28] For this reason every patient should have his or her blood pressure checked regularly (at least annually), particularly patients older than 60.

Uncontrolled high blood pressure can also affect the kidneys.[29-31] Kidney damage is the most common form of secondary hypertension. Such effects on the heart, kidneys, and brain are called *end-organ damage*.

Risk of heart disease, stroke, and end-organ damage can be eliminated or reduced if high blood pressure is treated early and effectively. Reduction of blood

FYI: Understanding Hypertension

Small arteries in the body, called arterioles, regulate blood pressure. The manner in which arterioles control blood pressure is sometimes compared with the way a nozzle regulates water pressure in a hose. If the nozzle is turned to make the opening larger, less pressure is needed to force the water through the hose. If the opening is smaller, the pressure in the hose increases.

Similarly, if the arterioles become narrower for any reason, blood cannot easily pass through. This increases blood pressure in the arteries and may overwork the heart. If the pressure increases above normal and stays there, the result is high blood pressure, or hypertension.

Uncontrolled high blood pressure adds to the workload of the heart and arteries. The heart, forced to work harder than normal over a long period, tends to enlarge. A slightly enlarged heart may function well, but a heart that is very much enlarged has a difficult time keeping up with the demands of the body.

As people grow older, the arteries and arterioles become hardened and less elastic. This process, atherosclerosis, takes place gradually, even in people who do not have high blood pressure. But high blood pressure tends to speed up the hardening.

Primary high blood pressure cannot be cured, but usually it can be controlled.

pressure can significantly reduce risk of heart disease and stroke in both men and women.[32]

Weight reduction and dietary interventions also contribute to the prevention and treatment of hypertension. A person with mild elevations of blood pressure often begins treatment with a program of weight reduction (if overweight) and salt (sodium) restriction before drugs are recommended.

Moderate elevations of blood pressure may be controlled by weight reduction and decreased sodium intake.[33] The optimal degree of sodium reduction has not yet been completely established. Table salt is 40% sodium. Removing the salt shaker from the table and not adding salt during food preparation can significantly reduce salt consumption. A physician's advice about weight reduction should also be obtained.

For persons with severe hypertension or mild to moderate hypertension not controlled by these measures, antihyper-

tensive drugs are likely to be required. If drug therapy is required, the drugs must be taken exactly as prescribed, and patients should be carefully monitored to ensure both compliance with therapy and effectiveness of the therapy in controlling hypertension.

Control of hypertension substantially decreases risk of stroke.[34,35] In the past systolic blood pressure was not thought to be a risk factor for stroke. New evidence has shown that systolic hypertension is a risk factor for stroke, particularly in the elderly.

High Blood Cholesterol Level

Cholesterol is manufactured by the body and is present in any animal products that we eat. It is found in especially large amounts in egg yolk and organ meats. Shrimp and lobster are moderately high in cholesterol, although low in saturated fat; hence they represent "better" eating choices than foods that are high in both cholesterol and saturated fat. Too much cholesterol can cause a buildup on artery walls, narrowing the passageway through which blood flows and leading to atherosclerosis, heart attack, and stroke.

Reducing Your Cholesterol

Current dietary guidelines from both the American Heart Association[39] and the National Cholesterol Education Program[40] recommend restricting consumption of fat to an upper limit of 30% of daily caloric intake.[41] In most people diets rich in saturated fats raise blood cholesterol levels. The major sources of saturated fats are meat, animal fats, some vegetable oils (palm kernel oil, coconut oil, cocoa butter, and heavily hydrogenated margarines and shortenings), dairy products (whole milk, cream, butter, ice cream, and cheese), and baked goods. Polyunsaturated fats and monounsaturated fats, on the other hand, tend to lower the level of cholesterol.

The goal is to keep saturated fat and total fat low. By partially substituting polyunsaturated and monounsaturated fats for saturated fat and by increasing the amount of complex carbohydrates in the diet, it is possible to achieve this goal.

The dietary recommendations of the AHA and the National Cholesterol Education Program are summarized as follows:

- For most meals, eat fish or poultry, and consume no more than 6 ounces per day. Do not eat the skin of poultry. When you prepare red meat (beef, pork, or lamb), use lean cuts, trim off excess fat, and serve small portions.

- Cook with limited amounts of liquid vegetable oils and polyunsaturated, nonhydrogenated margarines (for example, canola, corn, cottonseed, soybean, and safflower products). Olive oil is a monounsaturated fat source.

- Use skim milk products.

- Eat no more than 3 egg yolks per week. Use egg substitutes in place of eggs.

- Use low-fat cooking methods, such as baking, broiling, and roasting. Avoid fried foods.

A doctor can measure the amount of cholesterol in the blood with a simple test. Because the human body both manufactures cholesterol and consumes it (intake), a diet low in saturated fat and cholesterol will help lower the level of blood cholesterol if it is too high. Medications are also available to help maintain cholesterol levels within the normal range.

FYI: Cholesterol — Laying the Foundation for Atherosclerosis

Cholesterol is the main lipidlike (fat) component of atherosclerotic deposits in blood vessels. An elevation of the total blood cholesterol level (hypercholesterolemia) has been consistently associated with CAD.[36] Although hypercholesterolemia is sometimes a family trait, it is most often due to environmental factors, the most influential being diet. Studies in humans have shown that in most people the serum cholesterol level can be raised by ingestion of saturated fat and cholesterol and lowered by substantially reducing this intake.

The National Heart, Lung, and Blood Institute investigated the effect of cholesterol lowering on risk of CAD in men for 7 years in the Coronary Primary Prevention Trial.[37,38] Two groups were studied; both consumed a diet that lowered cholesterol by 4%. One group received the drug cholestyramine, which lowered cholesterol an additional 8.5%. The group with the lower cholesterol level had a 24% reduction in CAD and a 19% reduction in heart attacks. This is the first conclusive evidence that a reduction in cholesterol by drug treatment can decrease the incidence of CAD and heart attack. An elevation of serum triglycerides (the main fatty substance in the fluid portion of blood) is also associated with increased risk of CAD.

Changes in diet should never be drastic.[42,43] Elimination of essential foods can be harmful. Fad diets that totally exclude one type of food from the diet can lead to additional health problems. Moderate changes in diet and careful monitoring of cholesterol and saturated fat can usually keep blood cholesterol at acceptable levels.

It is generally accepted that atherosclerosis may begin in childhood, progress through young adulthood, and become manifest only in middle age or later. It is therefore recommended that children over the age of 2 years follow the same dietary guidelines recommended for adults.[43]

Physical Inactivity

Lack of exercise has been clearly established as a risk factor for heart attack, and regular exercise can reduce the risk of CAD.[44-46] When combined with overeating, lack of exercise may lead to excess weight, which is an additional contributing factor for heart attack. Persons over the age of 40 years should consult their physician before beginning an exercise program or significantly increasing their exercise level.

Regular exercise can increase cardiovascular functional capacity and may decrease myocardial oxygen demand for any given level of physical activity. The 1995 federal guidelines recommend 30 minutes of moderately intense physical activity most days of the week. The risk of vigorous physical activity may be reduced by appropriate medical evaluation.

Exercise

Exercise tones the muscles, stimulates circulation, helps prevent obesity, and promotes a general feeling of well-being. Exercise can help control blood lipid abnormalities and diabetes. There is evidence to suggest that the survival rate of heart attack victims is higher in those who have exercised regularly than in those who have not.

People of all ages should develop a physically active lifestyle as part of a comprehensive program to prevent heart

FYI: Cholesterol and Low- and High-Density Lipoproteins: the Good, the Bad, and the Ominous

The AHA recommends that the absolute numbers for total blood cholesterol and HDL (high-density lipoprotein) cholesterol be used to evaluate risk of heart disease and to determine appropriate treatment for patients. Additional information about risk can be gained by evaluating the LDL (low-density lipoprotein) and triglyceride level.

Total blood cholesterol is the most common measurement of blood cholesterol. The level of total blood cholesterol is used to classify risk of heart disease. Total blood cholesterol falls into 1 of 3 categories: desirable, borderline high risk, and high risk. Patients can lower their total cholesterol by lowering their intake of foods high in saturated fats.

About one third to one fourth of blood cholesterol is carried by **HDL**. HDL cholesterol is known as the "good" cholesterol because a high level of HDL cholesterol seems to protect against heart attack. Medical experts think that HDL tends to carry cholesterol away from the arteries and back to the liver, where it is passed from the body. Some experts believe that excess cholesterol is removed from atherosclerotic plaque by HDL, thus slowing the buildup.

Patients can help raise a low HDL level by not smoking, losing weight or maintaining a healthy weight, and being physically active for at least 30 to 60 minutes a day, at least 3 to 4 days every week.

LDL cholesterol is often called the "bad" cholesterol. Higher levels of LDL cholesterol reflect a higher risk of heart disease. When too much LDL cholesterol circulates in the blood, it can slowly build up in the walls of the arteries that feed the heart and brain. Together with other substances it can form plaque, a thick, hard deposit that can clog these arteries. Lower levels of LDL cholesterol reflect a lower risk of heart disease.

To lower LDL cholesterol, a physician may prescribe a diet low in saturated fat and cholesterol, regular exercise, and, if needed, a weight management program. Medications may also be prescribed to lower LDL cholesterol.

The triglyceride level can also be used to evaluate risk of heart disease. People with high blood triglycerides usually have lower HDL ("good") cholesterol and a higher risk of heart attack and (indirectly) stroke. Many people with high triglycerides have underlying diseases or genetic disorders.

To lower a high triglyceride level, the patient must change his or her lifestyle. The patient must reduce weight, eat foods low in saturated fat and cholesterol, exercise regularly, and stop smoking. Some patients may need to drink less alcohol. People with high triglyceride levels may also need to limit their carbohydrate intake to no more than 45% to 50% percent of total calories because carbohydrates raise triglycerides and lower HDL cholesterol.

The following table lists classifies blood cholesterol levels according to risk of heart disease.

Classification of Blood Cholesterol Levels and Risk of Heart Disease

Cholesterol	Desirable Level (mg/dL)	Borderline High-Risk Level (mg/dL)	High-Risk Level (mg/dL)
Total blood cholesterol	<200	200-239	≥240
LDL cholesterol	<130 Consider treatment if level is 100-129 in a patient with coronary heart disease)	130-159	≥160
HDL cholesterol	Normal: 40-50 (men) 50-60 (women)		<35
Triglyceride level	Normal: <200	200-400	400-1000 (>1000 is very high risk)

disease. Aerobic activities requiring movement of body weight over distance are especially valuable. Such activities include walking, climbing stairs, running, cycling, swimming, and similar activities. Improvements in cardiovascular fitness appear to result from regular exercise of moderate intensity (50% to 75% of capacity) performed 15 to 30 minutes at least every other day.

For high-risk patients, vigorous exercise should be prescribed with caution. Graded exercise tolerance tests, which may be used to help formulate an individual's exercise prescription, should be performed under medical supervision.

Strenuous and unaccustomed activity occasionally brings on a heart attack in an apparently healthy person who has undiagnosed heart disease. Persons over the age of 40 or with a known risk of cardiovascular disease should consult a physician before beginning an exercise program or engaging in heavy physical labor. An exercise test may be part of a physical examination.

Physical activity should be increased gradually in any exercise program. For someone evaluated as physically fit by his or her physician, the introduction of an enjoyable sport into one's life can be beneficial.

Diabetes

Diabetes is an independent risk factor for heart attack and stroke and is strongly correlated with high blood pressure.[47] Although diabetes is treatable, the diagnosis alone increases risk of stroke. People with diabetes often have high cholesterol and are overweight, further increasing their risk.

Diabetes appears most frequently during middle age and more often in people who are overweight. In its mild form diabetes can go undetected for many years, but it can sharply increase a person's risk of heart attack, making control of other risk factors even more important.

Diabetes, or a familial tendency toward diabetes, is associated with an increased

risk of CAD. The risk of CAD in diabetic men is twice that of nondiabetic men; in diabetic women risk of CAD is 3 times as great as that of nondiabetic persons. In diabetic women the death rate from CAD may be as great as that of nondiabetic men of the same age. Improved control of glucose levels reduces the vascular complications of diabetes.[48]

Control of Diabetes

A physician can detect diabetes and treat it by prescribing exercise and weight control programs, changes in eating habits, and drugs (if necessary). The diabetic patient should also be taught how to modify other commonly associated risk factors that may be present. These risk factors are hypercholesterolemia, hypertriglyceridemia, hypertension, and obesity.

Obesity

Obesity has recently been reclassified as a major, modifiable risk factor for coronary heart disease.[49] In most cases obesity is the result of eating too much and exercising too little. Obesity places a heavy burden on the heart.

Obesity is associated with an increased occurrence of CAD, particularly angina pectoris and sudden death, primarily because of its role in increasing blood pressure and blood cholesterol and precipitating diabetes.[50] There is also evidence that obesity may directly contribute to CAD. Few persons become obese without developing a less favorable coronary risk profile.

Most people reach their normal adult weight between the ages of 21 and 25. With each succeeding year, fewer calories are needed to maintain this weight. People in their 30s and 40s who eat as much as they did in their early 20s and who become physically less active will store excess calories as body fat.

Life expectancy may be shorter for people who are markedly overweight. Middle-aged men who are significantly overweight have about 3 times the risk of a fatal heart attack as do middle-aged men of normal weight.

Obesity also leads to a greater risk of hypertension and diabetes.

Eliminate Obesity

When the American Heart Association identified obesity as a major risk factor for heart disease, it issued a call to action for all healthcare providers.[49] To help patients lose weight, doctors usually recommend a program that combines exercise with a low-calorie diet.

There is no quick, easy way to lose weight. Extreme reducing diets should be avoided because they usually exclude foods essential to good health.

Weight reductions of 5% to 10% of body weight can decrease blood pressure and total blood cholesterol and improve glucose tolerance in diabetic patients (and those with impaired glucose tolerance). These are important advantages. However, even when extreme reducing diets do lower weight, they are not effective for maintaining lower weight unless they change patterns of eating. A physician should be consulted to determine the best weight for a patient of a given height and age and to help develop a plan for weight reduction.

Excessive Stress

A high level of stress is thought to contribute to risk of heart disease and stroke. But this factor is difficult to evaluate. It is virtually impossible to define and measure an individual's level of emotional and mental stress. All people feel stress, but they feel it in different amounts and react in different ways.

Excessive stress over a long period may create health problems in some people. Most doctors agree that reduction of emotional stress will benefit the health of the average person.

Risk Factors Specific to Stroke

A few risk factors are specific to stroke, including TIAs, heart attack, and high blood cell count.

TIAs

A TIA is a brief, reversible episode of focal neurologic dysfunction. It is one of the signs of atherosclerotic disease and a significant indicator of risk of stroke. Approximately one fourth of stroke patients have had a TIA.[34] The risk of stroke among patients with TIAs is approximately 5% within the first month. The risk increases to 12% at 1 year and an additional 5% for every year after that. Antiplatelet therapy inhibits the formation of clots and reduces risk of stroke as well as MI in patients with TIAs.[51]

Heart Disease

Heart disease significantly increases risk of stroke. Independent of blood pressure, people with CAD or heart failure have more than twice the risk of stroke as people with a normal heart. Elimination of cigarette smoking, reduction of elevated blood cholesterol, and treatment of high blood pressure reduce the risk of heart disease and thus the risk of stroke.

Atrial fibrillation is a significant modifiable risk factor for stroke, particularly in the elderly. The risk of thromboembolic stroke associated with atrial fibrillation can be reduced significantly through the use of anticoagulants, specifically warfarin. Aspirin may be prescribed for younger patients with atrial fibrillation but no other risk factors for stroke.[52]

High Red Blood Cell Count (Hypercoagulopathy)

A marked or even moderate increase in the red blood cell count is a risk factor for stroke because increased red blood cells thicken the blood, making clots more likely.[53] A high red blood cell count can be treated by removing blood and replacing it with intravenous fluid or by administering anticoagulants.

Sickle cell anemia (SCA) is an inherited condition associated with abnormal hemoglobin protein. When the patient with SCA becomes hypoxic, hypothermic, or dehydrated, the hemoglobin deforms, causing red blood cells to clump together and produce clots that obstruct blood flow

to tissues. These episodes, called *vaso-occlusive crises,* may produce organ failure or stroke. Although SCA cannot be eliminated, vaso-occlusive crises may be prevented in patients at risk by avoiding hypoxemia, hypothermia, and infection and maintaining hydration and oxygenation. The amount of abnormal hemoglobin can also be controlled through exchange transfusion.

Combined Risk Factors

Some low-level risk factors become significant when combined with certain other risk factors. For example, the use of oral contraceptives by young women who smoke cigarettes increases their risk of stroke considerably.[17,54] For further information about cardiovascular risk factors

FYI: Cardiovascular Risk Factors in Women

The major risk factors for coronary heart disease in women are

- Cigarette smoking (risk similar to that of men)

- Hypertension, including isolated systolic hypertension (benefits of antihypertensive therapy similar for women and men)

- Dyslipidemia (low level of HDL cholesterol is a risk factor for CAD in younger and older women and a stronger predictor of death in women than in men)

- Diabetes mellitus (stronger risk factor in women than in men)

- Obesity (abdominal adiposity is a particularly important risk factor for coronary heart disease in women)

- Sedentary lifestyle (as in men, a substantial reduction in risk of coronary heart disease results from even moderate activity)

- Poor nutrition

in women, see "FYI: Cardiovascular Risk Factors in Women."

Prudent Heart and Brain Living

Prudent heart and brain living is a lifestyle that minimizes the risk of future heart disease and stroke. This lifestyle includes weight control, physical fitness, sensible dietary habits, avoidance of cigarette smoking, reduction of serum cholesterol and triglycerides, and control of high blood pressure.

The AHA publishes a wide variety of educational materials about prudent heart and brain living that may provide additional information for the instructor and student. For more information, contact your local AHA.

A number of large studies have confirmed the effectiveness of risk factor modification in reducing cardiovascular morbidity and mortality. Most authorities believe that risk factor reduction is an important part of a comprehensive approach to reducing cardiovascular and cerebrovascular illness and death in the community, especially among children and young adults.

Millions of Americans begin endangering their hearts at a comparatively early age by acquiring poor living habits. Children begin to overeat and develop a taste for foods high in salt, cholesterol, and calories. Some are not encouraged to exercise, and watching television limits play activity. The smoking habit frequently begins during the early teen years, especially if parents smoke. By adulthood many Americans are overweight, lead sedentary lives, and smoke heavily. Many have high levels of cholesterol and triglycerides in their blood. High blood pressure is another prevalent risk factor.

Most of the scientific evidence available today indicates that reduction of risk factors may prevent many heart attacks and strokes. At the very least, reducing risk can result in good general health and physical fitness and can benefit every

TABLE 1. Major Controllable Risk Factors of Heart Attack and Stroke*

Factor	Explanation	Lifestyle to Reduce Risk
Cigarette smoking	Cigarette smoking is the most important single cause of preventable death in the United States. Smoking damages blood vessels and causes numerous other preventable diseases. Secondhand smoke can hurt your children, loved ones, and friends.	Stop smoking as soon as possible. Seek help from your physician. Pick a day now to quit. It is the greatest gift you can give yourself, your loved ones, and friends.
High blood pressure	Uncontrolled high blood pressure is associated with a greater risk of heart attack and is the single most important risk factor for stroke. High blood pressure can damage your blood vessels and even lead to a ruptured blood vessel in the brain.	Have your blood pressure checked frequently and seek treatment if high blood pressure is noted. Take your prescribed medications conscientiously.
High blood cholesterol	When excess cholesterol is deposited on the inner walls of the arteries, it can cause the arteries to narrow and obstruct blood flow to the heart or brain.	Have your doctor check your blood cholesterol levels regularly. Avoid a diet high in saturated fat.
Lack of exercise	A sedentary lifestyle can lead to heart attack, but vigorous exercise by persons who have not exercised regularly can be dangerous. Consult a physician before starting an exercise regimen.	Regular exercise (including walking) can stimulate circulation, prevent weight gain, and promote a general feeling of well being.
Obesity	Obesity increases the risk of high blood pressure, diabetes, and high blood cholesterol, therefore increasing the risk of heart attack and stroke.	Work with your physician to plan a healthy diet. Lose weight slowly. Fad diets are not successful in achieving long-term weight loss.
Heart disease	Heart disease is a major risk factor for stroke. A damaged pump or abnormal heart rhythms can cause blood clots to form and be released into the brain, leading to stroke.	Live a heart-healthy lifestyle and follow your doctor's instructions for treating all forms of heart and blood vessel disease.
Transient ischemic attacks (TIAs)	TIAs are strokelike symptoms that disappear in less than 24 hours. TIAs are strong predictors of stroke. They are usually treated with drugs that keep blood clots from forming.	If stroke symptoms occur, call 911 or the EMS system and seek immediate evaluation in the nearest Emergency Department

*Note: Other risk factors for heart attack and stroke include heredity, male gender, increasing age, diabetes, stress, and race (African Americans are at greater risk for heart attack and stroke). Contact your local AHA for more information on preventing heart attack and stroke.

TABLE 2. Indications of Risk of a Heart Attack

Are You at Risk for a Heart Attack?

The following factors increase the risk of heart attack. Check all that apply to you. If you have 2 or more risk factors, see a physician for a complete evaluation of your risk.

Men
❏ Are you more than 45 years old?

Women
❏ Are you more than 55 years old?
❏ Are you past menopause?
❏ Have your ovaries been removed and if so, you're not taking estrogen?

Both
❏ Did your father or brother have a heart attack before age 55?
❏ Did your mother or sister have a heart attack before age 65?
❏ Did your mother, father, sister, brother, or grandparent have a stroke?
❏ Do you smoke or live or work with others who smoke tobacco daily?
❏ Is your total cholesterol level 240 mg/dL or higher?
❏ You don't know your total cholesterol level?
❏ Is your high-density lipoprotein (HDL) ("good") cholesterol less than 35 mg/dL?
❏ You don't know your HDL level?
❏ Is your blood pressure 140/90 mm Hg or higher?
❏ Have you been told that your blood pressure is too high?
❏ You don't know your blood pressure?
❏ Do you exercise for less than 30 minutes on most days?
❏ Are you are 20 pounds or more overweight for your height and build?
❏ Is your fasting blood sugar level 128 mg/dL or higher?
❏ Do you need medicine to control your blood sugar level?
❏ Do you have coronary artery disease?
❏ Have you had a heart attack?
❏ Have you had a stroke or transient ischemic attack?

To learn more about preventing heart attack and stroke, phone your local American Heart Association (1-800-242-8721) or visit the AHA website at www.americanheart.org.

member of the family. Children benefit most of all by learning the habits of prudent heart living early in life.

Table 1 lists the major controllable risk factors of heart attack and stroke. Take a moment to review these risk factors and behaviors needed to achieve a heart-healthy and brain-healthy lifestyle.

Table 2 is a simple questionnaire that can help identify risk factors for heart attack. It may be useful for the healthcare provider to complete this questionnaire personally or to distribute it to his or her patients.

Summary of the Role of Prevention

As important as it is to provide emergency treatment to the victim of cardiac arrest and stroke, it is far more desirable to prevent these problems. Risk factor modification has clearly been shown to save lives. Education of the public is essential in the effort to decrease death from CAD and stroke. Control of recognized risk factors depends on both the education and willingness of the public to understand and actively participate in adopting a healthier lifestyle. Community-wide campaigns can be effective in reducing cardiovascular risk.

Educational efforts must also be directed toward overcoming patients' intrinsic denial of early evidence of cardiac disease and encouraging rapid entry into the EMS system when symptoms of CAD develop.

Summary of Key Concepts

↙ Knowledge of risk factors helps healthcare providers and BLS educators to evaluate their own risk, evaluate the risk of their patients and families, and use the information to obtain a history for patients in whom heart attack or stroke is suspected.

↙ Risk factors have a cumulative effect. A person with 2 major risk factors has a significantly greater risk of cardiovascular disease than a person with 1 major risk factor.

↙ Age, heredity, gender, and race are risk factors for heart attack and stroke that cannot be changed.

↙ Smoking, high blood pressure, and high blood cholesterol are risk factors for heart attack and stroke that can be controlled or modified.

↙ Secondhand smoke increases the risk of smoking-related diseases (cardiopulmonary disease, heart disease, cancer).

↙ Smoking increases the risk of sudden cardiac death.

↙ According to the American Heart Association, a cholesterol level less than 200 mg/dL and an HDL level greater than 35 mg/dL are desirable.

↙ Cessation of smoking will eventually reduce the risk of CAD to near that of a nonsmoker.

↙ TIAs, heart attack, and high red blood cell count are risk factors for stroke.

↙ An effective heart-healthy and brain-healthy lifestyle should include regular exercise, avoidance of cigarette smoking, a low-fat diet, control of weight and high blood pressure, and reduction in stress.

Review Questions

1. Joe and Tom are both 58 years old. Joe has high blood cholesterol (300 mg/dL), but he doesn't have high blood pressure and he doesn't smoke. Tom has high blood cholesterol (300 mg/dL) and high blood pressure, and he smokes 2 packs of cigarettes a day. Which of the following statements best describes the difference in risk for CAD between Joe and Tom?

   a. they are at equal risk because 1 risk factor is as bad as 3

   b. Tom is at greater risk because risk factors have a cumulative effect

   c. Tom's risk is only slightly greater because smoking is a minor risk factor

   d. Joe's risk is greater than Tom's because 1 risk factor blocks the effect of another

2. Mary is 78 years old. She was diagnosed with an MI 2 years ago. She has high blood pressure, and she smokes 2 packs of cigarettes a day. How many **total** risk factors for stroke does Mary have (both controllable and uncontrollable)?

   a. 1

   b. 2

   c. 3

   d. 4

3. Bill experienced a sudden onset of weakness on the left side of his body and difficulty speaking. These symptoms reversed in 8 hours. What risk factor for stroke is characterized by this presentation?

   a. MI

   b. TIA

   c. Atrial fibrillation

   d. Angina

4. Mary quit smoking several years ago. She is 60 years old and has no family history of heart disease and no other risk factors for cardiovascular disease. Which statement best describes her risk of sudden cardiac death?

   a. her risk of death has declined to almost that of people her age who have never smoked

   b. her risk of death remains as high as it was when she smoked because permanent damage to her myocardium has already occurred

   c. her risk of death may paradoxically increase because of the long-term damage to her myocardium

   d. the effect of quitting smoking in relation to the risk of sudden death is not understood

How did you do?

Answers: **1**, b; **2**, d; **3**, b; **4**, a.

References

1. *2000 Heart and Stroke Statistical Supplement.* Dallas, Tex: American Heart Association; 1999.

2. Gordon T, Kannel WB. Premature mortality from coronary heart disease: the Framingham Study. *JAMA.* 1971;215:1617-1625.

3. Gordon T, Kannel WB. Multiple risk functions for predicting coronary heart disease: the concept, accuracy, and application. *Am Heart J.* 1982;103:1031-1039.

4. Wu LL. Review of risk factors for cardiovascular diseases. *Ann Clin Lab Sci.* 1999;29:127-133.

5. Jacobs DR Jr, et al. Cigarette smoking and mortality risk: twenty-five-year follow-up of the Seven Countries Study. *Arch Intern Med.* 1999;159:733-740.

6. Gordon T, Kannel WB, McGee D, Dawber TR. Death and coronary attacks in men after giving up cigarette smoking: a report from the Framingham Study. *Lancet.* 1974;2:1345-1348.

7. Wilhelmsson C, Vedin JA, Elmfeldt D, Tibblin G, Wilhelmsen L. Smoking and myocardial infarction. *Lancet.* 1975;1:415-420.

8. Sparrow D, Dawber TR. The influence of cigarette smoking on prognosis after first myocardial infarction: a report from the Framingham Study. *J Chronic Dis.* 1978;31:425-432.

9. Castelli WP. Epidemiology of coronary heart disease: the Framingham Study. *Am J Med.* 1984;76(suppl 2A):4-12.

10. Kristein MM. 40 years of US cigarette smoking and heart disease and cancer mortality rates. *J Chronic Dis.* 1984;37:317-323.

11. Ockene JK, Kuller LH, Svendsen KH, Meilahn E. The relationship of smoking cessation to coronary heart disease and lung cancer in the Multiple Risk Factor Intervention Trial (MRFIT). *Am J Public Health.* 1990;80:954-958.

12. You RX, Thrift AG, McNeil JJ, Davis SM, Donnan GA. Ischemic stroke risk and passive exposure to spouses' cigarette smoking. *Am J Public Health.* 1999;89:572-575.

13. Gottlieb S. Study confirms passive smoking increases coronary heart disease. *BMJ.* 1999;318:891A.

14. Bailar JC III. Passive smoking, coronary heart disease, and meta-analysis. *N Engl J Med.* 1999;340:958-959.

15. He J, et al. Passive smoking and the risk of coronary heart disease: a meta-analysis of epidemiologic studies. *N Engl J Med.* 1999;340:920-926.

16. American Heart Association. Prevention Conference IV: prevention and rehabilitation of stroke. *Stroke.* 1997;28:1498-1526.

17. Farley TM, et al. Combined oral contraceptives, smoking, and cardiovascular risk. *J Epidemiol Community Health.* 1998;52:775-785.

18. Ockene IS, Miller NH, for the American Heart Association Task Force on Risk Reduction. Cigarette smoking, cardiovascular disease, and stroke: a statement for healthcare professionals from the American Heart Association. *Circulation.* 1997;96:3243-3247.

19. US Dept of Health and Human Services. *Reducing the Health Consequences of Smoking: 25 Years of Progress: A Report of the Surgeon General.* US Dept of Health and Human Services, Public Health Service, Centers for Disease Control, Center for Chronic Disease Prevention and Health Promotion, Office on Smoking and Health; 1989. DHHS Publication (CDC) 89-8411.

20. Kottke TE, Battista RN, DeFriese GH, Brekke ML. Attributes of successful smoking cessation interventions in medical practice: a meta-analysis of 39 controlled trials. *JAMA.* 1988;259:2883-2889.

21. Cohen SJ, Stookey GK, Katz BP, Drook CA, Smith DM. Encouraging primary care physicians to help smokers quit: a randomized controlled trial. *Ann Intern Med.* 1989;110:648-652.

22. Ockene JK, Kristeller J, Goldberg R, Amick TL, Pekow PS, Hosmer D, Quirk M, Kuplan K. Increasing the efficacy of physician-delivered smoking intervention: a randomized clinical trial. *J Gen Intern Med.* 1991;6:1-8.

23. Joseph AM, Norman SM, Ferry LH, Prochazka AV, Westman EC, Steele BG, Sherman SE, Cleveland M, Antonnucio DO, Hartman N, McGovern PG. The safety of transdermal nicotine as an aid to smoking cessation in patients with cardiac disease. *N Engl J Med.* 1996;335:1792-1798.

24. Hjalmarson A, Franzon M, Westin A, Wiklund O. Effect of nicotine nasal spray on smoking cessation: a randomized, placebo-controlled, double-blind study. *Arch Intern Med.* 1994;154:2567-2572.

25. Debusk RF, Miller NH, Superko HR, Dennis CA, Thomas RJ, Lew HT, Berger WE III, Heller RS, Rompf J, Gee D. A case-management system for coronary risk factor modification after acute myocardial infarction. *Ann Intern Med.* 1994;120:721-729.

26. Teunissen LL, Rinkel GJE, Algra A, van Gijn J. Risk factors for subarachnoid hemorrhage: a systematic review. *Stroke.* 1996;27:544-549.

27. MacMahon S, Rogers A. The epidemiological association between blood pressure and stroke: implications for primary and secondary prevention. *Hypertens Res.* 1994;17(suppl I):S23-S32.

28. Whisnant JP. Effectiveness versus efficacy of treatment of hypertension for stroke prevention. *Neurology.* 1996;46:301-307.

29. Stamler J, Stamler R, Neaton JD. Blood pressure, systolic and diastolic, and cardiovascular risks. *Arch Intern Med.* 1993;153:598-615.

30. Klag MJ, Whelton PK, Randall BL, Neaton JD, Brancati FL, Ford CE, Shulman NB, Stamler J. Blood pressure and end-stage renal disease in men. *N Engl J Med.* 1996;334:13-18.

31. Klag MJ, Whelton PK, Randall BL, Neaton JD, Brancati FL, Stamler J. End-stage renal disease in African-American and white men. *JAMA.* 1997;277:1293-1298.

32. Cook NR, Cohen J, Hebert P, Taylor JO, Hennekens CH. Implications of small reductions in diastolic blood pressure for primary prevention. *Arch Intern Med.* 1995;155:701-709.

33. Luft FC, Weinberger MH. Heterogeneous responses to changes in dietary salt intake: the salt-sensitivity paradigm. *Am J Clin Nutr.* 1997;65(suppl):612S-617S.

34. Feldmann E, Gorson N, Books JM, et al. Factors associated with early presentation of acute stroke. *Stroke.* 1993;24:1805-1809.

35. Hebert PR, Moser M, Mayer J, Glynn RJ, Hennekens CH. Recent evidence on drug therapy of mild to moderate hypertension and decreased risk of coronary heart disease. *Arch Intern Med.* 1993;153:578-581.

36. Stamler J, Wentworth D, Neaton JD. Is the relationship between serum cholesterol and risk of premature death from coronary heart disease continuous and graded? Findings in 356,222 primary screenees of the Multiple Risk Factor Intervention Trial (MRFIT). *JAMA.* 1986;256:2823-2828.

37. The Lipid Research Clinics Coronary Primary Prevention Trial results, I: reduction in incidence of coronary heart disease. *JAMA.* 1984;251:351-364.

38. The Lipid Research Clinics Coronary Primary Prevention Trial results, II: the relationship of reduction in incidence of coronary heart disease to cholesterol lowering. *JAMA.* 1984;251:365-374.

39. Krauss RM, Deckelbaum RJ, Ernst N, Fisher E, Howard BV, Knopp RH, Kotchen T, Lichtenstein AH, McGill HC, Pearson TA, Prewitt TE, Stone NJ, VanHorn L, Weinberg R. Dietary guidelines for healthy American adults. *Circulation.* 1996;94:1795-1800.

40. Summary of the second report of the National Cholesterol Education Program (NCEP) expert panel on detection, evaluation, and treatment of high blood cholesterol in adults (Adult Treatment Panel II). *JAMA.* 1993;269:3015-3023.

41. Lichtenstein AH, Van Horn L, for the Nutrition Committee. Very low fat diets. AHA advisory statement. *Circulation.* 1998;98:935-939.

42. Siguel EN, Lerman RH. Role of essential fatty acids: dangers in the US Department of Agriuulture dietary recommendations ('pyramid')

and in low-fat diets. *Am J Clin Nutr*. 1994;60: 973-974.

43. Olson RE. The dietary recommendations of the American Academy of Pediatrics. *Am J Clin Nutr*. 1995;61:271-273.

44. Smith SC Jr, Blair SN, Criqui MH, Fletcher GF, Fuster V, Gersh BJ, Gotto AM, Gould KL, Greenland P, Grundy SM, Hill MN, Hlatky MA, Houston-Miller N, Krauss RM, LaRosa J, Ockene IS, Oparil S, Pearson TA, Rappaport E, Starke RD, and the Secondary Prevention Panel. Preventing heart attack and death in patients with coronary disease. *Circulation*. 1995;92:2-4.

45. Wenger NK, Froelicher ES, Smith LK, Ades PA, Berra K, Blumenthal JA, Certo CM, Dattilo AM, Davis D, DeBusk RF, et al. *Cardiac Rehabilitation as Secondary Prevention. Clinical Practice Guideline No. 17.* Rockville, Md: US Dept of Health and Human Services, Public Health Service, Agency for Health Care Policy and Research, and the National Heart, Lung, and Blood Institute; October 1995. AHCPR publication No. 96-0672.

46. Paffenbarger RS Jr, Hyde RT, Wing AL, Hsieh CC. Physical activity, all-cause mortality, and longevity of college alumni. *N Engl J Med*. 1986;314:605-613.

47. Kannel WB, D'Agostino RB, Wilson PW, Belanger AJ, Gagnon DR. Diabetes, fibrinogen, and risk of cardiovascular disease: the Framingham experience. *Am Heart J*. 1990;120:672-676.

48. The Diabetes Control and Complications Trial Research Group. The effect of intensive treatment of diabetes on the development and progression of long-term complications in insulin-dependent diabetes mellitus. *N Engl J Med*. 1993;329:977-986.

49. Eckel RH, Krauss RM, for the AHA Nutrition Committee. American Heart Association call to action: obesity as a major risk factor for coronary heart disease. *Circulation*. 1998;97: 2099-2100.

50. Grundy SM, Balady GJ, Criqui MH, Fletcher G, Greenland P, Hiratzka LF, Houston-Miller N, Kris-Etherton P, Krumholz HM, LaRosa J, Ockene IS, Pearson TA, Reed J, Washington R, Smith SC Jr, for the American Heart Association Science Advisory and Coordinating Committee. Guide to primary prevention of cardiovascular diseases: a statement for health-care professionals from the Task Force on Risk Reduction. *Circulation*. 1997;95:2329-2331.

51. Antiplatelet Trialists' Collaboration. Collaborative overview of randomised trials of antiplatelet therapy, I: prevention of death, myocardial infarction, and stroke by prolonged antiplatelet therapy in various categories of patients. *BMJ*. 1994;308:81-106.

52. Miller VT, Pearce LA, Feinberg WM, et al. Differential effect of aspirin versus warfarin on clinical stroke types in patients with atrial fibrillation. *Neurology*. 1996;46:238-240.

53. Steinke W, Mangold J, Schwartz A, Hennerici M. Mechanisms of infarction in the superficial posterior cerebral artery territory. *J Neurol*. 1997;244:571-578.

54. Papademetriou V, Narayan P, Rubins H, Collins D, Robins S. Influence of risk factors on peripheral and cerebrovascular disease in men with coronary artery disease, low high-density lipoprotein cholesterol levels, and desirable low-density lipoprotein cholesterol levels. *Am Heart J*. 1998;136(4 pt 1):734-740.

You are part of an emergency response team in a physician's office building when Adam, a 55-year-old coworker, suddenly collapses on the floor next to you. You determine that he is unresponsive and immediately direct a coworker to phone the medical center emergency response number (to activate the emergency response team) and bring the emergency cart.

You open Adam's airway and look, listen, and feel for breathing. You detect no breaths, so you use a face shield that you carry with you and you deliver 2 slow rescue breaths. You note that the chest rises with each breath.

You then check for signs of circulation (a pulse, coughing, breathing, and movement). You cannot feel the carotid pulse, and you see no signs of coughing, breathing, or movement, so you begin chest compressions (at a rate of approximately 100 times per minute).

You provide chest compressions and rescue breathing at a ratio of 15:2. Within 2 minutes your coworkers arrive at the scene with emergency equipment, including a bag-mask system with oxygen and an AED. You continue chest compressions and rescue breathing until the AED pads are placed. You then stop compressions to allow the AED to analyze the victim's rhythm. The device recommends a shock. You deliver that shock and 2 more that are recommended immediately afterward. After the third shock the AED indicates *"no shock advised, check the victim."* You note that Adam has begun breathing and has signs of circulation, including a pulse. The medical center emergency response team arrives and transports Adam to the hospital.

A month later you enjoy participating in the "welcome back" staff party for Adam.

Adult CPR

Overview

BLS is a sequence of actions. These actions, taken during the first few minutes of an emergency, are critical to survival. The BLS sequence of actions includes the following:

- Prompt recognition of myocardial infarction and stroke and action to prevent respiratory and circulatory arrest

- Prompt action for any victim who is found to be suddenly unresponsive

- Rescue breathing for victims of respiratory arrest

- Chest compressions and rescue breathing for victims of cardiopulmonary arrest

- Defibrillation of ventricular fibrillation (VF) or tachycardia with an automated external defibrillator (AED)

- Recognition and relief of foreign-body airway obstruction

This chapter addresses the following aspects of BLS: (1) rescue breathing for victims of respiratory arrest and (2) chest compressions and rescue breathing for victims of cardiopulmonary arrest.

The chapter presents the ABCs of CPR (Airway, Breathing, and Circulation) for 1 and 2 rescuers and the "D" of defibrillation.

Learning Objectives

After reading this chapter and participating in the video segments and skills practice sessions, you should be able to

1. Define basic life support (BLS)

2. List the sequence of actions you should perform for an adult patient in respiratory and cardiac arrest

3. Describe situations when "phone fast" may be appropriate if you are a lone rescuer with an unresponsive adult

4. Describe and demonstrate 1- and 2-rescuer CPR

5. Describe and demonstrate the following adjuncts to ventilation:

   - Face shield
   - Pocket mask
   - Bag mask

6. Describe and demonstrate cricoid pressure (the Sellick maneuver)

BLS Response to Cardiopulmonary Emergencies

Phone First/Phone Fast

Most adults with sudden, nontraumatic cardiac arrest are found to be in VF when the initial electrocardiogram (ECG) is obtained.[1] For these victims the time from collapse to defibrillation is the single greatest determinant of survival.[1-12] The window of opportunity for successful defibrillation is small. Survival from cardiac arrest caused by VF declines by approximately 7% to 10% for each minute without defibrillation.[13] More than 12 minutes after collapse the cardiac arrest survival rate is only 2% to 5%.[1-14] Structured EMS systems that can be quickly accessed by calling 911 (or other emergency response number) improve survival from sudden cardiac death because they facilitate early defibrillation.[2,3,5,9,13,14] Because the data in adult victims is compelling, both trained and untrained bystanders should be instructed to phone 911 or other emergency response number as soon as they determine that an adult victim requires emergency care. This will hasten the arrival of EMS personnel with an AED at the victim's side. A greater reduction in time to defibrillation (with corresponding improvement in survival) has been shown when AEDs have been distributed throughout the community and lay rescuers have been trained in both CPR and use of an AED. Public access defibrillation programs are reviewed in Chapter 7.

In sharp contrast to causes of adult cardiac arrest, most causes of cardiopulmonary arrest in infants (less than 1 year of age) or children (1 to 8 years of age) are related to airway or ventilation problems rather than sudden cardiac arrest.[15] In these victims rescue support (especially rescue breathing) is essential and should be attempted first if the rescuer is trained and can use the appropriate technique.[16] This respiratory etiology of cardiopulmonary arrest in children provides the rationale for the "phone fast" approach to resuscitation in children — provide CPR for approximately 1 minute and then phone 911 or other emergency response number.

Exceptions to the phone first/phone fast rule include

■ Near-drowning: these victims require immediate rescue breathing, so you should phone fast (provide approximately 1 minute of rescue support before phoning 911 or other emergency response number) for both adults and children.

■ Cardiac arrest associated with trauma: these victims may develop respiratory arrest related to loss of consciousness and airway obstruction. Provide approximately 1 minute of rescue support and then phone fast for both adults and children.

■ Drug overdoses: respiratory arrest is a common complication when the victim is unresponsive, so provide approximately 1 minute of rescue support and then phone fast for both adults and children.

■ Children known to be at high risk for cardiac arrest: These children will benefit from the prompt arrival of a defibrillator (an AED if one is nearby). For this reason you should *phone first* when a child with known risk of cardiac arrest collapses suddenly, because sudden cardiac arrest is a likely cause. After making the call, return to the child and provide CPR until the defibrillator arrives.

The information above is appropriate in the so-called lone rescuer scenario, when the rescuer is the only person present to help the victim. In such a case the rescuer must choose between providing CPR and leaving the victim to phone 911 (or other emergency response number).

Of course, when a second rescuer is present, the issue of phone first versus phone fast is moot. When a victim is found to be unresponsive and a second rescuer is available, two things can happen simultaneously: the first rescuer should begin CPR while the second rescuer phones 911 or other emergency response number immediately. Healthcare providers will rarely find themselves performing resuscitation alone, so the 2-rescuer scenario is far more common than the lone-rescuer scenario.

Throughout this text, during performance of CPR an adult is defined as anyone 8 years of age or older.

Emergency Medical Dispatch

Emergency medical dispatch has evolved over the past 25 years to become a sophisticated and integral component of a comprehensive EMS response.[17-22] Emergency medical dispatchers (EMDs) provide the first link between the victim, bystanders, and emergency response personnel.[17-22] The National Association of EMS Physicians has stated that "prearrival instructions are a mandatory function of each emergency medical dispatcher in a medical dispatch center" and "standard medically approved telephone instructions by trained EMDs are safe to give and in many instances are a moral necessity."[23] All communities should provide formal training in emergency medical dispatch[24,25] and require the use of medical dispatch protocols, including prearrival telephone instructions for airway control, foreign-body airway obstruction, chest compressions, and use of an AED.[17-22,26,27]

Dispatchers are highly accurate in their identification of victims of cardiac arrest.[22]

The dispatcher can rapidly determine the patient's condition and activate the necessary emergency service by using written protocols to question the caller.[19,20,22,24,26] To dispatch the appropriate rescue personnel to the scene, the dispatcher will need to know that the victim is unresponsive and CPR is in progress or an AED is being used. If the rescuer does not know how to perform CPR or does not remember what steps to take, the EMD can instruct the rescuer in appropriate emergency interventions.[19,20,22,24,26]

Dispatch protocols are evolving as newer resuscitation science becomes available.[28] For example, to reduce the time to bystander intervention, some centers have simplified the dispatch-assisted CPR technique for untrained bystanders.[29,30] Dispatchers instruct the rescuer to locate the lower half of the sternum by placing their hands in the center of the chest at the nipple line.[29,30] In one study of dispatcher-assisted CPR in a system with a very short EMS response interval (approximately 4 minutes), chest compression–only CPR was associated with a survival rate equivalent to that for chest compressions plus ventilations for victims of witnessed arrest.[30] Several studies have shown that chest compressions alone are significantly better than no CPR at all for adult cardiac arrest, although they are not as good as CPR.[31-35] For these reasons chest compressions only instead of compression-ventilation CPR is recommended for use in dispatch-assisted CPR instructions, because the simplicity of this modified technique allows untrained bystanders to intervene rapidly. Further research is needed to evaluate simplified protocols and methods to encourage bystander CPR.

Studies have confirmed that dispatch-assisted CPR is practical and effective and can increase the percentage of cardiac arrests in which bystander CPR is performed.[22,24,26,27] Because dispatch instructions can be lifesaving, emergency medical dispatch assistance has rapidly become the standard of care in EMS systems.[17-22,24-27,29,36-38]

Although no scientific studies have documented improved survival with use of enhanced 911 systems (technology that automatically provides the EMD with the caller's location and telephone number), such systems expedite the EMD process and should be strongly encouraged.[17]

Indications for BLS

Respiratory Arrest

Respiratory arrest is present when respirations are completely absent or clearly inadequate to maintain effective oxygenation and ventilation. Healthcare providers should be able to identify respiratory arrest and should be able to determine when respirations are inadequate to maintain effective oxygenation or ventilation. When respirations are absent or inadequate, the healthcare provider must immediately establish a patent airway and provide rescue breathing to prevent cardiac arrest and hypoxic injury to the brain and other organs.

Respiratory arrest without cardiac arrest in the out-of-hospital setting can result from a number of causes, including submersion/near-drowning, stroke, foreign-body airway obstruction, smoke inhalation, epiglottitis, drug overdose, electrocution, suffocation, injuries, myocardial infarction, lightning strike, and coma of any cause. In the hospital, respiratory arrest without cardiac arrest may result from drug reaction, sedation, stroke, myocardial infarction, or coma of any cause. When primary respiratory arrest occurs, the heart and lungs can continue to oxygenate the blood for several minutes, and oxygen will continue to circulate to the brain and other vital organs.[39]

Cardiac Arrest

In cardiac arrest, circulation ceases and vital organs are deprived of oxygen. The victim will have no signs of circulation and no pulse. Signs of circulation include breathing, coughing, or movement in response to the rescue breaths delivered. Healthcare providers should be aware that victims in cardiac arrest often demonstrate "gasping" breathing efforts, called

agonal respirations. These gasps may occur early in cardiac arrest and do not constitute effective breathing. They are ineffective and will not maintain oxygenation or ventilation.[33,40,41]

Because lay rescuers assess the victim for breathing as a sign of circulation (absence of breathing and signs of circulation identify victims in cardiac arrest), they should be able to distinguish between breathing and agonal respirations. Lay rescuers are generally taught to look for "normal" breathing as one of the signs of circulation. Healthcare providers are taught to look for "breathing," with the assumption that they will be able to distinguish between agonal respirations and other inadequate respiratory efforts and effective spontaneous breathing.

Cardiac arrest may be accompanied by the following cardiac rhythms: VF, ventricular tachycardia, asystole, or pulseless electrical activity.

AED Use

The cardiac arrest rhythms of ventricular tachycardia and VF are treated most effectively with early defibrillation. Use of AEDs is now considered an important and lifesaving addition to BLS and provides the trained rescuer with the opportunity to implement the first 3 links in the Chain of Survival (early access, early CPR, and early defibrillation).[42,43] The sequence of action for a rescuer with training and access to an AED is identical to that of CPR except for the added step of attaching and using the AED. AEDs are effective and easy to use.[44] Chapter 7 presents the BLS use of automated external defibrillation.

The Sequence of BLS: Assess, Activate EMS, Perform ABCDs

The sequence of BLS includes the ABCs of CPR and the "D" of defibrillation. Each step of CPR includes both assessment and intervention. The assessment phases of BLS are crucial. No victim should undergo the more intrusive procedures of CPR (positioning, opening the

airway, rescue breathing, or chest compressions) until the need has been established by appropriate assessment. Assessment also involves a more subtle, constant process of observing the victim and the victim's response to rescue support. This assessment phase begins with assessment of responsiveness: if you find a victim suddenly unresponsive, activate the EMS system and perform the subsequent steps of CPR. The importance of the assessment phase should be stressed in CPR training.

Assess Responsiveness

The rescuer arriving at the side of the collapsed victim must quickly determine if the scene is safe, if the victim is responsive, and if there is any evidence that the victim sustained injuries. Tap or gently shake the victim and shout "Are you all right?" (See Figure 1A.)

If the victim has sustained trauma to the head and neck or if trauma is suspected, move the victim only if necessary to ensure safety or provide CPR. Improper movement may cause paralysis if the victim has a neck injury. If it is necessary to move a victim with suspected head and neck injuries, turn the head, neck, and torso as a unit ("log-roll" the victim) to avoid flexion or twisting of the neck or back.

Activate EMS

Activate the EMS system by phoning 911 or other emergency response number (see Figure 1B). This emergency number should be widely publicized in each community and workplace.

In hospitals and other medical facilities and some businesses or buildings, an established emergency medical response system provides a first or early response on-site. Such a response system notifies rescuers of the location of an emergency and the type of response needed. If a cardiopulmonary emergency occurs in a facility with an established medical response system, that system should be notified of the emergency because it

FIGURE 1. Check for unresponsiveness and activate EMS. **A,** Tap the victim's shoulder and ask "Are you all right?" **B,** If the victim does not respond, send someone to phone 911 or activate the emergency medical response system.

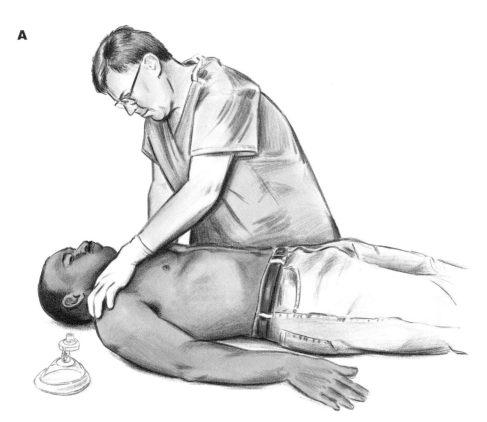

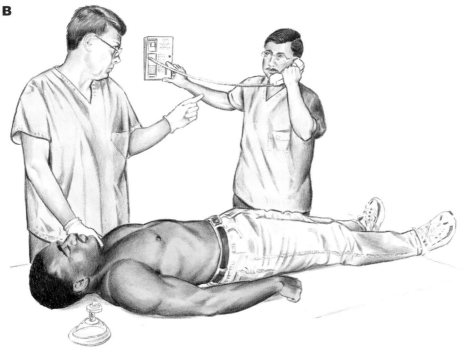

will provide a more rapid response than EMS personnel arriving from outside the facility. In such facilities the emergency medical response system should replace the EMS system in the sequences below.

The person who calls EMS or other emergency response system should be prepared to give the following information as calmly as possible[45]:

1. The location of the emergency (with names of cross streets or roads or office or room number if possible)

2. The telephone number from which the call is being made

3. What happened — heart attack, motor vehicle crash, etc

4. How many persons need help

5. Condition of the victim(s)

6. What aid is being given to the victim(s) (for example, "CPR is being performed" or "we're using an AED")

7. Any other information requested

To ensure that EMS personnel (or emergency response system operators) have no more questions, the caller should hang up only when instructed to do so by the EMD/emergency response system operator.

Airway

If the victim is unresponsive, you must determine if the victim is breathing adequately. In many instances this cannot be accurately ascertained unless the airway is opened. To assess breathing, the victim should be supine (lying on his or her back) with an open airway.

Position of the Victim

For resuscitative efforts and evaluation to be effective, the victim must be supine and on a firm, flat surface. If the victim is lying face down, you must roll the victim as a unit so that the head, shoulders, and torso move simultaneously without twisting. The head and neck should remain in the same plane as the torso, and the body should be moved as a unit. The nonbreathing patient should be supine, with arms alongside the body.

Position of the Rescuer

You should be at the victim's side, positioned to perform both rescue breathing and chest compression. You should anticipate the arrival of additional rescuers with an AED or manual defibrillator and should be prepared to operate the device when it arrives.

Opening the Airway

In the absence of sufficient muscle tone, the tongue and epiglottis may obstruct the pharynx (Figure 2A and B).[45-48] The tongue is the most common cause of airway obstruction in the unresponsive victim. Because the tongue is attached to the lower jaw, moving the lower jaw forward will lift the tongue away from the back of the throat and open the airway. The tongue or epiglottis[48] or both may also create an obstruction when inspiratory effort creates negative pressure in the airway, causing a valve-type mechanism to occlude the entrance to the trachea.

FYI: **Opening the Airway**

Lay Rescuers vs Healthcare Providers

The recommended technique for opening the airway must be simple, safe, easily learned, and effective. Because the head tilt–chin lift maneuver meets these criteria, it should be the method of choice for lay rescuers performing BLS. Lay rescuers should use this technique unless trauma is suspected. All rescuers are taught the head tilt–chin lift and jaw-thrust methods of opening the airway, but healthcare providers (BLS ambulance providers and others) should be proficient in both techniques.

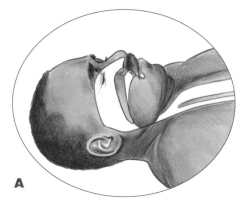
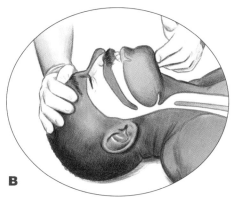

FIGURE 2. Obstruction of the airway in the unresponsive victim is relieved by head tilt–chin lift. **A,** Obstruction by the tongue and epiglottis. When a victim is unresponsive, the tongue and epiglottis can block the upper airway. **B,** The head tilt–chin lift maneuver lifts the tongue, relieving airway obstruction.

A

B

If there is no evidence of head or neck trauma, the rescuer should use the head tilt–chin lift maneuver to open the victim's airway as described below (see Figure 2B). Quickly remove any foreign material or vomitus that is visible in the mouth. Wipe liquids or semiliquids out of the mouth with the index and middle fingers of a gloved hand (or a hand covered by a piece of cloth). In the healthcare setting suction may be used. Extract solid material with a hooked index finger.

Head Tilt–Chin Lift Maneuver

To accomplish the head tilt–chin lift maneuver, place one hand on the victim's forehead and apply firm, backward pressure with the palm to tilt the head back. Place the fingers of the other hand under the bony part of the lower jaw near the chin. Lift the jaw upward to bring the chin forward and the teeth almost to occlusion. (See Figure 2B.) This maneuver supports the jaw and helps tilt the head back.

Do not press deep into the soft tissue under the chin because this might obstruct the airway. Do not use the thumb to lift the chin. The mouth should not be completely closed (unless mouth-to-nose breathing is the technique of choice for the victim).

When mouth-to-nose ventilation is indicated, apply increased force with the

hand that is already on the chin to close the mouth and provide effective mouth-to-nose ventilation.[48] If the victim's dentures are loose, head tilt–chin lift makes a mouth-to-mouth seal easier.[49] Remove the victim's dentures if they cannot be kept in place.

Jaw-Thrust Maneuver

This technique is recommended as an alternative method for opening the airway when trauma to the head or neck is present or suspected. This method should be taught to both lay rescuers and healthcare providers.

Place one hand on each side of the victim's head, resting your elbows on the

FIGURE 3. Jaw thrust without head tilt. The jaw is lifted without tilting the head. This is the airway maneuver of choice for a victim with a suspected cervical spine injury.

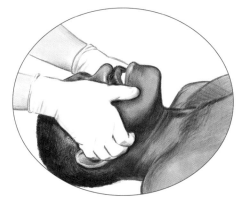

surface on which the victim is lying. Grasp the angles of the victim's lower jaw and lift with both hands, displacing the mandible forward (see Figure 3). If the lips close, retract the lower lip with your thumb. If mouth-to-mouth breathing is necessary while you maintain the jaw thrust, close the victim's nostrils by placing your cheek tightly against them. This technique is very effective for opening the airway,[50] but it is fatiguing and technically difficult.[49]

The jaw-thrust technique without head tilt is the safest initial approach to opening the airway of the victim with suspected neck injury because it can usually be accomplished without extending the neck. The head should be carefully supported without tilting it backward or turning it from side to side.

Breathing

Assessment: Determine Absent or Inadequate Breathing

To assess breathing, place your ear near the victim's mouth and nose while maintaining an open airway (see Figure 4). Then while observing the victim's chest (1) *look* for the chest to rise and fall, (2) *listen* for air escaping during exhalation, and (3) *feel* for the flow of air. If the chest does not rise and fall and no air is exhaled, the victim is not breathing. This evaluation procedure should take no more than 10 seconds.

Most victims with respiratory or cardiac arrest have no signs of breathing. Some victims will demonstrate apparent respiratory efforts with signs of upper airway obstruction. These victims may resume effective breathing when you open the airway.

Some victims will make weak, inadequate attempts to breathe. In addition, reflex gasping respiratory efforts (agonal respirations) may occur early in the course of primary cardiac arrest. Both absent and inadequate respirations require rapid intervention with rescue breathing. If you are

FIGURE 4. Check for breathing. If no trauma is suspected, open the airway with a head tilt–chin lift, place your face near the victim's nose and mouth, and look, listen, and feel for breathing.

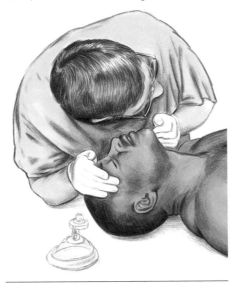

not *confident* that respirations are adequate, proceed immediately with rescue breathing.

If a victim resumes breathing and regains signs of circulation (pulse, normal breathing, coughing, or movement) during or after resuscitation, continue to help the victim maintain an open airway until he or she is sufficiently alert to protect his or her own airway. Place the victim in the recovery position if he or she maintains adequate breathing and signs of circulation.

Recovery Position

The recovery position is used in the management of victims who are unresponsive but breathing with signs of circulation.

When an unresponsive victim is breathing spontaneously, the airway may become obstructed by the tongue, mucus, or vomitus. These problems may be prevented when the victim is placed on his or her side, because fluid can drain easily from the mouth.

Some compromise is needed between the ideal position to maintain airway patency and the optimal position to allow monitoring and support with good body alignment. A modified lateral position is used because a true lateral position tends to be unstable, involves excessive lateral flexion of the cervical spine, and results in less free drainage of secretions or vomit from the mouth. A near-prone position, on the other hand, can hinder adequate ventilation owing to splinting of the diaphragm and reduction in pulmonary and thoracic compliance.[51] Many different versions of the recovery position exist, each with its own advocates, but none is perfect. When deciding which position to use, consider the following 6 principles[52]:

- The victim should be in as near a true lateral position as possible, with the head dependent to allow free drainage of fluid.

- The position should be stable.

- Avoid any pressure on the chest that impairs breathing.

- It should be possible to turn the victim onto his or her side and to return to the back easily and safely, without flexion or rotation of the back, neck, or spine.

FIGURE 5. Recovery position. This stable, modified lateral position maintains alignment of the back and spine while allowing the rescuer to observe and maintain access to the victim.

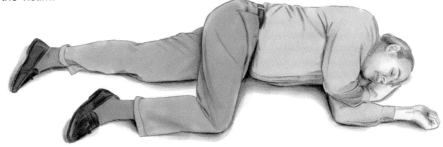

■ Good observation of and access to the airway should be possible.

■ The position itself should not cause an injury to the victim.

It is particularly important to protect the spine when turning the victim.[53,54] If trauma is present or suspected, move the victim only if an open airway cannot otherwise be maintained or if CPR is needed. The victim in the recovery position must still be closely monitored, with emphasis on airway and breathing and assessment of perfusion to the lowermost arm.[55,56]

If the victim is to remain in the recovery position for more than 30 minutes, turn the victim to the opposite side. Although no single specific recovery position can be recommended, the one illustrated in Figure 5 is suitable for training purposes. For complete details about placement of a victim in the recovery position, see the FYI box "The Recovery Position."

Provide Rescue Breathing

Rescue breathing requires that the rescuer inflate the victim's lungs adequately with each breath.

Mouth-to-Mouth Breathing

Mouth-to-mouth rescue breathing is a quick, effective way to provide oxygen to the victim.[57] The rescuer's exhaled air contains enough oxygen to supply the victim's needs.[57] To provide rescue breaths, hold the victim's airway open, pinch the nose closed with your thumb and index finger (using the hand on the forehead). When you pinch the nose closed, you prevent air that you deliver into the victim's mouth from escaping through the victim's nose. Take a deep breath and seal your lips around the victim's mouth, creating an airtight seal (see Figure 6). Give slow breaths, delivering each breath over 2 seconds, making sure the victim's chest rises with each breath.

Gastric inflation frequently develops during mouth-to-mouth ventilation.[58,59] Gastric inflation can result in serious

---

FYI: The Recovery Position (for the Unresponsive Victim Who Is Breathing Normally)

If there is no evidence of trauma and the victim is unresponsive but breathing, place the victim on his or her side in the recovery position. The recovery position keeps the airway open. To place the victim in the recovery position:

1. Kneel beside the victim and straighten the victim's legs.

2. Place the victim's arm that is nearest you in a "waving goodbye" position (extend the victim's arm to the side, bend the arm at the elbow, and lay the forearm so that it is parallel with the head and the palm is facing up. The arm will be at a right angle to the victim's body.)

3. Place the victim's other arm across the chest so that the back of the hand can be held against the victim's cheek near you.

4. Use one hand to grasp the back of the victim's far-side thigh a few inches above the knee, and pull the thigh up toward the victim's body.

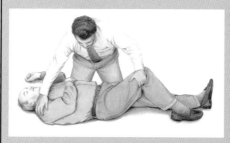

5. Place your other hand over the victim's far-side shoulder, and roll the victim toward you onto his or her side. Move the victim's uppermost hand toward the victim's nearest cheek (the hand must not be trapped under the body).

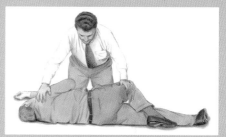

6. Adjust the upper leg of the knee you are holding so that both the hip and knee are bent at right angles.

7. Tilt the victim's head back to keep the airway open. Place the back of the victim's uppermost hand under his or her cheek. Use this hand to maintain head tilt. Use chin lift if necessary.

Continue to check the victim:

8. Check breathing frequently (look, listen, and feel).

9. If the victim stops breathing, turn the victim onto his or her back, phone 911 (or other emergency response number), and get the AED if available (or be sure someone else does), and begin CPR.

10. ***Memory aid: Victim is waving goodbye while taking a nap.***

Figure 6. Mouth-to-mouth rescue breathing.

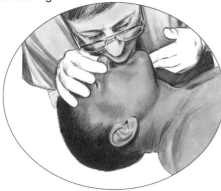

complications, such as regurgitation,[60-62] aspiration,[63] or pneumonia.[64] Stomach inflation may also increase intragastric pressure,[58,59,65-68] elevate the diaphragm, restrict lung movements, and thereby decrease respiratory system compliance.[58,69,70] Gastric inflation occurs when the pressure in the esophagus exceeds the lower esophageal sphincter opening pressure, causing the sphincter to open so that air delivered during rescue breaths enters the stomach instead of the lungs.[58,69-74] During cardiac arrest the likelihood of gastric inflation increases because the lower esophageal sphincter relaxes.[71] Factors that contribute to gastric inflation during rescue breathing include short inspiratory time, large tidal volume, and high peak airway pressure.[58,69-74]

The 1992 ECC Guidelines[75] recommended that adult rescue breaths provide a tidal volume of 800 to 1200 mL, delivered over 1 to 2 seconds. Provision of a smaller tidal volume can reduce the likelihood of gastric inflation but will not maintain adequate arterial oxygen saturation unless supplemental oxygen is delivered with a face mask or bag mask.[76,77]

To reduce the risk of gastric inflation during mouth-to-mouth ventilation, deliver slow breaths at the lowest tidal volume that will still make the chest visibly rise with each ventilation. For mouth-to-mouth ventilation in most adults, this volume will be approximately 10 mL/kg (approximately 700 to 1000 mL) and should be delivered over 2 seconds.

This recommendation represents a slightly decreased range of tidal volume and uses the upper limit of inspiratory time compared with the 1992 guidelines. This new recommendation is intended to reduce the risk of gastric inflation (and its serious consequences) while maintaining adequate arterial oxygen saturation during respiratory and cardiac arrest.

The rescuer should take a deep breath before delivering each rescue breath to optimize exhaled gas composition and ensure provision of maximal oxygen to the victim.[78] You are providing adequate ventilation if you see the victim's chest rise and fall and hear and feel the air escape during exhalation. When possible (for example, during 2-rescuer CPR), keep the airway patent between rescuer breaths to allow unimpeded exhalation.

If initial (or subsequent) attempts to ventilate the victim are unsuccessful, reposition the victim's head and reattempt rescue breathing. Improper chin and head positioning is the most common cause of difficulty with ventilation. If the victim cannot be ventilated after repositioning the head, the *healthcare provider* should proceed with maneuvers to relieve foreign-body airway obstruction in the unresponsive victim (see Chapter 8, "Adult Foreign-Body Airway Obstruction"). The lay rescuer should proceed with chest compressions.

Mouth-to-Nose Breathing

The mouth-to-nose method of ventilation is recommended when it is impossible to ventilate through the victim's mouth, the mouth cannot be opened (trismus), the mouth is seriously injured, or a tight mouth-to-mouth seal is difficult to achieve.[79] Mouth-to-nose breathing may be the best method of providing ventilation while rescuing a submersion victim from the water. The rescuer's hands are often used to support the victim's head and shoulders during rescue. The mouth-to-nose technique may enable the rescuer to begin rescue breathing as soon as the victim's head is out of the water.

To provide mouth-to-nose breathing, tilt the victim's head back with one hand on the forehead. Use the other hand to lift the victim's mandible (as in head tilt–chin lift) and close the victim's mouth. Take a deep breath, seal your lips around the victim's nose, and exhale into the victim's nose. Then remove your lips from the victim's nose, allowing passive exhalation (see Figure 7). It may be necessary to open the victim's mouth intermittently and separate the lips with the thumb to allow free exhalation, particularly if nasal obstruction is present.[80]

Figure 7. Mouth-to-nose rescue breathing.

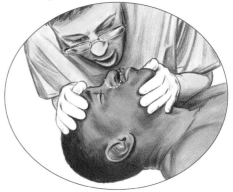

Mouth-to-Stoma Breathing

A tracheal stoma is a permanent opening at the front of the neck (see Figure 8A).[81] When a person with a tracheal stoma requires rescue breathing, perform direct mouth-to-stoma breathing by making an airtight seal around the stoma and blowing until the victim's chest rises (see Figure 8B). Then remove your lips from the patient, allowing passive exhalation (Figure 8C).

A tracheostomy tube may be present in the tracheal stoma. This tube must be patent for successful spontaneous breathing or rescue breathing to occur. If the tube is not patent and you are unable to clear an obstruction or secretions, remove and replace the tube. If a second tube is unavailable and the original tube is obstructed, remove the tube and provide rescue breathing through the stoma. If a significant volume of air escapes through the victim's nose and mouth during ven-

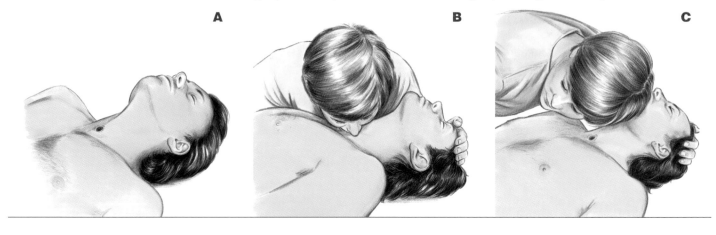

FIGURE 8. Mouth-to-stoma rescue breathing. **A,** Stoma. **B,** Mouth-to-stoma breathing. **C,** Allowing air to excape between breaths.

tilation through the tracheostomy, seal the victim's mouth and nose with your hand or a tightly fitting face mask to prevent leakage of air through the nose and mouth when you deliver air into the tracheostomy tube. The problem of air escape is alleviated if the tracheostomy tube has an inflated cuff.

Mouth-to–Barrier Device Breathing

Healthcare providers should be able to provide mouth-to-mouth breathing, mouth-to-nose breathing, and mouth-to-stoma breathing. In the workplace, however, they will use barrier devices or bag-mask systems during ventilation.

The Occupational Safety and Health Administration (OSHA) requires that universal precautions be used when there is any exposure to blood or bodily fluids (eg, saliva). Universal precautions include the use of barrier devices during rescue breathing, so these must be available in the workplace for rescuers who are expected to perform CPR.

Two broad categories of barrier devices are available: face shields and mouth-to-mask devices. Face shields usually have no exhalation valve, and the victim's expired air escapes between the shield and the victim's face. Mouth-to-mask devices typically have a 1-way valve so that exhaled air does not enter the rescuer's mouth. Barrier devices should have a low resistance to gas flow to keep the user from tiring from excessive effort.

Mouth-to–Face Shield Rescue Breathing

Unlike mouth-to-mask devices, face shields have only a clear plastic or silicone sheet that separates the rescuer and victim. Place the opening of the face shield over the mouth of the victim. In some models a short (1- to 2-inch) tube is part of the shield. Insert the tube into the mouth over the tongue. Pinch the nose closed and seal your mouth around the center opening of the face shield. Provide slow breaths (2 seconds) through a 1-way valve or filter in the center of the face shield. The patient's exhaled air will escape between the shield and the victim's face when you remove your mouth from the shield (see Figure 9).

The face shield should remain on the victim's face during performance of chest compressions. If the victim begins to vomit during rescue efforts, remove the face shield and clear the airway.

Because the efficacy of face shields has not been documented conclusively, healthcare professionals and those with a duty to respond should also be instructed in the use of mouth-to-mask and/or bag-mask devices.[82,83] Proximity to the victim's face and the possibility of contamination if the victim vomits are major disadvantages of face shields.[84,85]

Rescuers should use face shields only as a substitute for mouth-to-mouth breathing and replace them with mouth-to-mask or bag-mask devices at the first opportunity.

Tidal volumes and inspiratory times provided during mouth-to-mouth breathing with a face shield should be the same as during mouth-to-mouth breathing without a face shield (tidal volume of approximately 10 mL/kg or 700 to 1000 mL in an adult delivered over 2 seconds and sufficient to make the chest rise clearly).

Mouth-to-Mask Rescue Breathing

In mouth-to-mask breathing a transparent mask is used with or without a 1-way valve. The 1-way valve directs the rescuer's breath into the victim while diverting the victim's exhaled air away from the rescuer. Some masks have an oxygen inlet that permits administration of supplemental oxygen.

Effective use of the mask barrier device requires instruction and supervised

FIGURE 9. Face shield. The shield is placed over the victim's mouth and nose, with the opening at the center of the shield placed over the victim's mouth. The technique of rescue breathing is the same as that used for mouth-to-mouth breathing.

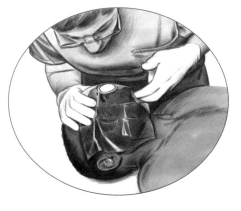

practice. Effective mouth-to–mask ventilation can be easier to perform than mouth-to–face shield ventilation because the rescuer can use both hands to open the airway and seal the mask to the victim's face. During 2-person CPR the mask can be used in a variety of ways. The most appropriate method will depend on the experience of personnel and the equipment available. The 2 most common techniques for using the mouth-to-mask device are the lateral and cephalic techniques. In the *lateral technique* the rescuer is positioned at the victim's side and uses a head tilt–chin lift to open the victim's airway. This position is ideal for performing 1-rescuer CPR because the rescuer can use the same position for both rescue breathing and chest compressions.

When the *cephalic technique* is used, the rescuer is positioned above the victim's head. This technique uses a jaw thrust and has the advantage of having the rescuer face the victim's chest during rescue breathing (so that the rescuer can monitor chest rise with rescue breathing). This technique can be used by 1 rescuer for rescue breathing alone when the patient is in respiratory arrest or during 2-rescuer CPR. This technique is *not* the preferred technique for the lone rescuer, who must also perform cardiac compressions.

Lateral Technique

Position yourself beside the victim's head in a location that will facilitate both rescue breathing and chest compressions:

■ Place the mask on the victim's face, using the bridge of the nose as a guide for correct position.

■ Seal the mask by placing the index and thumb of your hand closest to the top of the victim's head along the border of the mask and placing the thumb of your other hand along the lower margin of the mask.

■ Place the remaining fingers of your hand closest to the victim's feet along the bony margin of the jaw and lift the jaw. If no cervical spine injury is sus-

pected, perform a head tilt–chin lift (see Figure 10).

■ Compress firmly completely around the outside margin of the mask to provide a tight seal.

■ Provide slow rescue breaths while observing for chest rise.

FIGURE 10. Mouth-to-mask ventilation, lateral technique. The lateral technique allows the rescuer to perform 1-rescuer CPR from a position at the victim's side. A head tilt–chin lift is performed to open the airway.

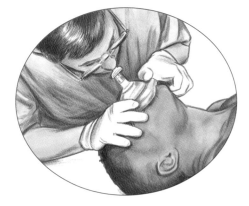

Cephalic Technique

Position yourself directly above the victim's head:

■ Apply the mask to the victim's face, using the bridge of the nose as a guide for correct position.

■ Place your thumbs and thenar eminence (portion of the palm at the base of the thumb) along the lateral edges of the mask.

■ Place the index fingers of both hands under the victim's mandible and lift the jaw into the mask. Place the remaining fingers of your hand under the angle of the victim's jaw (see Figure 11A). If no head or cervical spine injury is suspected, perform a head tilt to facilitate airway opening.

■ While lifting the jaw, squeeze the mask with your thumbs and thenar eminence to achieve an airtight seal (see jaw thrust).

■ Provide slow rescue breaths (2 seconds each) while observing for chest rise.

Another way to hold the mask in place is the E-C technique. Using the thumb and index finger of each hand to make a "C," press around the edges of the mask. Use the remaining fingers to lift the angles of the jaw (3 fingers form an "E") and open the airway (Figure 11B).

With either variation of the cephalic technique, the rescuer uses both hands to hold the mask and open the airway. For victims with suspected cervical spine injury, lift the mandible at the angles of the jaw without tilting the head.

Oral airways and cricoid pressure may be used with mouth-to-mask and any other form of rescue breathing for the unresponsive victim.

If oxygen is unavailable, tidal volumes and inspiratory times used for mouth-to-mask rescue breathing should be the same as those used for mouth-to-mouth breathing (tidal volume of approximately 10 mL/kg or 700 to 1000 mL in an adult delivered over 2 seconds and sufficient to make the chest rise clearly). Of course, during rescue breathing it is impossible to quantify the tidal volume. The tidal volume should be sufficient to make the chest clearly rise.

If supplemental oxygen is provided with the face mask (a minimum oxygen flow rate of 10 L/min providing an inspired concentration of oxygen greater than or equal to 40%),[86] lower tidal volumes may be used (tidal volume of approximately 6 to 7 mL/kg or 400 to 600 mL given over 1 to 2 seconds until the chest rises). Lower tidal volumes reduce the risk of gastric inflation[58,59] and its serious consequences.[58,60-64,69,70] However, these smaller tidal volumes are effective for maintaining adequate arterial oxygen saturation *only if* supplemental oxygen is delivered to the device.[76] These lower tidal volumes may not maintain normocarbia, particularly during prolonged arrest, and the resultant hypercarbia may produce acidosis.[87]

Bag-Mask Device

Bag-mask devices consist of a bag and a non-rebreathing valve attached to a face mask. These devices are the most common method of providing positive-pressure ventilation in the EMS and hospital settings. Most commercially available adult bag-mask units have a volume of approximately 1600 mL, which is usually adequate for lung inflation. In several studies, however, many rescuers were unable to deliver adequate tidal volumes to unintubated manikins with the bag and mask.[88-92] Adult bag-mask ventilation may provide a smaller tidal volume than mouth-to-mouth or mouth-to-mask ventilation because the lone rescuer may have difficulty obtaining a leak-proof seal

FIGURE 11. Mouth-to-mask cephalic technique. **A,** Use thumb and thenar eminance on top of the mask to hold the mask in place. Use the second and third fingers of both hands to lift the jaw. **B,** Alternative cephalic E-C technique of holding mask. Circle the thumb and first finger around the top of the mask (forming a "C") while using the third, fourth, and fifth fingers of each hand (forming an "E") to lift the jaw.

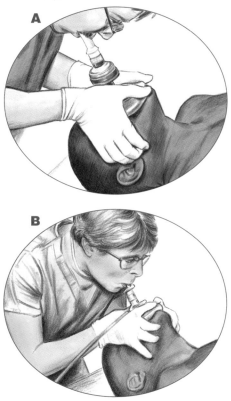

A

B

FIGURE 12. Two-rescuer use of the bag mask. The rescuer at the victim's head uses the E-C technique, with the thumb and first finger of each hand creating a "C" to provide a complete seal around the edges of the mask. The rescuer uses the remaining 3 fingers (the "E") to lift the mandible and extend the neck while observing chest rise. The second rescuer slowly squeezes the bag (over 2 seconds) until the chest rises.

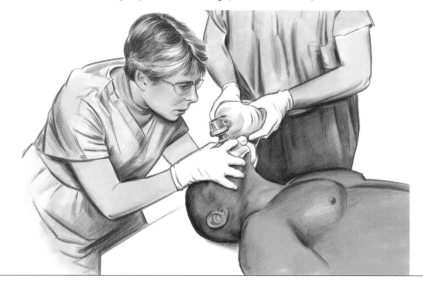

to the face while squeezing the bag and maintaining an open airway. For this reason, self-inflating bag-mask units are most effective when 2 trained and experienced rescuers work together, one sealing the mask to the face and the other squeezing the bag slowly over 2 seconds (see Figure 12).

The use of small tidal volumes during resuscitation has significant advantages, although small tidal volumes increase the risk of hypoxia and hypercarbia and related complications.[87] The use of small tidal volumes with oxygen supplementation during resuscitation has been evaluated in laboratory[59,66,93] and clinical[67,93] settings, particularly in the setting of respiratory arrest.[67] With smaller tidal volumes, airway pressure does not exceed the victim's lower esophageal sphincter pressure,[58,69-71] so lower tidal volumes will reduce gastric inflation and its potential consequences, including regurgitation,[60-62] aspiration,[63] and pneumonia.[64] The use of supplemental oxygen with smaller tidal volumes has been shown to maintain oxygen saturation in patients with respiratory arrest.[67,76]

If supplemental oxygen (at a minimum flow rate of 8 to 12 L/min with oxygen concentration greater than or equal to 40%) is available, the rescuer who is skilled in bag-mask ventilation should attempt to deliver a smaller tidal volume (6 to 7 mL/kg or approximately 400 to 600 mL) over 1 to 2 seconds. Of course, in the clinical setting the actual tidal volume delivered is impossible to determine. Tidal volume should be titrated to provide sufficient ventilation to produce visible chest expansion. If ventilation with this small tidal volume is successful, the chest should rise and oxygen saturation will be maintained in the patient with effective systemic perfusion.[67]

If chest rise is *not* seen during ventilation with the smaller tidal volume, adjust the face mask to eliminate air leak, reposition the head and neck (unless trauma is present), and use the jaw-thrust maneuver to open the airway and prevent obstruction. If necessary, administer a larger tidal volume. If circulation is present, monitoring of arterial oxygen saturation may be helpful for evaluating the efficacy of ventilation during ventilation. In one small study of prolonged cardiopulmonary arrest, this smaller tidal volume was associated with development of hypercarbia.[87]

If oxygen is unavailable, attempt to deliver the same tidal volume recommended for mouth-to-mouth ventilation (10 mL/kg, 700 to 1000 mL) over 2 seconds. This tidal volume should result in very obvious chest rise.[77]

An adult bag-mask device should have the following features:

- A nonjamming valve system that allows a maximum oxygen inlet flow of 30 L/min

- Either no pressure relief valve or a pressure relief valve that can be closed/inactivated

- Standard 15-mm/22-mm patient connectors

- An oxygen reservoir to allow delivery of high concentrations of oxygen[94]

- A non-rebreathing valve, which cannot be obstructed by foreign material

- Ability to function satisfactorily under common environmental conditions and extremes of temperature

Technique of Bag-Mask Ventilation

The bag-mask ventilation technique requires instruction and practice. You should be able to use the equipment effectively in a variety of situations. If you are providing respiratory support only, position yourself at the top of the victim's head. If there is no neck injury, tilt the victim's head back and raise it with a towel or pillow to achieve the sniffing position.

Apply the mask to the face with one hand, using the bridge of the nose as a guide for correct position. Place the third, fourth, and fifth fingers along the bony portion of the mandible and the thumb and index fingers of the same hand on the mask. Maintain head tilt and jaw thrust to obtain airway patency and mask fit (see Figure 13).

Compress the bag with your other hand and observe the victim's chest to ensure that ventilation is adequate. Deliver each

breath over 2 seconds (use 1 to 2 seconds when you deliver smaller tidal volumes with oxygen supplementation). You may want to compress the bag against your body to achieve the selected tidal volume. It is critical to maintain an airtight seal during the delivery of each breath.

Provision of effective ventilation is more likely when 2 rescuers use the bag-mask system: 1 rescuer holds the mask and 1 rescuer squeezes the bag (see Figure 12). Techniques for holding the mask are the same as those for the mouth-to-mask devices described above. If a third rescuer is available, cricoid pressure may be applied.

Bag-mask ventilation is an essential skill that requires considerable practice to master. Accordingly, the use of alternative airway devices such as the laryngeal mask airway and the esophageal-tracheal Combitube are being introduced within the scope of BLS for healthcare providers.

These devices are generally easier to insert than tracheal tubes, and the technique of providing ventilation is similar to that used for the intubated patient. These devices may provide an alternative to bag-mask ventilation for healthcare providers with adequate training and experience in their use.

Cricoid Pressure

Cricoid pressure, or the Sellick technique, is the application of pressure to the *unresponsive* victim's cricoid cartilage. The pressure pushes the trachea posteriorly, compressing the esophagus against the cervical vertebra during rescue breathing. Cricoid pressure is effective for preventing gastric inflation during positive-pressure ventilation of *unresponsive* victims. A reduction in gastric inflation, in turn, reduces the risk of regurgitation and aspiration.[95-98]

Cricoid pressure should be applied only when the victim is unresponsive. Proper use of the cricoid pressure technique requires an additional rescuer to provide cricoid pressure alone, without assisting in other resuscitative activities. The technique should be used only by healthcare professionals when an extra rescuer is present who is not required to assist with rescue breathing, chest compressions, or defibrillation. This means that if cricoid pressure is to be used during 2-rescuer CPR, 3 rescuers would actually be required: 1 rescuer to provide rescue breathing, 1 rescuer to perform chest compressions, and 1 rescuer to apply cricoid pressure.

The technique for applying cricoid pressure is as follows:

FIGURE 13. One-rescuer use of the bag mask. The rescuer circles the top edges of the mask with her thumb and index finger and lifts the jaw with the remaining fingers (the E-C technique). She squeezes the bag while observing chest rise. Mask seal is the key to successful use of the bag mask.

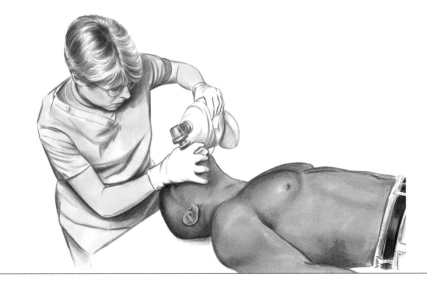

FIGURE 14. Cricoid pressure (Sellick maneuver).

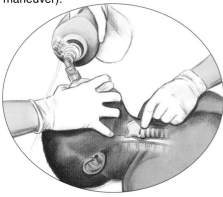

1. Locate the thyroid cartilage (Adam's apple) with your index finger.

2. Slide your index finger to the base of the thyroid cartilage and palpate the prominent horizontal ring below the thyroid cartilage (this is the cricoid cartilage).

3. Using the tips of your thumb and index finger, apply firm backward pressure to the cricoid cartilage (see Figure 14).

Recommendations for Rescue Breathing

To provide rescue breathing, deliver 2 breaths slowly (2 seconds each), allowing complete exhalation between breaths to diminish the likelihood of exceeding the esophageal opening pressure. This technique should result in less gastric inflation, regurgitation, and aspiration. If rescue breathing alone is provided, deliver approximately 10 to 12 breaths per minute (1 breath every 4 to 5 seconds).

When both compressions and ventilations are delivered, provide 15 compressions to 2 ventilations for both 1- and 2-rescuer CPR until the patient is intubated. The rescuer performing the chest compressions should pause after every 15th chest compression to deliver (or allow the second rescuer to deliver) 2 slow breaths. Chest compressions can be started immediately after the second inflation. Once the patient is intubated, it will not be necessary to pause during chest compressions to provide ventilations.

Circulation

Assessment: Check for Signs of Circulation (Lay Rescuer)

Cardiac arrest results in the absence of signs of circulation, including the absence of a pulse. The pulse check has been the "gold standard" usually relied on by professional rescuers to determine if the heart is or is not beating (cardiac arrest). Absence of a pulse has been used to indicate the need to place AED leads and initiate chest compressions.

Unfortunately the pulse check is neither rapid nor reliable for detecting the presence or absence of circulation, particularly when used by laypersons. Since 1992 several published studies have called into question the validity of the pulse check as a test for cardiac arrest, particularly when used by laypersons.[99-108] This research has used manikin simulation,[104] unresponsive patients undergoing cardiopulmonary bypass,[108] unresponsive mechanically ventilated patients,[105] and responsive "test persons."[100,105] The conclusions from this pulse check research are as follows[103]:

1. Rescuers require far too much time to perform the pulse check. The majority of all rescue groups, including laypersons, medical students, paramedics, and physicians take much longer than the recommended 5 to 10 seconds to check for the carotid pulse. In one study half of the rescuers required more than 24 seconds to decide whether a pulse was present.

   With survival from VF falling by 7% to 10% for every minute defibrillation is delayed, the time allotted to determine the presence or absence of circulation must be brief. Only 15% of the participants confirmed a pulse within 10 seconds, the maximum time currently allotted for a pulse check.[108]

2. When considered as a diagnostic test, the pulse check is surprisingly inaccurate. This accuracy can be expressed in a classic 2×2 matrix from a representative study.[108] (See Table.) This data indicates that

   a. Specificity (the ability to correctly identify victims who have no pulse and *are* in cardiac arrest) is only 90%. When subjects were pulseless, rescuers thought a pulse was present approximately 10% of the time. By mistakenly thinking a pulse *is* present when it is not, rescuers will fail to provide chest compressions and will not attach an AED for 10 of every 100 people in cardiac arrest. The consequences of such errors would be death without possibility of resuscitation for 10 of every 100 victims of cardiac arrest.

   b. Sensitivity (ability to correctly recognize victims who *have* a pulse and *are not* in cardiac arrest) was only 55%. When a pulse was *present,* rescuers assessed it as being *absent* approximately 45% of the time. By erroneously thinking a pulse was absent, rescuers would provide chest compressions for approximately 40 of 100 potential victims who do not need them and would unnecessarily use an AED if available.

3. Overall accuracy was only 65%, leaving an error rate of 35%.

On review of this data as well as data indicating the need to simplify CPR education, the experts and delegates at the 1999 Evidence Evaluation Conference and the International Guidelines 2000 Conference concluded that the pulse check could not be recommended as a tool for lay rescuers to identify victims of cardiac arrest in the CPR sequence. If rescuers use the pulse check to identify victims of cardiac arrest, they will "miss" true cardiac arrest at least 10 of 100 times. In addition, rescuers will provide unnecessary chest compressions and may use an AED for many victims who are not in cardiac arrest and do not require such intervention. This error is less serious but still undesirable. The more serious error is clearly the potential failure to intervene with victims of cardiac arrest who require immediate intervention to survive.

Therefore, the lay rescuer should not rely on the pulse check to determine the need for chest compressions or use of an AED. Lay rescuers should not perform the pulse check and will not be taught the pulse check in CPR courses. Instead lay rescuers will be taught to assess for signs of circulation, including normal breathing, coughing, or movement in response to 2 rescue breaths. This guideline recommendation applies to victims of any age.

Healthcare providers, however, should continue to use the pulse check as one of several signs of circulation. Other signs of circulation include normal breathing, coughing, or movement.

It is expected that this guideline change will result in more rapid and accurate identification of victims of cardiac arrest. It should eliminate delays in provision of

chest compressions and use of the AED. Most important, it should decrease missed opportunities to provide CPR and early defibrillation for victims of cardiac arrest.

Assessment: Check for Signs of Circulation (Healthcare Provider)

For laypersons, assessment of signs of circulation means the following: deliver 2 rescue breaths and evaluate the victim for normal breathing, coughing, or movement in response to the rescue breaths. The lay rescuer looks, listens, and feels for breathing while scanning the victim for signs of other movement. Lay rescuers are instructed to look for normal breathing to minimize confusion with agonal respirations.

When healthcare providers assess for signs of circulation, they quickly perform a pulse check while simultaneously evaluating the victim for breathing, coughing, or movement. Professional rescuers are instructed to look for "breathing" because

they are trained to differentiate agonal breathing from forms of ventilation not associated with cardiac arrest.

In practice, the assessment for signs of circulation for the *lay rescuer* is performed as follows:

1. Provide initial 2 rescue breaths to the unresponsive, nonbreathing victim.

2. Look for signs of circulation:

   a. With your ear near the victim's mouth, look, listen, and feel for normal breathing or coughing.

   b. Quickly scan the victim for any signs of movement.

3. If the victim is not breathing normally, coughing, or moving, immediately begin chest compressions or attach an AED if available.

This assessment should take no more than 10 seconds.

TABLE. Sensitivity, Specificity, and Reliability of Pulse Check: Performance of Pulse Check as a Diagnostic Test

	Pulse Is Present	Pulse Is Absent	Totals
Rescuer thinks pulse is present	81 (Sensitivity: correct positive result of pulse check ÷ all times a pulse was actually present) — a	6 — b	87 (No. of times rescuer thought pulse present = a+b)
Rescuer thinks pulse is absent	66 — c	53 (Specificity: correct negative result of pulse check ÷ all times there actually was no pulse) — d	119 (No. of times rescuer thought pulse absent = c+d)
Totals	147 (Total number of study opportunities where a pulse was actually present = a+c)	59 (Total number of study opportunities where a pulse was actually absent = b+d)	206 (Total study opportunities = a+b+c+d)

Calculations derived from above:
  a. Positive predictive value: Of the total times the rescuer thinks a pulse is present (total = 87 times), a pulse *is* present = 81/87 times = 93%.
  b. Negative predictive value: Of the total times the rescuer thinks a pulse is absent (total = 119 times), a pulse *is* absent = 53/119 times = 45%.
  c. Sensitivity: Rescuer's ability to detect a pulse when one actually is present = 81/147 = 55%.
  d. Specificity: Rescuer's ability to recognize that a pulse is absent when a pulse actually is absent = 53/59 = 90%.
  e. Accuracy = "rescuer correct"/total = (81 pulse correctly found + 53 pulse correctly thought absent)/206 = 65%.
Modified from Cummins RO, Hazinski MF. Cardiopulmonary resuscitation techniques and instruction: when does evidence justify revision? *Ann Emerg Med.* 1999;34:780-784.
Based on data from Eberle B, Dick WF, Schneider T, Wisser G, Doetsch S, Tzanova I. Checking the carotid pulse: diagnostic accuracy of first responders in patients with and without a pulse. *Resuscitation.* 1996;33:107-116.

Healthcare providers should perform a pulse check with assessment (above) for other signs of circulation. If you are not confident that circulation is present, start chest compressions or attach the AED.

To perform a pulse check in the adult, the healthcare provider typically attempts to palpate a carotid pulse.[99] As an alternative, the femoral artery pulse may be palpated. Pulses will persist in these arteries even when hypotension and poor perfusion cause peripheral pulses to disappear.

To locate the carotid artery pulse, maintain a head tilt with one hand on the victim's forehead and locate the trachea, using 2 or 3 fingers of the other hand (see Figure 15A). Slide these 2 or 3 fingers into the groove between the trachea and the muscles at the side of the neck, where the carotid pulse can be felt (see Figure 15B). Use only gentle pressure to palpate rather than compress the artery. This technique is often easier and requires less pressure to perform on the side nearer the rescuer.

Chest Compressions

The chest compression technique consists of serial, rhythmic applications of pressure over the lower half of the sternum.[109] These compressions create blood flow by increasing intrathoracic pressure or directly compressing the heart.[110,111]

When rescue breathing is provided and blood is circulated to the lungs by chest compressions, the victim will likely receive enough oxygen to maintain oxygenation of the brain and other vital organs for several minutes until defibrillation can be performed.

Human data,[118,119] animal data,[110,114-118] and theoretical models,[112,113] all support a chest compression rate of more than 80 compressions per minute to achieve optimal forward flow during CPR. A rate of 100 compressions per minute is recommended. The compression rate refers to the speed of compressions and not the number of compressions actually delivered in 1 minute.

A compression rate of 100 per minute will actually result in delivery of fewer than 100 compressions per minute by the lone rescuer who must interrupt chest compressions to perform ventilations. The actual number of chest compressions delivered per minute is determined by the accuracy and consistency of the rate of chest compressions and the number and duration of pauses for ventilation.

The previous version of the ECC guidelines recommended a ratio of 15 compressions to 2 ventilations provided by a lone rescuer and a ratio of 5 compressions to 1 ventilation provided by 2 rescuers.[52,75] A compression-ventilation ratio of 15:2 provides more chest compressions per minute (approximately 64 vs 50) than a ratio of 5:1.[120]

There is evidence to suggest that adult cardiac arrest victims are more likely to be resuscitated if a higher number of chest compressions are delivered per minute during CPR, even if the victims receive fewer ventilations per minute.[35,121] The quality of rescue breathing and chest compressions is not affected by the compression-ventilation ratio.[120]

During cardiac arrest, coronary perfusion pressure gradually rises with the performance of sequential chest compressions.[121] Coronary perfusion pressure is higher after 15 uninterrupted chest compressions than it is after 5 chest compressions.[121] Therefore, after each pause for ventilation, several compressions must be performed before optimal brain and coronary perfusion pressures are reestablished.[121]

For these reasons, a ratio of 15 compressions to 2 ventilations is recommended for 1 *or* 2 rescuers of adult victims until the airway is secured. Research is ongoing to determine the benefits of further increasing the number of compressions between ventilations during CPR. When the airway is protected with a cuffed tracheal tube (inserted by ACLS rescuers), compressions may be continuous at a rate of approximately 100 per minute and ventilations are asynchronous at a rate of 10 to 12 per minute.

FIGURE 15. Checking the carotid pulse. **A,** Locate the trachea. **B,** Gently feel for the carotid pulse.

A

B

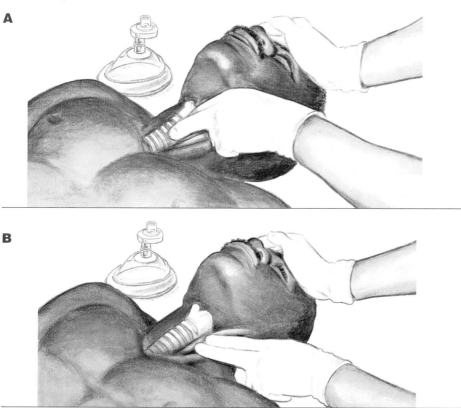

In reality, rescuers often compress at a rate slower than 100 per minute.[121,122] During teaching and performance of CPR, some form of audio timing prompt may help the rescuer achieve the recommended compression rate of approximately 100 per minute.[123,124]

The victim must be in the horizontal (supine) position during chest compressions, because blood flow to the brain is reduced even with properly performed compressions. If the head is elevated above the heart, blood flow to the brain is further reduced or eliminated, so the head should not be elevated. If the victim cannot be removed from bed, place a board or other rigid surface, preferably the full width of the bed, under the victim's back to avoid diminished effectiveness of chest compression.

Proper Hand Position

Proper hand placement is established by identifying the lower half of the sternum. The guidelines below may be used, or the rescuer may choose alternative techniques to identify the lower half of the sternum.

1. The rescuer uses 2 or 3 fingers from the hand nearest the victim's feet to locate the lower margin of the victim's rib cage on the side next to the rescuer (see Figure 16A).

2. The fingers of this first hand are then moved up the rib cage to the notch where the ribs meet the lower sternum in the center of the lower part of the chest (the xiphoid process).

3. The heel of the second hand is placed on the lower half of the sternum (see Figure 16B), and the first hand is placed on top of the second on the sternum so that the hands are parallel (see Figure 16C). The long axis of the heel of the rescuer's hand should be placed on the long axis of the sternum. This will keep the main force of compression on the sternum and decrease the chance of rib fracture.

4. The fingers may be either extended or interlaced but should be kept off the chest.

If you have difficulty generating force during compressions, an acceptable alternative hand position is to grasp the wrist of the hand on the chest with the hand locating the lower end of the sternum. This technique is helpful for rescuers whose hands and wrists are arthritic.

A simplified method of achieving correct hand position has also been used in various settings for teaching the chest compression technique to laypersons.[22,23,29,38,125-130] To find a position on the lower half of the sternum, place the heel of one hand in the center of the chest between the nipples (see Figure 17). This method has been used with success for over 10 years in dispatch-instruction CPR and other settings.[22,23,29,38,125-130]

Proper Compression Technique

Effective compressions are accomplished by using the following guidelines:

FIGURE 16. Location of proper hand position over the lower half of the sternum for chest compressions.
A, Locate the margin of the ribs, using the first and second fingers of the hand closer to the victim's feet.
B, Follow the rib margin to the base of the sternum (xiphoid process) and place your hand above the fingers of the first hand, on the lower half of the victim's sternum.
C, Place the other hand on top of the hand on the sternum.

B

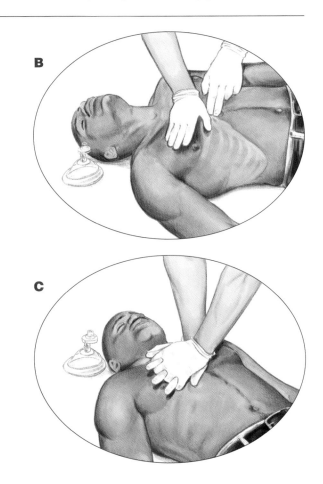

A

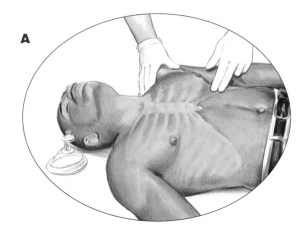

C

FIGURE 17. Simplified technique for location of proper hand position. Place your hands on the sternum at the nipple line.

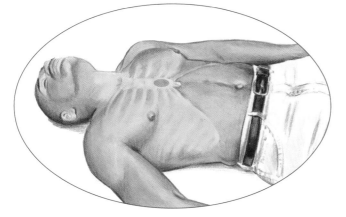

1. The elbows are locked in position, arms straightened, and the rescuer's shoulders positioned directly over his or her hands so that the thrust for each chest compression is straight down on the sternum (see Figure 18). If the thrust is not in a straight downward direction, the victim's torso has a tendency to roll, part of the force is lost, and the chest compression may be less effective.

2. The compressions should depress the victim's sternum approximately 1½ to 2 inches (4 to 5 cm) if the victim is a normal-sized adult. Rarely, in very slight persons lesser degrees of compression may be enough to generate a palpable carotid or femoral pulse. In some persons 1½ to 2 inches (4 to 5 cm) of sternal compression may be inadequate, and a slightly greater degree of chest compression may be needed to generate a carotid or femoral pulse.

Note: Optimal sternal compression is best gauged by using the compression force that generates a palpable carotid or femoral pulse.[39] However, palpation of a pulse during chest compressions requires the presence of at least 2 professional rescuers. Furthermore, detection of a pulse during CPR does not necessarily mean that there is optimal or even adequate blood flow, because a compression wave may be felt without a good forward flow of blood. The lone rescuer should follow the sternal compression guideline of 1½ to 2 inches (4 to 5 cm).

3. Release pressure on the chest to allow blood to flow into the chest and heart. The pressure must be released completely and the chest allowed to return to its normal position after each compression (although the rescuer's hands should continue to touch the victim's sternum to maintain proper hand position). Chest compressions should be performed at a rate of 100 compressions per minute.

4. Effective cerebral and coronary perfusion has been shown to occur when 50% of the duty cycle is allotted to the chest compression phase and 50% to the chest relaxation phase.[112,122,131,132] This is a ratio that rescuers find reasonably easy to achieve with practice.[122]

5. To maintain correct hand position, do not lift your hands from the chest and do not change hand position in any way during compressions. Allow the chest to return to its normal position after each compression.

Rescue breathing and chest compression must be combined for effective resuscitation of the victim of cardiopulmonary arrest. Research over the past 40 years has helped identify the mechanisms for blood flow during chest compression. In both animal models and human patients, blood flow during CPR probably results from manipulation of intrathoracic pressure (thoracic pump mechanism) as well as from direct cardiac compression.[109-111] The duration of CPR affects the mechanism of blood flow during CPR.[133-137] When CPR duration is short, blood flow is generated more by the cardiac pump than the thoracic pump mechanism. When the duration of cardiac arrest or the efforts of CPR are prolonged, the heart becomes less compliant. In this setting the thoracic pump mechanism dominates, and the cardiac output generated by chest compression is significantly decreased.[133-137]

Over the past 20 years there has been important research in various techniques and devices to improve blood flow during CPR, including pneumatic vest CPR,[138] interposed abdominal compression CPR (IAC-CPR),[139-141] and active compression-decompression CPR.[142-147] Recent evaluation of these devices in humans[131,138-148] has resulted in more specific recommendations for their use. These interventions are well beyond the scope of BLS. They are reviewed in great detail in the ACLS textbook and the ACLS Provider Manual.

During cardiac arrest properly performed chest compressions can produce systolic arterial blood pressure peaks of 60 to 80 mm Hg, but diastolic blood pressure is low.[137] Mean blood pressure in the carotid

FIGURE 18. Position of the rescuer during chest compressions.

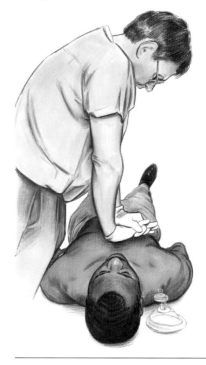

artery seldom exceeds 40 mm Hg.[137] Cardiac output resulting from chest compressions is probably only one fourth to one third of normal, and it decreases during prolonged standard CPR.[137] Vascular pressure during chest compression can be optimized by using the recommended chest compression force and duration and maintaining a chest compression rate of 100 compressions per minute.[131]

Airway-breathing-circulation (ABC) is the specific sequence used to initiate CPR in the United States and many other countries. In the Netherlands, however, circulation-airway-breathing (CAB) is the common protocol for implementation of CPR, with resuscitation outcomes similar to those reported for the ABC protocol in the United States.[149] No human studies have compared the ABC technique with CAB. Hence, a statement of relative efficacy cannot be made and a change in present teaching is not warranted. Both techniques are effective.

Compression-Only Resuscitation

Surveys of professional and lay rescuers have identified a substantial reluctance to perform mouth-to-mouth ventilation if barrier devices are unavailable, because of fear of transmittable infections.[150-154] If a rescuer is unwilling or unable to perform mouth-to-mouth ventilation, he or she should initiate chest compression–only resuscitation immediately.

Current evidence suggests that the outcome of chest compressions without mouth-to-mouth ventilation is significantly better than *no resuscitation attempt at all* in witnessed adult cardiac arrest.[31-35] Some evidence in animal models and limited adult clinical trials suggests that positive-pressure ventilation was not essential during the first few minutes of resuscitation when prompt ACLS is provided. The Cerebral Resuscitation Group of Belgium also showed no difference in outcome of resuscitation whether or not mouth-to-mouth ventilation was performed in addition to chest compression.[35]

Several mechanisms may account for the effectiveness of chest compression alone. Studies have shown that spontaneous gasping can maintain near-normal minute ventilation, $PaCO_2$, and PaO_2 during short periods of CPR without positive-pressure ventilation.[33,155] Because the cardiac output generated during chest compression is only 25% of normal, there is also a reduced requirement for ventilation to maintain optimal ventilation-perfusion relationships.[156,157]

Chest compression–only resuscitation is *not* a consideration for the healthcare provider in the healthcare setting because barrier devices and bag-mask ventilation equipment should be readily available. Chest compression–only resuscitation is recommended *only* in the following circumstances:

1. When a rescuer is unwilling or unable to perform mouth-to-mouth rescue breathing or

2. In dispatch-assisted CPR instructions, in which the simplicity of this modified technique allows untrained bystanders to quickly intervene.

Cough CPR

Self-initiated chest compression is possible. Its use is limited to clinical situations in which the patient has a monitored cardiac arrest, the arrest is recognized before loss of responsiveness, and the patient can cough forcefully.[133-136] The increase in intrathoracic pressure that occurs with coughing will generate blood flow to the brain and maintain responsiveness for a prolonged period. The opportunity for cough CPR exists for only the first 10 to 15 seconds of the cardiac arrest.

1- and 2-Rescuer CPR
1-Rescuer CPR

Laypersons other than those specifically trained to respond to emergencies (eg, lifeguards and police officers) should be taught only 1-rescuer CPR because laypersons in rescue situations seldom use the 2-rescuer technique. When 2 rescuers

are present, they can alternate performing 1-rescuer CPR. One-rescuer CPR should be performed as follows:

1. **Assessment of responsiveness:** tap or gently shake the victim and shout "Are you OK?" If the victim is unresponsive:

2. **Activate the EMS system or other emergency response system.**

3. **Airway:** Position the victim and open the airway with the head tilt–chin lift or jaw-thrust maneuver.

4. **Breathing:** Look, listen, and feel for normal breathing.

   a. If the victim is unresponsive but breathing normally with no signs of trauma, place the victim in the recovery position and maintain an open airway.

   b. If the adult victim is unresponsive and not breathing, provide rescue breathing by giving 2 initial breaths with mouth-to-mouth, mouth-to–barrier device, or bag-mask ventilation. If breaths are effective, the victim's chest will rise with each breath. If you are unable to give 2 effective breaths, reposition the victim's head and reattempt ventilation. If ventilation is still unsuccessful, follow the sequence for foreign-body airway obstruction in the unresponsive victim. The *lay rescuer* should continue the sequence below, providing chest compressions.

   c. After signs of circulation are checked, if the victim has signs of circulation but is not breathing, continue rescue breathing, giving 1 breath every 4 to 5 seconds (10 to 12 breaths per minute) without chest compressions.

   d. If adequate spontaneous breathing is restored and signs of circulation are present, maintain an open airway and place the victim in a recovery position.

5. **Circulation:** Assess for signs of a pulse and signs of circulation. After

delivery of the 2 effective initial breaths, look for normal breathing, coughing, or movement by the victim. At the same time, attempt to feel for a carotid pulse — take no more than 10 seconds to do this. If there are no signs of circulation, begin chest compressions:

a. Locate proper hand position.

b. Perform 15 chest compressions at a rate of 100 per minute. Depress the chest 1½ to 2 inches (4 to 5 cm) each time. Make sure the chest is allowed to rebound to its normal position after each compression by removing all pressure from the chest (while still maintaining contact with the sternum and proper hand position). Count "1 and, 2 and, 3 and, 4 and, 5 and, 6 and, 7 and, 8 and, 9 and, 10 and, 11 and, 12 and, 13 and, 14 and, 15." (Any mnemonic that accomplishes the same compression rate is acceptable.)

c. Open the airway and deliver 2 slow rescue breaths (of 2 seconds each).

d. Return your hands to the chest, over the lower half of the sternum. Find the proper hand position and begin 15 more compressions at a rate of 100 per minute.

e. Perform 4 complete cycles of 15 compressions and 2 ventilations, and recheck for signs of breathing and circulation.

6. **Reassessment:** After 4 cycles of compressions and ventilations (15:2 ratio), reevaluate the victim, checking for signs of circulation. Take no more than 10 seconds to do this.

a. If signs of circulation are absent, resume CPR, beginning with chest compressions.

b. If signs of circulation are present, check for breathing.

(1) If breathing is present, place the victim in the recovery position and monitor breathing and circulation.

(2) If breathing is absent, provide rescue breathing at a rate of approximately 1 breath every 4 to 5 seconds (approximately 10 to 12 times per minute) and monitor circulation closely.

If CPR is continued, stop and check for signs of circulation and spontaneous breathing every few minutes. Do not interrupt CPR except in special circumstances.

Entrance of a Second Rescuer to Replace the First Rescuer

When another rescuer is available at the scene, the second rescuer should activate the EMS system (if not done previously) and perform 1-rescuer CPR when the first rescuer, who initiated CPR, becomes fatigued. Do this with as little interruption as possible. When the second rescuer arrives, reassess breathing and pulse before resuming CPR.

2-Rescuer CPR

All professional rescuers (BLS ambulance providers, healthcare professionals, and appropriate laypersons such as lifeguards) should learn both the 1-and 2-rescuer techniques. When possible, airway adjunct methods such as mouth-to-mask ventilation should be used.

In 2-rescuer CPR, one person is positioned at the victim's side and performs chest compressions. The other professional rescuer remains at the victim's head, maintains an open airway, monitors the carotid pulse for adequacy of chest compressions, and provides rescue breathing.

The compression rate for 2-rescuer CPR is approximately 100 compressions per minute. The compression-ventilation ratio is 15:2, with a pause for ventilation of 2 seconds each until the airway is secured. Once the airway is secured (ie, the patient is intubated), compressions and ventilations are asynchronous. The compression rate will be approximately 100 per minute and the ventilation rate

approximately 10 to 12 per minute (1 breath every 5 seconds). Exhalation occurs in between the 2 breaths and during the first chest compression of the next cycle.

When the person performing chest compressions becomes fatigued, the rescuers should exchange positions with minimal delay (see Figure 19).

Monitoring the Victim

Rescuers must monitor the victim's condition to assess the effectiveness of the rescue effort. The person ventilating the patient assumes responsibility for monitoring signs of circulation and breathing.

To assess the effectiveness of the lay rescuer's chest compressions, the professional rescuer should check the pulse during compressions. To determine if the victim has resumed spontaneous breathing and circulation, chest compressions must be stopped for 5 seconds at about the end of the first minute and every few minutes thereafter.

— End of BLS Sequence —

Unique Situations in CPR

Changing Location During CPR

A victim should not be moved for convenience from a cramped or busy location until effective CPR has been provided and the victim has a spontaneous pulse or until help arrives so that CPR can be performed without interruption. If the location is unsafe, such as a burning building, the victim should be moved to a safe area and CPR then started immediately.

Stairways

In some instances a victim must be transported up or down a flight of stairs. It is best to perform CPR at the head or foot of the stairs and, at a predetermined signal, to interrupt CPR and move as quickly as possible to the next level, where CPR should be resumed. Interruptions should be brief and must be avoided if possible.

FIGURE 19. Two-rescuer CPR. The first rescuer is performing mouth-to-mask ventilation using a barrier device with supplemental oxygen. The first rescuer is responsible for ensuring that the chest rises with each ventilation and should periodically check to ensure that chest compressions are producing a palpable carotid pulse. The second rescuer is performing chest compressions. Chest compressions and ventilations should be interrupted after approximately 1 minute and then every few minutes to see if normal breathing or signs of circulation have returned. The rescuers should change positions when either rescuer becomes fatigued.

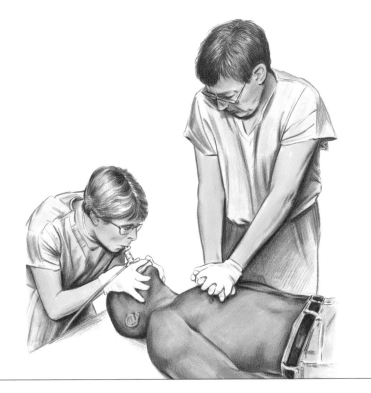

Litters

Do not interrupt CPR while transferring a victim to an ambulance or other mobile emergency care unit. With a low-wheeled litter, the rescuer can stand alongside the victim, maintaining the locked-arm position for compression. With a high-wheeled litter or bed, the rescuer may have to kneel beside the victim on the bed or litter to gain the needed height over the victim's sternum.

Generally CPR should be interrupted only when tracheal intubation is being performed by trained personnel, an AED is being attached or used, or when there are problems with transportation. If the rescuer is alone, a momentary delay of CPR is necessary to activate the EMS system.[26]

Pitfalls and Complications of BLS

CPR is most effective in supporting life when performed properly, but even properly performed CPR has been known to result in complications.[158] Fear of complications should not prevent potential rescuers from providing CPR to the best of their ability.

Rescue Breathing

Rescue breathing frequently causes gastric inflation, particularly if large ventilation volumes are delivered with rapid flow rates.[58,59] Gastric inflation is a common complication of CPR in children.[59,66-69] It can be minimized by maintaining an open airway and limiting ventilation volumes to the point at which the chest rises adequately and by not exceeding esophageal opening pressure.[73] This is

best achieved by delivering each rescue breath slowly (2 seconds per breath).

Marked inflation of the stomach may promote regurgitation[60-62] and reduce lung volume by elevating the diaphragm.[58,69-70] If the stomach becomes inflated during rescue breathing, the airway should be rechecked and repositioned, the rise and fall of the chest observed, and excessive airway pressure avoided. Slow rescue breathing should be continued without attempting to expel the stomach contents. Experience has shown that attempting to relieve stomach inflation by manual pressure over the victim's upper abdomen is almost certain to cause regurgitation if the stomach is full.

If regurgitation does occur, the rescuer should turn the victim's entire body to the side, wipe out the mouth, return the body to the supine position, and continue CPR. Gastric inflation can be further minimized by ensuring that the airway remains open during inspiration and expiration. Unfortunately this is difficult in 1-rescuer CPR, but it can be achieved during 2-rescuer CPR.

Chest Compression

Proper CPR techniques lessen the possibility of complications, but even properly performed chest compressions can cause rib fractures in adult patients.[159] Rib fractures and other injuries are uncommon in infants and children.[160,161] Other complications may occur despite proper CPR technique, including fracture of the sternum, separation of the ribs from the sternum, pneumothorax, hemothorax, lung contusions, lacerations of the liver and spleen, and fat emboli.[158] These complications may be minimized by use of proper hand position during performance of chest compressions, but they cannot be entirely prevented.

Concern for injuries that may result from properly performed CPR should not impede prompt and energetic application of CPR. The only alternative to timely initiation of effective CPR for the cardiac arrest victim is death.

The "D" of Defibrillation (AEDs)

Most adults with sudden, witnessed, non-traumatic cardiac arrest are found to be in VF.[1] For these victims the time from collapse to defibrillation is the single greatest determinant of survival.[1-4,12] Survival from VF cardiac arrest declines by approximately 7% to 10% for each minute without defibrillation.[13] Therefore, healthcare providers should be trained and equipped to provide defibrillation at the earliest possible moment for victims of sudden cardiac arrest.

Early defibrillation in the community is defined as a shock delivered within 5 minutes of receipt of the call to EMS. This 5-minute call-to-defibrillation interval in the community is an important goal to achieve.

Early defibrillation must also be provided in hospitals and medical facilities. First responders in medical facilities should be able to provide early defibrillation in all areas of the hospital and ambulatory care facilities to patients who have collapsed in VF. In these areas healthcare providers should be able to deliver a shock within 3 minutes ±1 minute of arrest for a high percentage of patients. To achieve these goals, BLS providers must be trained and equipped to use defibrillators and must practice on the defibrillator present in their clinical area.

Chapter 7 reviews the use of an AED and its integration with CPR.

Summary of Adult BLS

Rescue breathing and chest compressions are the critical skills of BLS that maintain delivery of oxygenated blood to vital organs until defibrillation and ACLS can restore circulation and stabilize the victim of sudden cardiac death. Remember the ABCs of CPR — airway, breathing, and circulation — followed by the "D" of defibrillation, and let them be your guide in the management of sudden cardiac death.

Summary of Key Concepts

- Open the airway with the head tilt–chin lift (or jaw thrust without head tilt for patients in whom spinal injury is suspected).

- For victims in respiratory arrest, initially provide 2 slow rescue breaths followed by 1 breath every 4 to 5 seconds (10 to 12 breaths per minute).

- Forceful or excessive ventilation during CPR may cause gastric inflation, regurgitation, and aspiration.

- A tidal volume of approximately 10 mL/kg (approximately 700 to 1000 mL) is delivered over 2 seconds until observing well-defined chest rise for mouth-to-mouth breathing or mouth-to-mask breathing without oxygen.

- When supplemental oxygen is available and oxygen saturation is monitored, a tidal volume of 6 to 7 mL/kg (approximately 400 to 600 mL) can be delivered over 1 to 2 seconds until observing chest rise when using a bag-mask or mouth-to-mask device.

- Cricoid pressure is helpful for preventing gastric inflation in the unresponsive victim but requires the presence of an additional rescuer.

- Healthcare providers perform a pulse check while looking for signs of circulation (normal breathing, coughing, or movement).

- The ratio of 15 compressions to 2 ventilations is recommended for both 1- and 2-rescuer adult CPR for the victim with an unprotected (non-intubated) airway.

- The compression rate for 1- and 2-rescuer adult CPR is approximately 100 compressions per minute.

- Chest compression–only resuscitation is recommended only in the following circumstances: (1) when a rescuer is unwilling or unable to perform mouth-to-mouth rescue breathing or (2) for use in dispatch-assisted CPR instructions in which the simplicity of this modified technique allows untrained bystanders to intervene rapidly.

- Use the recovery position in the management of victims who are unresponsive, breathing, and have signs of circulation (unless spinal injury is suspected).

- The BLS sequence of action for cardiac arrest:

  1. Assess responsiveness

  2. Phone 911 or other emergency response number

  3. Open the airway (head tilt–chin lift or, if trauma is present, jaw thrust)

  4. Assess breathing (look, listen, and feel)

  5. Provide rescue breathing (2 initial breaths, each delivered slowly over 2 seconds)

  6. Check for signs of circulation (pulse check, breathing, coughing, or movement)

  7. If there are no signs of circulation, provide chest compressions (at a rate of approximately 100 compressions per minute with a compression-ventilation ratio of 15:2).

Review Questions

1. You are in the cafeteria when you hear a patient cry out from one of the small dining rooms. You enter the room and find the patient, wearing a hospital gown and armband, collapsed on the floor. An anxious relative is nearby. What should be your first step in the BLS sequence of action?

   a. check for breathing

   b. check for signs of circulation

   c. check for responsiveness

   d. open the airway

2. While at work you discover someone lying unconscious in the hallway. You first establish that the victim is unresponsive. Which of the following is the correct sequence of actions for you to take?

   a. phone the emergency response number, check for signs of circulation, open the airway, then give rescue breaths if needed

   b. open the airway, give rescue breaths if needed, check for signs of circulation, then phone 911 if no signs of circulation

   c. phone 911 or the emergency response number, open the airway, give rescue breaths if needed, then check for signs of circulation

   d. give rescue breaths, check for signs of circulation, phone 911, then begin chest compressions

3. You find a patient who is unresponsive. You send a colleague to phone the emergency response number. You perform a head tilt–chin lift and look, listen, and feel for breathing. If the victim is not breathing, what should you do next?

   a. give 2 rapid breaths

   b. give 2 slow breaths

   c. give 1 slow breath

   d. give 1 rapid breath

   e. begin chest compressions

4. You have found a person who is unresponsive. You open the airway and find that the victim is not breathing. You provide 2 rescue breaths and you now check for signs of circulation. Where should you feel for the pulse of an unresponsive adult victim?

   a. the radial pulse

   b. the carotid pulse

   c. the femoral pulse

   d. the brachial pulse

5. You arrive at the side of a victim in respiratory arrest. Another rescuer is already performing rescue breathing using a pocket mask and tells you that someone has already phoned the emergency response number. What action can you take to assist the other rescuer and help reduce the chances of gastric inflation?

   a. provide pressure on the gastric area

   b. encourage the other rescuer to breathe faster

   c. assist in opening the airway

   d. apply cricoid pressure

6. You are caring at the scene for a woman who fell 20 feet from a rooftop. She is unresponsive, and you direct bystanders to phone 911. Your next step in the BLS sequence of action should be to

   a. perform jaw thrust without head tilt

   b. check for signs of circulation

   c. perform head tilt–chin lift

   d. begin chest compressions

7. A coworker suddenly collapses to the floor next to you. You establish unresponsiveness and direct bystanders to phone 911. You look, listen, and feel for breathing. The victim is not breathing. You give 2 slow breaths and check for signs of circulation. There are no signs of circulation. Which compression-ventilation ratio should you use for 1-rescuer CPR?

   a. 15 compressions to 2 ventilations

   b. 10 compressions to 2 ventilations

   c. 5 compressions to 2 ventilations

   d. 5 compressions to 1 ventilation

8. You are performing rescue breathing for a victim of respiratory arrest. You ensure that you are delivering a proper rescue breath by

   a. seeing a change in the victim's color

   b. checking the victim for signs of circulation regularly

   c. seeing the victim's chest rise during rescue breathing

   d. checking the airway frequently

How did you do?

Answers: 1, c; **2,** c; **3,** b; **4,** b; **5,** d; **6,** a; **7,** a; **8,** c.

References

1. Bayes de Luna A, Coumel P, Leclercq JF. Ambulatory sudden cardiac death: mechanisms of production of fatal arrhythmia on the basis of data from 157 cases. *Am Heart J.* 1989; 117:151-159.

2. Cummins RO, Ornato JP, Thies WH, Pepe PE. Improving survival from sudden cardiac arrest: the "chain of survival" concept. A statement for health professionals from the Advanced Cardiac Life Support Subcommittee and the Emergency Cardiac Care Committee, American Heart Association. *Circulation.* 1991;83: 1832-1847.

3. Calle PA, Verbeke A, Vanhaute O, Van Acker P, Martens P, Buylaert W. The effect of semi-automatic external defibrillation by emergency medical technicians on survival after out-of-hospital cardiac arrest: an observational study in urban and rural areas in Belgium. *Acta Clinica Belgica.* 1997;52:72-83.

4. Mosesso VN Jr, Davis EA, Auble TE, Paris PM, Yealy DM. Use of automated external defibrillators by police officers for treatment of out-of-hospital cardiac arrest. *Ann Emerg Med.* 1998;32:200-207.

5. Weaver WD, Hill D, Fahrenbruch CE, Copass MK, Martin JS, Cobb LA, Hallstrom AP. Use of the automatic external defibrillator in the management of out-of-hospital cardiac arrest. *N Engl J Med.* 1988;319:661-666.

6. Cummins RO, Graves JR. Critical results of standard CPR: prehospital and inhospital. In: Kaye W, Bircher NG, eds. *Cardiopulmonary Resuscitation: Clinics in Critical Care Medicine.* New York, NY: Churchill-Livingstone; 1989:87-102.

7. Cummins RO, Eisenberg MS. Prehospital cardiopulmonary resuscitation: is it effective? *JAMA.* 1985;253:2408-2412.

8. Cummins RO, Eisenberg MS, Hallstrom AP, Litwin PE. Survival of out-of-hospital cardiac arrest with early initiation of cardiopulmonary resuscitation. *Am J Emerg Med.* 1985;3: 114-119.

9. Ladwig KH, Schoefinius A, Danner R, Gurtler R, Herman R, Koeppel A, Hauber P. Effects of early defibrillation by ambulance personnel on short- and long-term outcome of cardiac arrest survival: the Munich experiment. *Chest.* 1997; 112:1584-1591.

10. Sweeney TA, Runge JW, Gibbs MA, Raymond JM, Schafermeyer RW, Norton HJ, Boyle-Whitesel MJ. EMT defibrillation does not increase survival from sudden cardiac death in a two-tiered urban-suburban EMS system. *Ann Emerg Med.* 1998;31:234-240.

11. Kellermann AL, Hackman BB, Somes G, Kreth TK, Nail L, Dobyns P. Impact of first-responder defibrillation in an urban emergency medical services system. *JAMA.* 1993;270: 1708-1713.

12. Shuster M, Keller JL. Effect of fire department first-responder automated defibrillation. *Ann Emerg Med.* 1993;22:721-727.

13. Cummins RO. From concept to standard-of-care? Review of the clinical experience with automated external defibrillators. *Ann Emerg Med.* 1989;18:1269-1275.

14. White RD, Hankins DG, Bugliosi TF. Seven years' experience with early defibrillation by police and paramedics in an emergency medical services system. *Resuscitation.* 1998;39: 145-151.

15. Zaritsky A, Nadkarni V, Getson P, Kuehl K. CPR in children. *Ann Emerg Med.* 1987;16: 1107-1111.

16. American Heart Association, International Liaison Committee on Resuscitation (ILCOR). Guidelines 2000 for cardiopulmonary resuscitation and emergency cardiovascular care. International Consensus on Science. *Circulation.* 2000;102(suppl):I-1-I-384.

17. Becker LB, Pepe PE. Ensuring the effectiveness of community-wide emergency cardiac care. *Ann Emerg Med.* 1993;22(2 pt 2): 354-365.

18. Zachariah BS, Pepe PE. The development of emergency medical dispatch in the USA: a historical perspective. *Eur J Emerg Med.* 1995;2: 109-112.

19. Rossi R. The role of the dispatch centre in pre-clinical emergency medicine. *Eur J Emerg Med.* 1994;1:27-30.

20. Nemitz B. Advantages and limitations of medical dispatching: the French view. *Eur J Emerg Med.* 1995;2:153-159.

21. Pepe PE, Zachariah BS, Sayre MR, Floccare D. Ensuring the chain of recovery for stroke in your community: Chain of Recovery Writing Group. *Prehosp Emerg Care.* 1998;2:89-95.

22. Bang A, Biber B, Isaksson L, Lindqvist J, Herlitz J. Evaluation of dispatcher-assisted cardiopulmonary resuscitation. *Eur J Emerg Med.* 1999;6:175-183.

23. National Association of EMS Physicians. Emergency medical dispatching. *Prehosp Disaster Med.* 1989;4:163-166.

24. Calle PA, Lagaert L, Vanhaute O, Buylaert WA. Do victims of an out-of-hospital cardiac arrest benefit from a training program for emergency medical dispatchers? *Resuscitation.* 1997;35:213-218.

25. Nordberg M. NAEMD (National Academy of Emergency Medical Dispatch) strives for universal certification. *Emerg Med Serv.* 1999;28: 45-46.

26. Curka PA, Pepe PE, Ginger VF, Sherrard RC, Ivy MV, Zachariah BS. Emergency medical services priority dispatch. *Ann Emerg Med.* 1993;22:1688-1695.

27. Clawson JJ, Sinclair B. "Medical Miranda" — improved emergency medical dispatch information from police officers. *Prehosp Disaster Med.* 1999;14:93-96.

28. Nordberg M. Emergency medical dispatch: a changing profession. *Emerg Med Serv.* 1998; 27:25-26,28-34.

29. *Standard Practice for Emergency Medical Dispatch.* Philadelphia, Pa: American Society for Testing and Materials; 1990. Publication F1258-90.

30. Hallstrom A, Cobb L, Johnson E, Copass M. Cardiopulmonary resuscitation by chest compression alone or with mouth-to-mouth ventilation. *N Engl J Med.* 2000;342:1546-1553.

31. Berg RA, Kern KB, Sanders AB, Otto CW, Hilwig RW, Ewy GA. Bystander cardiopulmonary resuscitation: is ventilation necessary? *Circulation.* 1993;88:1907-1915.

32. Chandra NC, Gruben KG, Tsitlik JE, Brower R, Guerci AD, Halperin HH, Weisfeldt ML, Permutt S. Observations of ventilation during resuscitation in a canine model. *Circulation.* 1994;90:3070-3075.

33. Tang W, Weil MH, Sun SJ, Kette D, Kette F, Gazmuri RJ, O'Connell F. Cardiopulmonary resuscitation by precordial compression but without mechanical ventilation. *Am J Resp Crit Care Med.* 1994;150:1709-1713.

34. Noc M, Weil MH, Tang W, Turner T, Fukui M. Mechanical ventilation may not be essential for initial cardiopulmonary resuscitation. *Chest.* 1995;108:821-827.

35. Van Hoeyweghen RJ, Bossaert LL, Mullie A, Calle P, Martens P, Buylaert WA, Delooz H. Quality and efficiency of bystander CPR: Belgian cerebral resuscitation. *Resuscitation.* 1993;26:47-52.

36. National Heart Attack Alert Program Coordinating Committee, Access to Care Subcommittee. Emergency medical dispatching: rapid identification and treatment of acute myocardial infarction. *Am J Emerg Med.* 1995;13: 67-73.

37. Porteous GH, Corry MD, Smith WS. Emergency medical services dispatcher identification of stroke and transient ischemic attack. *Prehosp Emerg Care.* 1999;3:211-216.

38. Clawson JJ, Hauert SA. Dispatch life support: establishing standards that work. *J Emerg Med Serv JEMS.* 1990;15:82-84,86-88.

39. Mackenzie GJ, Taylor SH, McDonald AH, Donald KW. Haemodynamic effects of external cardiac compression. *Lancet.* 1964;1: 1342-1345.

40. Noc M, Weil MH, Sun SJ, Tang W, Bisera J. Spontaneous gasping during cardiopulmonary resuscitation without mechanical ventilation. *Am J Resp Crit Care Med.* 1994;150:861-864.

41. Clark JJ, Larsen MP, Culley LL, Graves JR, Eisenberg MS. Incidence of agonal respirations in sudden cardiac arrest. *Ann Emerg Med.* 1992;21:1464-1467.

42. Weisfeldt ML, Kerber RE, McGoldrick RP, Moss AJ, Nichol G, Ornato JP, Palmer DG, Riegel B, Smith SC Jr. American Heart Association report on the Public Access Defibrillation Conference, December 8-10, 1994. Automatic External Defibrillation Task Force. *Circulation.* 1995;92:2740-2747.

43. Weisfeldt ML, Kerber RE, McGoldrick RP, Moss AJ, Nichol G, Ornato JP, Palmer DG, Riegel B, Smith SC Jr. Public access defibrillation: a statement for healthcare professionals from the American Heart Association Task Force on Automatic External Defibrillation. *Circulation.* 1995;92:2763.

44. Gundry JW, Comess KA, DeRook FA, Jorgenson D, Bardy GH. Comparison of naive sixth-grade children with trained professionals in the use of an automated external defibrillator. *Circulation.* 1999;100:1703-1707.

45. Chandra NC, Hazinski MF, Stapleton E. *Instructor's Manual for Basic Life Support.* Dallas, Tex: American Heart Association; 2000.

46. Safar P. Ventilatory efficacy of mouth-to-mouth artificial respiration: airway obstruction during manual and mouth-to-mouth artificial respiration. *JAMA.* 1958;167:335-341.

47. Safar P, Escarraga LA, Chang F. Upper airway obstruction in the unconscious patient. *J Appl Physiol.* 1959;14:760-764.

48. Ruben HM, Elam JO, Ruben AM, Greene DG. Investigation of upper airway problems in resuscitation: studies of pharyngeal x-rays and performance by laymen. *Anesthesiology.* 1961; 22:271-279.

49. Guildner CW. Resuscitation — opening the airway: a comparative study of techniques for opening an airway obstructed by the tongue. *JACEP.* 1976;5:588-590.

50. Elam JO, Greene DG, Schneider MA, Ruben HM, Gordon AS, Hustead RF, Benson DW, Clements JA, Ruben A. Head-tilt method of oral resuscitation. *JAMA.* 1960;172:812-815.

51. Safar P, Escarraga LA. Compliance in apneic anesthetized adults. *Anesthesiology.* 1959;20: 283-289.

52. Handley AJ, Becker LB, Allen M, van Drenth A, Kramer EB, Montgomery WH. Single-rescuer adult basic life support: an advisory statement from the Basic Life Support Working Group of the International Liaison Committee on Resuscitation (ILCOR). *Resuscitation.* 1997;34:101-108.

53. Turner S, Turner I, Chapman D, Howard P, Champion P, Hatfield J, James A, Marshall S, Barber S. A comparative study of the 1992 and 1997 recovery positions for use in the UK. *Resuscitation.* 1998;39:153-160.

54. Doxey J. Comparing 1997 Resuscitation Council (UK) recovery position with recovery position of 1992 European Resuscitation Council guidelines: a user's perspective. *Resuscitation.* 1998;39:161-169.

55. Fulstow R, Smith GB. The new recovery position: a cautionary tale. *Resuscitation.* 1993;26: 89-91.

56. Rathgeber J, Panzer W, Gunther U, Scholz M, Hoeft A, Bahr J, Kettler D. Influence of different types of recovery positions on perfusion indices of the forearm. *Resuscitation.* 1996;32: 13-17.

57. Wenzel V, Idris AH, Banner MJ, Fuerst RS, Tucker KJ. The composition of gas given by mouth-to-mouth ventilation during CPR. *Chest.* 1994;106:1806-1810.

58. Wenzel V, Idris AH, Banner MJ, Kubilis PS, Band R, Williams JL, Lindner KH. Respiratory system compliance decreases after cardiopulmonary resuscitation and stomach inflation: impact of large and small tidal volumes on calculated peak airway pressure. *Resuscitation.* 1998;38:113-118.

59. Idris AH, Wenzel V, Banner MJ, Melker RJ. Smaller tidal volumes minimize gastric inflation during CPR with an unprotected airway. *Circulation.* 1995;92:I-759. Abstract.

60. Morton HJV, Wylie WD. Anaesthetic deaths due to regurgitation or vomiting. *Anaesthesia.* 1951;6:192-205.

61. Ruben A, Ruben H. Artificial respiration: flow of water from the lung and the stomach. *Lancet.* 1962;1:780-781.

62. Stone BJ, Chantler PJ, Baskett PJ. The incidence of regurgitation during cardiopulmonary resuscitation: a comparison between the bag valve mask and laryngeal mask airway. *Resuscitation.* 1998;38:3-6.

63. Lawes EG, Baskett PJF. Pulmonary aspiration during unsuccessful cardiopulmonary resuscitation. *Intensive Care Med.* 1987;13:379-382.

64. Bjork RJ, Snyder BD, Campion BC, Loewenson RB. Medical complications of cardiopulmonary arrest. *Arch Intern Med.* 1982;142:500-503.

65. Spence AA, Moir DD, Finlay WE. Observations on intragastric pressure. *Anaesthesia* 1967;22:249-256.

66. Wenzel V, Idris AH, Banner MJ, Kubilis PS, Williams JL. Influence of tidal volume on the distribution of gas between the lungs and stomach in the nonintubated patient receiving positive-pressure ventilation. *Crit Care Med.* 1998;26:364-368.

67. Wenzel V, Keller C, Idris AH, Dörges V, Lindner KH, Brimacombe JR. Effects of smaller tidal volumes during basic life support ventilation in patients with respiratory arrest: good ventilation, less risk? *Resuscitation.* 1999;43:25-29.

68. Weiler N, Heinrichs W, Dick W. Assessment of pulmonary mechanics and gastric inflation pressure during mask ventilation. *Prehosp Disaster Med.* 1995;10:101-105.

69. Cheifetz IM, Craig DM, Quick G, McGovern JJ, Cannon ML, Ungerleider RM, Smith PK, Meliones JN. Increasing tidal volumes and pulmonary overdistention adversely affect pulmonary vascular mechanics and cardiac output in a pediatric swine model. *Crit Care Med.* 1998;26:710-716.

70. Berg MD, Idris AH, Berg RA. Severe ventilatory compromise due to gastric distension during pediatric cardiopulmonary resuscitation. *Resuscitation.* 1998;36:71-73.

71. Bowman FP, Menegazzi JJ, Check BD, Duckett TM. Lower esophageal sphincter pressure during prolonged cardiac arrest and resuscitation. *Ann Emerg Med.* 1995;26:216-219.

72. Melker RJ. Recommendations for ventilation during cardiopulmonary resuscitation: time for change? *Crit Care Med.* 1985;13:882-883.

73. Baskett P, Nolan J, Parr M. Tidal volumes which are perceived to be adequate for resuscitation. *Resuscitation.* 1996;31:231-234.

74. Guidelines for the basic management of the airway and ventilation during resuscitation: a statement by the Airway and Ventilation Management Working Group of the European Resuscitation Council. *Resuscitation.* 1996;31: 187-200.

75. Guidelines for cardiopulmonary resuscitation and emergency cardiac care. Emergency Cardiac Care Committee and Subcommittees, American Heart Association. *JAMA.* 1992;268: 2171-2295.

76. Idris AH, Gabrielli A, Caruso L. Smaller tidal volume is safe and effective for bag-valve-ventilation, but not for mouth-to-mouth ventilation: an animal model for basic life support. *Circulation.* 1999;100(suppl 1):I-644. Abstract.

77. Dörges V, Ocker H, Hagelberg S, Wenzel V, Idris AH, Schmucker P. Smaller tidal volumes with room air are not sufficient to ensure adequate oxygenation during basic life support. *Resuscitation.* 2000;44:37-41.

78. Htin KJ, Birenbaum DS, Idris AH, Banner MJ, Gravenstein N. Rescuer breathing pattern significantly affects O_2 and CO_2 received by patient during mouth-to-mouth ventilation. *Crit Care Med.* 1998;26:(suppl 1)A56.

79. Ruben H. The immediate treatment of respiratory failure. *Br J Anaesth.* 1964;36:542-549.

80. Safar P, Redding J. The "tight jaw" in resuscitation. *Anesthesiology.* 1959;20:701-702.

81. International Association of Laryngectomees. First Aid for (Neck Breathers) *Laryngectomees.* New York, NY: American Cancer Society; 1971.

82. Simmons M, Deao D, Moon L, Peters K, Cavanaugh S. Bench evaluation: three face-shield CPR barrier devices. *Respir Care.* 1995; 40:618-623.

83. Exhaled-air pulmonary resuscitators (EAPRs) and disposable manual pulmonary resuscitators (DMPRs). *Health Devices.* 1989;18:333-352.

84. Figura N. Mouth-to-mouth resuscitation and *Helicobacter pylori* infection. *Lancet.* 1996; 47:1342.

85. Heilman KM, Muschenheim C. Primary cutaneous tuberculosis resulting from mouth-to-mouth respiration. *N Engl J Med.* 1965;273: 1035-1036.

86. Johannigman JA, Branson RD. Oxygen enrichment of expired gas for mouth-to-mask resuscitation. *Respir Care.* 1991;36:99-103.

87. Langhelle A, Sunde K, Wik L, Steen PA. Arterial blood gases with 500- versus 1000-mL tidal volume during out-of-hospital CPR. *Resuscitation.* 2000;45:27-33.

88. Elling R, Politis J. An evaluation of emergency medical technicians' ability to use manual ventilation devices. *Ann Emerg Med.* 1983;12: 765-768.

89. Hess D, Baran C. Ventilatory volumes using mouth-to-mouth, mouth-to-mask, and bag-valve-mask techniques. *Am J Emerg Med.* 1985;3:292-296.

90. Cummins RO, Austin D, Graves JR, Litwin PE, Pierce J. Ventilation skills of emergency medical technicians: a teaching challenge for emergency medicine. *Ann Emerg Med.* 1986; 15:1187-1192.

91. Johannigman JA, Branson RD, Davis K Jr, Hurst JM. Techniques of emergency ventilation: a model to evaluate tidal volume, airway pressure, and gastric insufflation. *J Trauma.* 1991;31:93-98.

92. Fuerst RS, Banner MJ, Melker RJ. Gastric inflation in the unintubated patient: a comparison of common ventilating devices. *Ann Emerg Med.* 1992;21:636.

93. Dörges V, Sauer C, Ocker H, Wenzel V, Schmucker P. Airway management during cardiopulmonary resuscitation: a comparative study of bag-valve-mask, laryngeal mask airway and combitube in a bench model. *Resuscitation.* 1999;41:63-69.

94. Elam JO. Bag-valve-mask O_2 ventilation. In: Safer P, Elam JO, eds. *Advances in Cardiopulmonary Resuscitation: The Wolf Creek Conference on Cardiopulmonary Resuscitation.* New York, NY: Springer-Verlag Inc; 1977:73-79.

95. Sellick BA. Cricoid pressure to control regurgitation of stomach contents during induction of anesthesia. *Lancet.* 1961;2:404-406.

96. Dailey RH, Simon B, Young GP, Steward RD. *The Airway: Emergency Management.* St. Louis, Mo: Mosby Year Book; 1992.

97. Salem MR, Joseph NJ, Heyman HJ, Belani B, Paulissian R, Ferrara TP. Cricoid pressure is effective in obliterating the esophageal lumen in the presence of a nasogastric tube. *Anesthesiology.* 1985;4:443-446.

98. Petito SP, Russell WJ. The prevention of gastric inflation — a neglected benefit of cricoid pressure. *Anaesth Intensive Care.* 1988;16:139-143.

99. Mather C, O'Kelly S. The palpation of pulses. *Anaesthesia.* 1996;51:189-191.

100. Bahr J, Klingler H, Panzer W, Rode H, Kettler D. Skills of lay people in checking the carotid pulse. *Resuscitation.* 1997;35:23-26.

101. Ochoa FJ, Ramalle-Gomara E, Carpintero JM, Garcia A, Saralegui I. Competence of health professionals to check the carotid pulse. *Resuscitation.* 1998;37:173-175.

102. Flesche CW, Zucker TP, Lorenz C, Nerudo B, Tarnow J. The carotid pulse check as a diagnostic tool to assess pulselessness during adult basic life support. *Euroanaesthesia.* 1995. Abstract.

103. Cummins RO, Hazinski MF. Cardiopulmonary resuscitation techniques and instruction: when does evidence justify revision? *Ann Emerg Med.* 1999;34:780-784.

104. Flesche CW, Neruda B, Breuer S, Tarnow J. Basic cardiopulmonary resuscitation skills: a comparison of ambulance staff and medical students in Germany. *Resuscitation.* 1994; 28:S25.

105. Flesche CW, Neruda B, Neotges T, Tarnow J. Do cardiopulmonary resuscitation skills among medical students meet current standards and patients' needs? *Resuscitation.* 1994;28:S25.

106. Monsieurs KG, De Cauwer HG, Bossaert LL. Feeling for the carotid pulse: is five seconds enough? *Resuscitation.* 1996;31:S3.

107. Flesche CW, Breuer S, Mandel LP, Breivik H, Tarnow J. The ability of health professionals to check the carotid pulse. *Circulation.* 1994; 90(suppl 1):288.

108. Eberle B, Dick WF, Schneider T, Wisser G, Doetsch S, Tzanova I. Checking the carotid pulse check: diagnostic accuracy of first responders in patients with and without a pulse. *Resuscitation.* 1996;33:107-116.

109. Kouwenhoven WB, Jude JR, Knickerbocker GG. Closed-chest cardiac massage. *JAMA.* 1960;173:1064-1067.

110. Maier GW, Tyson GS Jr, Olsen CO, Kernstein KH, Davis JW, Conn EH, Sabiston DC Jr, Rankin JS. The physiology of external cardiac massage: high-impulse cardiopulmonary resuscitation. *Circulation.* 1984;70:86-101.

111. Rudikoff MT, Maughan WL, Effron M, Freund P, Weisfeldt ML. Mechanisms of blood flow during cardiopulmonary resuscitation. *Circulation.* 1980;61:345-352.

112. Fitzgerald KR, Babbs CF, Frissora HA, Davis RW, Silver DI. Cardiac output during cardiopulmonary resuscitation at various compression rates and durations. *Am J Physiol.* 1981;241:H442-H448.

113. Babbs CF, Thelander K. Theoretically optimal duty cycles for chest and abdominal compression during external cardiopulmonary resuscitation. *Acad Emerg Med.* 1995;2:698-707.

114. Maier GW, Newton JR, Wolfe JA, Tyson GS, Olsen CO, Glower DD, Spratt JA, Davis JW, Feneley MP, Rankin JS. The influence of manual chest compression rate on hemodynamic support during cardiac arrest: high-impulse cardiopulmonary resuscitation. *Circulation.* 1986;74:IV-51-IV-59.

115. Feneley MP, Maier GW, Kern KB, Gaynor JW, Gall SA, Sanders AB, Raessler K, Muhlbaier LH, Rankin JS, Ewy GA. Influence of compression rate on initial success of resuscitation and 24 hour survival after prolonged manual cardiopulmonary resuscitation in dogs. *Circulation.* 1988;77: 240-250.

116. Wolfe JA, Maier GW, Newton JR, Glower DD, Tyson GS, Spratt JA, Rankin JS, Olsen CO. Physiologic determinants of coronary blood flow during external cardiac massage. *J Thoracic Cardiovasc Surg.* 1988;95:523-532.

117. Sanders AB, Kern KB, Fonken S, Otto CW, Ewy GA. The role of bicarbonate and fluid loading in improving resuscitation from prolonged cardiac arrest with rapid manual chest compression CPR. *Ann Emerg Med.* 1990; 19:1-7.

118. Swenson RD, Weaver WD, Niskanen RA, Martin J, Dahlberg S. Hemodynamics in humans during conventional and experimental methods of cardiopulmonary resuscitation. *Circulation.* 1988;78:630-639.

119. Kern KB, Sanders AB, Raife J, Milander MM, Otto CW, Ewy GA. A study of chest compression rates during cardiopulmonary resuscitation in humans. *Arch Intern Med.* 1992;152:145-149.

120. Wik L, Steen PA. The ventilation-compression ratio influences the effectiveness of two rescuer advanced cardiac life support on a manikin. *Resuscitation.* 1996;31:113-119.

121. Kern KB, Hilwig RW, Berg RA, Ewy GA. Efficacy of chest compression–only BLS CPR in the presence of an occluded airway. *Resuscitation.* 1998;39:179-188.

122. Handley AJ, Handley JA. The relationship between rate of chest compression and compression:relaxation ratio. *Resuscitation.* 1995;30:237-241.

123. Berg RA, Sanders AB, Milander M, Tellez D, Liu P, Beyda D. Efficacy of audio-prompted rate guidance in improving resuscitator performance of cardiopulmonary resuscitation on children. *Acad Emerg Med.* 1994;1:35-40.

124. Milander MM, Hiscok PS, Sanders AB, Kern KB, Berg RA, Ewy GA. Chest compression and ventilation rates during cardiopulmonary resuscitation: the effects of audible tone guidance. *Acad Emerg Med.* 1995;2:708-713.

125. Aufderheide T, Stapleton ER, Hazinski MF, Cummins RO. *Heartsaver AED for the Lay Rescuer and First Responder*. Dallas, Tex: American Heart Association; 1999.

126. Emergency Cardiac Care Committee, American Heart Association. *Heartsaver ABC*. Dallas, Tex: American Heart Association; 1999.

127. Emergency Cardiac Care Committee, American Heart Association. *Heartsaver CPR in Schools*. Dallas, Tex: American Heart Association; 1999.

128. Clawson JJ. Dispatch priority training: strengthening the weak link. *J Emerg Med Serv.* 1981;6:32-36.

129. Clawson JJ. Telephone treatment protocols: reach out and help someone. *J Emerg Med Serv.* 1986;11:43-46.

130. Culley LL, Clark JJ, Eisenberg MS, Larsen MP. Dispatcher-assisted telephone CPR: common delays and time standards for delivery. *Ann Emerg Med.* 1991;20:362-366.

131. Halperin HR, Tsitlik JE, Guerci AD, Mellits ED, Levin HR, Shi AY, Chandra N, Weisfeldt ML. Determinants of blood flow to vital organs during cardiopulmonary resuscitation in dogs. *Circulation.* 1986;73:539-550.

132. Swart GL, Mateer JR, DeBehnke DJ, Jameson SJ, Osborn JL. The effect of compression duration on hemodynamics during mechanical high-impulse CPR. *Acad Emerg Med.* 1994;1:430-437.

133. Criley JM, Blaufuss AH, Kissel GL. Cough-induced cardiac compression: self-administered form of cardiopulmonary resuscitation. *JAMA.* 1976;236:1246-1250.

134. Petelenz T, Iwinski J, Chlebowczyk J, Czyz Z, Flak Z, Fiutowski L, Zaorski K, Petelenz T, Zeman S. Self-administered cough cardiopulmonary resuscitation (c-CPR) in patients threatened by MAS events of cardiovascular origin. *Wiad Lek.* 1998;51:326-336.

135. Saba SE, David SW. Sustained consciousness during ventricular fibrillation: case report of cough cardiopulmonary resuscitation. *Cathet Cardiovasc Diagn.* 1996;37:47-48.

136. Miller B, Cohen A, Serio A, Bettock D. Hemodynamics of cough cardiopulmonary resuscitation in a patient with sustained torsades de pointes/ventricular flutter. *J Emerg Med.* 1994;12:627-632.

137. Paradis NA, Martin GB, Goetting MG, et al. Simultaneous aortic, jugular bulb, and right atrial pressures during cardiopulmonary resuscitation in humans: insights into mechanisms. *Circulation.* 1989;80:361-368.

138. Guerci AD, Chandra NC, Gelfand MI, et al. Vest CPR increases aortic pressure in humans. *Circulation.* 1989;80(suppl II):II-496. Abstract.

139. Sack JB, Kesselbrenner MB, Bregman D. Survival from in-hospital cardiac arrest with interposed abdominal counterpulsation during cardiopulmonary resuscitation. *JAMA.* 1992; 267:379-385.

140. Sack JB, Kesselbrenner MB, Jarrad A. Interposed abdominal compression-cardiopulmonary resuscitation and resuscitation outcome during asystole and electromechanical dissociation. *Circulation.* 1992;86:1692-1700.

141. Barranco F, Lesmes A, Irles JA, Blasco J, Leal J, Rodriguez J, Leon C. Cardiopulmonary resuscitation with simultaneous chest and abdominal compression: comparative study in humans. *Resuscitation.* 1990;20: 67-77.

142. Cohen TJ, Tucker KJ, Lurie KG, Redberg RF, Dutton JP, Dwyer KA, Schwab TM, Chin MC, Gelb AM, Scheinman MM, et al. Active compression-decompression: a new method of cardiopulmonary resuscitation. *JAMA.* 1992;267:2916-2923.

143. Plaisance P, Lurie K, Vicaut E, Adnet F, Petit JL, Epain D, Ecollan P, Gruat R, Cavagna P, Biens J, Payen D. Comparison of standard cardiopulmonary resuscitation and active compression decompression for out-of-hospital cardiac arrest. *N Engl J Med.* 1999;341: 569-575.

144. Plaisance P, Adnet F, Vicaut E, Hennequin B, Magne P, Prudhomme C, Lambert Y, Cantineau JP, Leopold C, Ferracci C, Gizzi M, Payen D. Benefit of active compression-decompression cardiopulmonary resuscitation as a prehospital advanced cardiac life support: a randomized multicenter study. *Circulation.* 1997;95:955-961.

145. Lurie KG, Barnes T, Sukhum P, Detloff B, McKnite S, Zielinkski T, Mulligan K. Evaluation of a prototypic inspiratory impedance threshold valve designed to enhance the efficiency of cardiopulmonary resuscitation. *Resp Care.* Submitted 1999.

146. Lurie KG, Coffeen PR, Shultz JJ, McKnite SH, Detloff B, Mulligan K. Improving active compression-decompression cardiopulmonary resuscitation with an inspiratory impedance valve. *Circulation.* 1995;91:1629-1632.

147. Lurie KG, Mulligan K, McKnite S, Detloff B, Lindstrom P, Lindner K. Optimizing standard cardiopulmonary resuscitation with an inspiratory threshold valve. *Chest.* 1998;113:1084-1090.

148. Mauer D, Schneider T, Dick W, Withelm A, Elich D, Mauer M. Active compression-decompression resuscitation: a prospective, randomized study in a two-tiered EMS system with physicians in the field. *Resuscitation.* 1996;33:125-134.

149. Simoons ML, Kimman GP, Ivens EMA, Hartman JAM, Hart HN. Follow up after out-of-hospital resuscitation. Read before the XIIth Annual Congress of the European Society of Cardiology; Stockholm, Sweden: September 16-20, 1990.

150. Ornato JP, Hallagan LF, McMahan SB, Peeples EH, Rostafinski AG. Attitudes of BCLS instructors about mouth-to-mouth resuscitation during the AIDS epidemic. *Ann Emerg Med.* 1990;19:151-156.

151. Brenner BE, Van DC, Cheng D, Lazar EJ. Determinants of reluctance to perform CPR among residents and applicants: the impact of experience on helping behavior. *Resuscitation.* 1997;35:203-211.

152. Hew P, Brenner B, Kaufman J. Reluctance of paramedics and emergency medical technicians to perform mouth-to-mouth resuscitation. *J Emerg Med.* 1997;15:279-284.

153. Brenner BE, Kauffman J. Reluctance of internists and medical nurses to perform mouth-to-mouth resuscitation. *Arch Intern Med.* 1993;153:1763-1769.

154. Locke CJ, Berg RA, Sanders AB, Davis MF, Milander MM, Kern KB, Ewy GA. Bystander cardiopulmonary resuscitation: concerns about mouth-to-mouth contact. *Arch Intern Med.* 1995;155:938-943.

155. Berg RA, Kern KB, Hilwig RW, Berg MD, Sanders AB, Otto CW, Ewy GA. Assisted ventilation does not improve outcome in a porcine model of single-rescuer bystander cardiopulmonary resuscitation. *Circulation.* 1997;95:1635-1641.

156. Weil MH, Rackow EC, Trevino R, Grundler W, Falk JL, Griffel MI. Difference in acid-base state between venous and arterial blood during cardiopulmonary resuscitation. *N Engl J Med.* 1986;315:153-156.

157. Sanders AB, Otto CW, Kern KB, Rogers JN, Perrault P, Ewy GA. Acid-base balance in a canine model of cardiac arrest. *Ann Emerg Med.* 1988;17:667-671.

158. Krischer JP, Fine EG, Davis JH, Nagel EL. Complications of cardiac resuscitation. *Chest.* 1987;92:287-291.

159. Scholz KH, Tebbe U, Herrmann C, Wojcik J, Lingen R, Chemnitius JM, Brune S, Kreuzer H. Frequency of complications of cardiopulmonary resuscitation after thrombolysis during acute myocardial infarction. *Am J Cardiol.* 1992;69:724-728.

160. Bush CM, Jones JS, Cohle SD, Johnson H. Pediatric injuries from cardiopulmonary resuscitation. *Ann Emerg Med.* 1996;28: 40-44.

161. Spevak MR, Kleinman PK, Belanger PL, Primack C, Richmond JM. Cardiopulmonary resuscitation and rib fractures in infants: a postmortem radiologic-pathologic study. *JAMA.* 1994;272:617-618.

You are a healthcare provider on the medical-surgical floor of a hospital. You have been asked to bring the "code" cart and the AED to a patient's room. When you get there, you find a 52-year-old man collapsed on the floor. He is unresponsive and not breathing, with no pulse. One nurse is providing bag-mask ventilation, another is providing chest compressions.

The nurses ask you to operate the AED. You place it by the victim's left ear, turn it on, and attach the electrodes to the patient. You "clear" the patient and analyze the rhythm.

The AED advises a shock. You "clear" the patient and deliver a shock. After the shock the AED analyzes the rhythm again and gives a "no shock advised" message. The patient has a pulse, is moving slightly, and is breathing adequately. The code team arrives and assumes responsibility for the patient's care.

The patient is sent to the electrophysiology lab to receive an ICD. You visit him that evening and meet his family. They thank you for saving the man's life.

Automated External Defibrillation

Overview

The interval from collapse to defibrillation is the most important determinant of survival from cardiac arrest.[1-16] Lay rescuer AED programs are a public health initiative that aims to shorten this interval by placing AEDs in the hands of trained laypersons throughout the community. It provides the opportunity to defibrillate victims within a few minutes of collapse. This initiative has the potential to be the single greatest advance in the treatment of sudden cardiac arrest since the development of CPR. Extraordinary survival rates — as high as 49%[17,18] — have been achieved with the use of AEDs by trained lay rescuers.[17-24] These survival rates are twice as high as previously reported survival rates involving the most effective EMS systems.[25]

The AED is a remarkable example of new technology that is contributing to this dramatic increase in survival from sudden cardiac arrest. AEDs are sophisticated, computerized devices that are reliable and simple to operate, allowing almost anyone to attempt defibrillation.[26] Flight attendants,[23,24] security personnel,[27] police officers,[17-22] firefighters, lifeguards, family members,[28] school-age children,[26] and many other trained laypersons have used AEDs successfully. AEDs may be located in airports,[29] airplanes,[23,30] casinos,[27] high-rise office buildings, housing complexes, recreational facilities, sports arenas,[31] shopping malls, golf courses, and numerous other public places. Healthcare professionals

have also embraced the use of AEDs[32,33]; AEDs are used by BLS ambulance providers and in hospitals,[34-38] dental clinics, and physicians' offices.

With the inclusion of AED use in BLS skills, BLS is now defined by the first 3 links in the Chain of Survival: early

access, early CPR, and early defibrillation.[39] Widely used by the public and distributed throughout the community, AEDs significantly advance the concept proposed by the American Heart Association more than 2 decades ago: the community should become the ultimate coronary care unit.[40]

Learning Objectives

At the end of this chapter you will be able to

1. Discuss the importance of early defibrillation

2. Discuss lay rescuer AED programs

3. Describe the purpose of an AED

4. List the steps common to the operation of all AEDs

5. Describe the proper procedure for attaching the AED electrode pads in the correct positions on the victim's chest

6. Explain why no one should touch the victim while the AED is analyzing, charging, or shocking the victim

7. List at least 3 special conditions that may require you to modify your actions when using an AED

8. Describe the proper actions to take when the AED gives a *"no shock indicated"* (or *"no shock advised"*) message

9. List the 3 clinical findings that indicate the need to provide chest compressions and attach an AED

10. Assign roles for 3 rescuers who arrive at the scene of a cardiac arrest with an AED

11. Demonstrate how to manage the following collapsed victims with an AED:

    ■ No shock advised, no pulse

    ■ Shock advised, 1 shock, return of pulse and breathing

    ■ Shock advised, 3 shocks in a row, CPR for 1 minute, return of pulse after the fourth shock

12. Discuss how to maintain an AED

Principle of Early Defibrillation

Early defibrillation is critical for victims of sudden cardiac arrest for the following reasons:

■ The most frequent initial rhythm in witnessed sudden cardiac arrest is ventricular fibrillation (VF)

■ The most effective treatment for VF is electrical defibrillation

■ The probability of successful defibrillation diminishes rapidly over time

■ VF tends to convert to asystole within a few minutes

Many adult patients in VF arrest can survive neurologically intact even if defibrillation is performed as late as 6 to 10 minutes after sudden cardiac arrest.[25,41-50] Performance of CPR while awaiting the arrival of the AED appears to prolong VF and preserve heart and brain function.[43,44] CPR alone, however, will not convert VF to a normal rhythm.

The interval between collapse and defibrillation is the critical determinant of survival from VF cardiac arrest.[42-58] With every minute that defibrillation is delayed, the chance of survival from VF cardiac arrest declines by 7% to 10%[56] (Figure 1). The survival rate is also affected by bystander CPR, which improves survival at any given collapse-to-defibrillation interval.

A survival rate of 70% to 90% has been reported[47-50] in outpatient cardiac rehabilitation units when defibrillation was accomplished within the first minute of collapse. When defibrillation is delayed, survival decreases, falling to approximately 50% when defibrillation is performed at 5 minutes after collapse, 30% at 7 minutes, 10% at between 9 and 11 minutes, and 2% to 5% beyond 12 minutes.[25,41-56] One recent observational study with a historic control suggests that survival from VF arrest may be improved if first responders perform CPR for 1 minute *before* defibrillation. This is applicable only when defibrillation is delayed for 4 minutes or longer (in this

FIGURE 1. Survival to hospital discharge: Effect of collapse-to-CPR interval and collapse-to-defibrillation interval on survival. The graph displays the probability of survival-to-hospital discharge in relation to 4 intervals from collapse to start of CPR (1, 5, 10, and 15 minutes) and collapse to defibrillation (5, 10, 15, and 20 minutes). To determine the probability of survival for an individual patient, identify the curve indicating the interval between collapse and CPR, and then identify the point on that curve that corresponds to the interval from collapse to defibrillation (see horizontal axis). The probability of survival is then indicated on the vertical axis. Based on data from King County, Washington (N=1667 witnessed VT/VF arrests),[45] with additional cases from Tucson, Arizona (N=205 witnessed VT/VF arrests).[53]

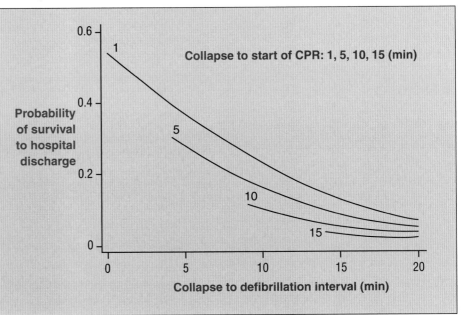

study the median time to defibrillation was 11 minutes) and no bystander CPR is performed.[57]

Survival rates from VF cardiac arrest can be remarkably high if the event is witnessed and both early CPR and early defibrillation are provided. For example, when patients in supervised cardiac rehabilitation programs experience a witnessed cardiac arrest, defibrillation is usually performed within minutes; in 4 studies of cardiac arrest in this setting, 90 of 101 victims (89%) were successfully resuscitated.[47-50] This is the highest survival rate reported for a defined out-of-hospital population. High success rates (50% or greater) have been reported for resuscitation after witnessed collapse when early CPR and early defibrillation were performed by police,[17-19] on airplanes and in airports,[23,29,30] and in casinos.[27]

Communities with no out-of-hospital ACLS providers have reported improved

survival rates for cardiac arrest when first-responder defibrillation programs were established.[51-55] When defibrillators were placed in the hands of basic EMS personnel, the most impressive results were reported in King County, Washington, where the survival rate of patients with VF improved from 7% to 26%,[51] and in rural Iowa, where the survival rate rose from 3% to 19%.[52] More modest results have been observed in rural communities in southeastern Minnesota,[53] northeastern Minnesota,[54] and Wisconsin.[55]

The earlier defibrillation occurs, the higher the survival rate.[45,56,58-61] Emergency personnel have only a few minutes after the victim's collapse to reestablish a perfusing rhythm. CPR can sustain a patient for a short time but cannot directly restore an organized rhythm. Restoration of a perfusing rhythm requires immediate bystander CPR followed by defibrillation within a few minutes of the initial arrest.

Figure 2[41] displays the sequence of events that must occur for successful resuscitation from cardiac arrest. The use of AEDs increases the variety of personnel who can perform CPR and attempt defibrillation, thus shortening the time between collapse and defibrillation.[29,45,51-55,58-61] This exciting prospect explains the addition of this intervention as an integral component of BLS.

Early defibrillation (within 5 minutes of EMS call receipt to shock) is recommended as a high-priority goal in the ECC Guidelines 2000. Every community should assess its capability to provide this intervention and institute whatever measures are necessary to make this recommendation a reality.

Structure and Function of AEDs

AEDs are automated external defibrillators. The word *automated* actually means *semiautomated*, because most commercially available AEDs will "advise" the operator that a shock is indicated but will not deliver a shock without an action by the rescuer (ie, the rescuer must push the SHOCK button). Fully automated defibrillators (ie, AEDs that deliver a shock as soon as they are attached and turned on, without further operator intervention) are

used only in special circumstances and are not discussed further in this chapter.

The AED is attached to the patient with adhesive electrodes. The device is equipped with a proprietary microprocessor-based rhythm analysis system that analyzes the rhythm. If ventricular tachycardia (VT) or VF is detected, the shock-advisory system "advises" a shock through visual or voice prompts.[62,63] Most AEDs operate in the same way and have similar components (Figure 3). The common aspects of AED function and operation are presented below with information about troubleshooting.

Automated Analysis of Cardiac Rhythms

AEDs are highly sophisticated, microprocessor-based devices that record and then analyze the ECG signal to determine if it is consistent with VF or pulseless VT. The AED samples the victim's cardiac rhythm through a bandwidth amplifier that is very narrow when compared with the broad bandwidth amplifiers used to record diagnostic-quality 12-lead ECGs. The narrow bandwidth filters out radio transmission, interference from 60-cycle current flow, and artifactual signals that result from loose electrodes and poor

electrode contact. Some intermittent radio transmissions can produce an ECG artifact if a transmitter or receiver is used within 6 feet of a patient during rhythm analysis. Some devices are programmed to detect spontaneous movement by the patient or movement of the patient by others.[62,63]

Most AEDs analyze multiple features of the surface ECG signal, including frequency, amplitude, and some mathematical integration of frequency and amplitude (such as slope or wave morphology) to determine if the rhythm is consistent with VF or VT. The AED confirms VF on the basis of additional features such as low amplitude and the absence of a flat baseline. Normal sinus rhythm, for example, is characterized by a flat line between complexes. The AED then advises a shock when an ECG signal consistent with these characteristics is detected. Because the AED is attached to a victim who has no signs of circulation (for healthcare providers, this includes no pulse), the AED presumes the absence of a pulse. If the patient has a wide QRS with a fast signal rate (for example, more than 180 beats per minute [bpm] in an adult), the AED "detects" pulseless VT and recommends a shock (see Figure 4).

FIGURE 2. Sequence of events and key intervals that occur with cardiac arrest.[41] EMS indicates emergency medical services system.

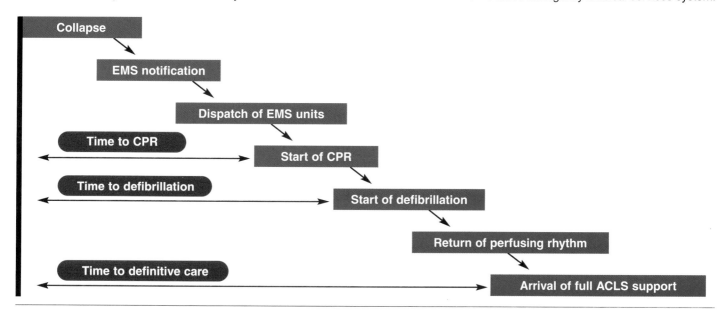

AEDs have been extensively tested, both in vitro against libraries of recorded cardiac rhythms[64] and clinically in numerous field trials.[65-72] Their accuracy in rhythm analysis is high.[67-69] The rare errors noted in field trials have been almost entirely errors of omission in which the AED failed to recognize low-amplitude VF or tachycardia or when the operator failed to follow the recommended operating procedures, such as analyzing the rhythm despite movement by the patient.[73]

Inappropriate Shocks or Failure to Shock

AEDs should be placed in the analysis mode only when cardiac arrest has been confirmed and only when all movement, particularly patient transport, has ceased. AED analysis can be affected by movement of the patient (eg, seizures and agonal respirations), repositioning of the patient, or artifactual signals.[65-73] Agonal respiration poses a problem because some devices "lock out" analysis if the patient continues to have gasping respirations.

Failure to follow the manufacturer's instructions for use of a fully automatic external defibrillator has in rare instances (less than 0.1%) resulted in delivery of inappropriate electrical countershocks.[12] The use of radio receivers and transmitters should be avoided during rhythm analysis. The major errors reported in clinical trials have been occasional failures to deliver shocks to rhythms that may benefit from electrical therapy, such as fine VF.[67,69,73]

Occasionally the analysis and treatment cycles of implanted and automated defibrillators conflict.[67,69,73,74] How to use AEDs for patients with implantable defibrillators *(automatic implantable cardioverter-defibrillators, or ICDs or AICDs)* is presented later in this chapter.

Ventricular Tachycardia

Although AEDs are not designed to deliver synchronized shocks, all AEDs will recommend a shock for monomorphic and polymorphic VT if the rate exceeds preset values (more than 180 bpm for most AEDs). AEDs should be attached *only* to

---

FIGURE 3. Schematic drawing of AED attached to patient.

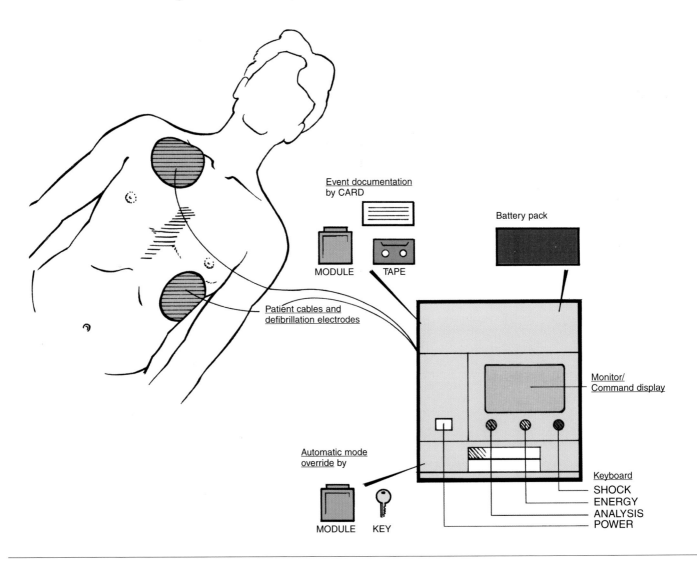

FIGURE 4. Features of surface ECG analyzed by AED.

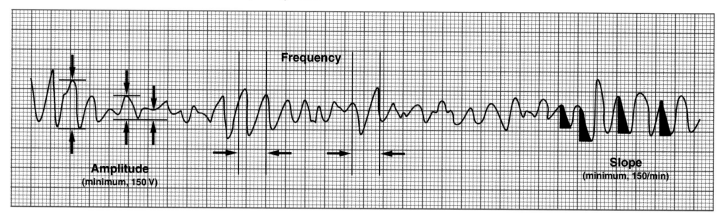

patients who are unresponsive, not breathing normally, and have no signs of circulation (and no pulse if circulation is assessed by the healthcare provider). This will avoid a recommendation by the AED to shock a victim with VT with effective circulation (perfusing VT).

The rescuer/AED operator serves as a second verification system for cardiac arrest. The rescuer should confirm that the patient has suffered a cardiac arrest (no response, no breathing, no signs of circulation) before attaching the AED. In an unresponsive, apneic patient without signs of circulation, electrical shocks are indicated whether the rhythm is supraventricular tachycardia (SVT), VT, or VF. There have been rare reports of shocks delivered to responsive patients with perfusing ventricular or supraventricular arrhythmias.[12,67] These are operator errors, not device errors, which are preventable with proper training and good patient assessment skills.[70]

AED Operation

AEDs should be used only when patients have the following 3 clinical findings:

- Unresponsiveness
- No effective breathing
- No signs of circulation

Throughout this chapter, *for the health-care professional* the term *signs of circulation* includes a pulse or signs of normal breathing, coughing, or movement. Signs of circulation are present if the patient

has a pulse or is breathing normally, coughing, or moving. Signs of circulation are absent if the patient has no pulse and is not breathing normally, coughing, or moving. The word *breathing* is used to indicate *effective* respirations; the patient with agonal respirations is *not* breathing, because agonal breaths are not effective breaths.

Throughout this chapter, *for the lay rescuer* the term *signs of circulation* includes normal breathing, coughing, or movement. Signs of circulation are absent if the patient is not breathing normally, is not coughing, and has no movement. Normal breathing is noted so that lay rescuers will not mistakenly think that agonal breathing indicates the presence of effective breathing.

Before attaching the AED, the operator should first determine whether special situations exist that require additional actions before the AED is used or that contraindicate its use altogether.

Special Situations

The following 4 situations may require the operator to take additional actions before using an AED or during its operation:

- The victim is less than 8 years of age (or weighs less than approximately 25 kg).
- The victim is immersed in water or water is covering the victim's chest.
- The victim has an implanted pacemaker (ICD or AICD).

- A transdermal medication patch or other object is located on the surface of the victim's skin where the AED electrode pads are placed.

Children Less Than 8 Years Old

Cardiac arrest is less common in children than in adults, and respiratory arrest is a far more common cause of arrest in children than sudden cardiac death.[86-89] Approximately 50% of pediatric cardiac arrests occur in infants less than 1 year old.[86] In the first months of life, sudden infant death syndrome and respiratory disease are the major causes of arrest.[90,91] Beyond the neonatal period, unintentional injuries, including trauma and submersion, are the major causes of cardiac arrest.[91]

The most common terminal rhythm observed in patients 17 years of age and younger is asystole or pulseless electrical activity.[86,88-89,92-96] When pediatric cardiac arrest rhythms are reported, estimates of VF range from 7% to 15%.[86,88,92-94,96] The frequency of VF varies with the population included or excluded from the study, whether or not the arrest was witnessed, and the interval between EMS call and rhythm assessment.

In some studies pediatric patients who have VF and receive defibrillation at the scene have a higher initial resuscitation rate and are more likely to be discharged from the hospital with a good neurologic outcome.[88,92,97] For this reason it is important to identify pediatric victims of cardiac arrest with VT/VF to enable rapid provision of defibrillation.

In the prehospital setting AEDs are commonly used for adults in sudden collapse. When attached to the victim with adhesive electrodes, the AED evaluates the victim's ECG to determine if a "shockable" rhythm is present, charges to an appropriate dose, and when activated by the rescuer, delivers a shock. AEDs use voice prompts to assist the operator.

Several manufacturers now market AEDs that accommodate both adult electrode pads and pediatric cable-pad systems that attenuate the delivered energy to a dose more appropriate for children under the age of 8 years. Clinical experience with these devices has yet to be published.

Data from two recent, large studies of the effectiveness of the AED rhythm analysis algorithms in pediatric patients have been published since the ECC Guidelines 2000 were drafted.[98,99]

The following conclusions are part of an advisory statement that has been prepared to revise the ECC Guidelines 2000 recommendation for use of AEDs in children under the age of 8 years.[100]

- AEDs may be used for children 1 to 8 years of age with no signs of circulation after 1 minute of CPR. Ideally the device should deliver a child dose. The arrhythmia detection algorithm used in the device should demonstrate high specificity for pediatric shockable rhythms (ie, will not recommend shock delivery for nonshockable rhythms): *Class IIb.*

- Currently there is insufficient evidence to support a recommendation for or against the use of AEDs in infants <1 year of age.

- For a single rescuer responding to a child without signs of circulation, 1 minute of CPR continues to be recommended before any other action, such as activating EMS or attaching an AED.

- Defibrillation is recommended for documented VF/pulseless VT: *Class I.*

FYI: AED Waveforms and Energy Levels

Defibrillators should be set to deliver the lowest effective energy needed to terminate VF. If energy and current are too low, the shock will not terminate the arrhythmia; if energy and current are too high, myocardial damage may result.[75-79] There is no clear relation between body size and energy requirements for defibrillation in adults.

Modern AEDs use 1 of 2 types of waveforms: monophasic or biphasic. Monophasic waveforms deliver current in 1 direction and vary the speed of voltage increase to maximum and voltage decrease to zero. The voltage decrease to zero can be gradual.

Biphasic waveforms deliver current that flows in a positive direction for a specified duration. In the second phase the direction of current is reversed so that it flows in a negative, "opposite" direction.

In a prospective, out-of-hospital study of 175-J and 320-J monophasic shocks delivered by a manual defibrillator, defibrillation rates and survival to hospital discharge were identical in patients who received shocks of 175 J and 320 J.[80]

The recommended first-shock energy for monophasic waveform defibrillation is 200 J; the recommended second shock is 200 or 300 J; the recommended third shock is 360 J.[80] The intent of this escalating energy dosage protocol is to maximize shock success (termination of VF) while minimizing shock toxicity.[75-79] The patient receives the higher shock energy only if lower doses fail to convert the arrhythmia.

The first biphasic waveform for use in an AED was approved in the United States in 1996. The impedance-compensating biphasic truncated exponential (BTE) waveform was incorporated into an AED that delivered nonescalating 150-J shocks. In-hospital testing showed that the BTE waveform with low-energy shocks of 115 J and 130 J was as effective for treatment of short-duration VF as 200-J shocks with the monophasic dampened sine (MDS) waveform.[81,82] Experience with the biphasic defibrillator for treatment of out-of-hospital cardiac arrest has also been positive.[17-19]

Other versions of biphasic waveforms have been introduced and have undergone initial evaluation in the electrophysiology laboratory during implantation and testing of ICDs. Experience with short-duration VF in which a low-energy (120 to 170 J) constant-current, rectilinear biphasic waveform was used has recently been reported.[83] This waveform is also effective in terminating atrial fibrillation during elective cardioversion with energies as low as 70 J.[84]

The available data indicates that biphasic waveform shocks of relatively low energy (200 J or less) are safe and have equivalent or higher efficacy for termination of VF compared with higher-energy escalating monophasic waveform shocks.[85] No prospective trial, however, has directly compared biphasic and monophasic devices. Therefore, any benefit of one waveform over the other (as yet unproved) is unlikely to equal the magnitude of benefit derived from significantly decreasing the time from collapse to defibrillation.

The steps for AED use are as follows (also see Figure 13):

- POWER ON the AED (turn it on).

- Attach the AED pads/electrodes to the victim's chest (right upper sternal border, left chest under the arm at the level of the left nipple).

- "Clear" the victim and analyze the rhythm.

- If a shock is indicated, "clear" the victim and deliver a shock.

For children under 8 years of age, use a child pad-cable system if available. Children under 8 years of age weigh less than 25 kg and are usually less than 50 inches (128 cm) in length, based on a Broselow color-coded tape.[104] Do not use child pads for an adult victim because they will likely deliver an inadequate defibrillation dose for the adult.

In summary, although VF is not a common arrhythmia in children, the frequency with which it occurs in pediatric arrests[86,88,92-94,96,97] is enough to recommend the use of AEDs out-of-hospital in children 1 to 8 years and older (weighing 9 to 25 kg or more). The AHA does not recommend for or against the use of AEDs in infants less than 1 year old (weighing less than about 9 kg) because there is limited data about safety, efficacy, and dose.

Healthcare providers who routinely care for children at risk for arrhythmia and cardiac arrest (eg, in hospital) should continue to use defibrillators capable of appropriate energy adjustment. The initial priorities for cardiac arrest in infants and children less than 8 years old are airway support, oxygenation, and ventilation.

Water

Water is a good conductor of electricity. A shock delivered to a victim in water could be conducted from the AED through the water to rescuers and bystanders. Rescuers or bystanders could receive a shock or minor burns if they are in an AED-water-rescuer pathway. It is more likely that water on the skin of the victim's chest will provide a direct path of energy from one electrode pad to the other, bypassing the heart. This prevents the delivery of

Critical Concepts: Pad Placement

Practice choosing the correct size (adult or child) electrode pad and opening the package while your partner performs CPR. When you are ready to apply the electrode pads, remove the adhesive backing of the first pad. Then ask your partner to briefly stop chest compressions. Quickly apply the pads directly to the skin of the victim's chest and allow the AED to analyze the rhythm. Be sure to caution your partner and any bystanders to avoid touching the patient during this analysis. With some AEDs you may have to press the ANALYZE button. Other AEDs will automatically analyze as soon as the electrode pads are properly attached.

You may receive a voice prompt or alarm if the electrode pads are not securely attached to the chest or if the cables are not fastened properly. The voice warning will prompt you to *"check pads"* or *"check electrodes,"* or words to that effect. *This voice prompt means that* *there is a poor connection somewhere between the patient's skin and the AED.*

Troubleshoot by checking the following:

1. If the victim has a hairy chest, briskly remove the pads and reapply a new set of pads. You may want to clip the chest hair or shave the chest (see "The Hairy Chest Problem").

2. If the victim is wet or diaphoretic, remove the pads, wipe the chest dry with a cloth, and attach a new set of pads.

3. Be sure the pads stick firmly and evenly to the skin of the chest.

4. Verify connections: Be sure the cables are correctly connected to the AED.

5. Verify connections: Be sure the cables are correctly connected to the adhesive electrode pads.

When the problem is corrected, most AEDs will automatically go into the analyze mode.

Foundation Facts: The Hairy Chest Problem

If the victim has a hairy chest, the adhesive electrode pads may stick to the hair of the chest rather than the skin of the chest, preventing solid contact with the skin. This will lead to a *"check electrodes"* or *"check electrode pads"* message from the AED. If you receive such a message, try the following:

- Press down firmly on each pad. This may produce sufficient adhesion between the pad and the skin to solve the problem.

- If unsuccessful, briskly pull off the electrode pads. This will remove much of the chest hair.

- Wipe the area and if a lot of hair remains, shave the area for electrode pad placement with a few strokes of the prep razor in the AED carrying case. Open and apply a new set of electrode pads.

Plastic disposable razors should be packed in the AED storage case with 2 extra sets of electrode pads. Hospital personnel should keep razors and extra sets of AED electrodes with the resuscitation equipment.

adequate current to the heart, reducing the likelihood of defibrillation.

If the victim's chest is covered with water, remove the victim from the water and quickly dry the chest before attaching the AED electrodes. If the victim is lying on snow or in a small puddle, you may use the AED if the chest is dry. If the rescue involves a diving injury or other possible cause of spinal injury, take care to maintain cervical immobilization while moving the victim.

Implanted Pacemakers/ICDs

Defibrillators that deliver low-energy shocks directly to the myocardium are implanted in patients with a history of malignant arrhythmias, who are at risk for sudden death. These devices can be immediately identified because they create a hard lump beneath the skin of the upper chest or abdomen (usually on the victim's left side). The lump is half the size of a deck of cards, with a small overlying scar. If an AED electrode pad is placed directly over an implanted medical device, the device may block delivery of the shock to the heart.[105]

If an implanted defibrillator is identified, place the AED electrode pad at least 1 inch (2.5 cm) to the side of the implanted device. Then follow the normal steps for operating an AED.[105] However, if the ICD is delivering shocks to the patient (the patient's muscles contract in a manner like that observed during external defibrillation), allow 30 to 60 seconds for the ICD to complete the treatment cycle before delivering a shock from the AED. Occasionally the analysis and shock cycles of AICDs and AEDs will conflict.[74]

Transdermal Medication Patches

AED electrodes should not be placed directly on top of a medication patch (eg, a patch of nitroglycerin, nicotine, pain medication, hormone replacement therapy, or antihypertensive medication). The medication patch may transfer energy from the electrode pad to the heart and may cause small burns to the skin.[106] The only reported problems associated with shocks delivered through a transdermal patch have involved medication patches with a metal backing. Because medication

FYI: Guidelines for AED Use in Patients With Implantable Defibrillators

A properly functioning automatic implantable cardioverter-defibrillator (AICD) will analyze VF and VT accurately and deliver therapy more effectively than an external defibrillator. In only rare circumstances should an AICD be disabled. To disable the device, place a pacemaker ("doughnut") magnet over it. Most newer devices will be disabled while the magnet is in place and will return to programmed function when the magnet is removed.

Effects of Magnet Application

- Suspends overdrive pacing for tachycardias
- Allows sensing and pacing if programmed for bradycardias
- Suspends detection and treatment of VF and VT
- Suspends functions only while the magnet is in place

Assessment and Treatment of Patients With an AICD Who Are in Cardiac Arrest or Hemodynamically Unstable

- **Cardiac arrest — patient in presumed VF or VT**
  - *If AICD is not delivering a shock:*
    - Treat immediately as if there is no implanted device (ACLS VF/VT protocol)
  - *If AICD is delivering shocks but shocks are ineffective:*
    - Apply magnet to turn off AICD
    - Treat as if there is no AICD (ACLS VF/VT protocol)

- **Cardiac arrest — patient *not* in presumed VF or VT:**
  - *If AICD is not delivering a shock:*
    - Treat immediately as if there is no implanted device (ACLS rhythm-appropriate protocols)
  - *If AICD shocks are inappropriate:*
    - Apply magnet to turn off AICD
    - Treat as if there is no AICD (ACLS rhythm-appropriate protocols)

- **No cardiac arrest — patient *not* in VF or VT**
  - *If AICD shocks are inappropriate (for example, rhythm is SVT, atrial fibrillation or flutter, lead fracture or displacement)*
    - Apply magnet to stop inappropriate therapy
    - Treat as if there is no AICD (ACLS rhythm-appropriate protocols)

The doughnut-shaped deactivating magnet is now routinely carried as emergency equipment by many advanced life support units in urban areas. In the ECC Guidelines 2000 these magnets are classified as a critical item for Emergency Departments, hospital critical care units, and acute coronary care units. The AHA recommends that these devices be made immediately available to providers of out-of-hospital advanced care. Reasonable exceptions are recognized, the most cogent reason being low levels of anticipated use, for example, in rural areas, physicians' offices, or areas where a physician is not available to insert a pacemaker.

clavicle) and the other lateral to the left nipple, with the top margin of the pad a few inches below the axilla (Figure 6). The correct position of the electrode pads is often displayed on the pads or another part of the AED. To facilitate quick and correct attachment of pads, stop CPR just before attaching the pads.

If the victim is noticeably diaphoretic, dry the chest with a cloth or towel before attaching the electrode pads. If the victim has a hairy chest, the adhesive electrode pads may stick to the hair on the chest, preventing effective contact with the skin of the chest. This creates high transthoracic impedance,[107] leading to a *"check electrodes"* or *"check electrode pads"* message from the AED. If this error message occurs, briskly remove the pads (thereby removing the hair attached to

the pad). Wipe the chest. If a lot of hair still remains, shave the chest in the area of the pads before attaching a new set of electrodes.

Step 3: "Clear" the Victim and Analyze the Rhythm

"Clear" rescuers and bystanders from the victim — this means that you must ensure that no one is touching the victim before proceeding. Avoid all movement affecting the patient during analysis to ensure that artifact error does not occur.[12,56] Some AEDs require the operator to press an ANALYZE button to initiate analysis, whereas other devices automatically begin analysis when the electrode pads are attached to the chest. Rhythm assessment takes from 5 to 15 seconds, depending on the brand of AED. If VT/VF is present, the device will announce

it through a written message, visual or auditory alarm, or a voice-synthesized statement that a shock is indicated.

Step 4: "Clear" the Victim and Press the SHOCK Button

Before pressing the SHOCK button, ensure that no one is touching the victim. Always loudly state a *"Clear the patient"* message, such as *"I'm clear, you're clear, everybody's clear"* or simply *"Clear."* At the same time, perform a visual check to ensure that no one is in contact with the patient. Most AEDs begin charging the capacitors automatically if a treatable ("shockable") rhythm is detected. A tone, voice-synthesized message, or light indicates that charging has started. Delivery of a shock should occur only after the victim is cleared.[108] The shock will produce a sudden contraction of the patient's musculature (like that seen with a conventional defibrillator).

After the first shock, do not restart CPR. Instead, immediately press the ANALYZE button if needed; some AEDs will automatically start another rhythm analysis cycle. If VT/VF persists, the AED will indicate it, and the *"charging"* and *"shock indicated"* sequence will repeat for the second and third shocks. The goal is to quickly analyze the patient for persistent VT/VF rhythm and quickly deliver up to 3 shocks if needed. If a third shock is provided, the AED will prompt the rescuer to check the patient immediately after that shock whether or not defibrillation has occurred. The healthcare provider should check for signs of circulation, including a pulse.

The universal steps for AED operation are reviewed in the Critical Concepts box.

Outcomes and Actions After Defibrillation

"Shock Indicated" Message: Recurrent VF

If signs of circulation do not return after 3 shocks, rescuers without immediate ACLS backup should resume CPR for 60 seconds.

Critical Concepts:
The Universal Steps for AED Operation

1. **POWER ON the AED** first (this activates voice prompts for guidance in all subsequent steps).

   - Open the carrying case or top of the AED.

   - Turn the power on (some devices will "power on" automatically when you open the lid or case).

2. **ATTACH electrode pads** to the victim's bare chest (stop chest compressions just before attaching the pads).

   - Choose correct pad (adult vs child) for size/age of victim. Use child pads for children less than 8 years of age if available. Do not use child pads for adult victims.

   - Peel the backing away from the electrode pads. Stop CPR.

   - Attach the adhesive electrode pads to the victim's bare chest.

   - Attach the AED connecting cables to the AED box (some are pre-connected).

3. "Clear" the patient and **ANALYZE the rhythm.**

   - Press the ANALYZE button to start rhythm analysis (some AEDs do not require this step).

   - Always "clear" the victim during analysis. Be sure that no one is touching the victim, not even the person in charge of rescue breathing.

4. "Clear" the patient and **PRESS the SHOCK button if shock is indicated.**

   - Clear the victim before delivering the shock: be sure no one is touching the victim. Turn oxygen off or direct flow away from the patient's chest.

   - Press the SHOCK button to deliver the shock when — and only when — the AED signals a shock is indicated AND no one is touching the victim.

patches are no longer manufactured with metal backing, this problem has disappeared. To prevent the medication from blocking delivery of energy, however, remove the patch and wipe the area clean before attaching the AED electrode pad.

The Universal AED: Common Steps to Operate All AEDs

The AHA recommends that AEDs used in PAD programs (eg, large buildings, shopping malls, or homes) be stored beside a telephone. This allows the rescuer to activate the EMS system (phone 911 or other emergency response number) and get the AED quickly. In some locations notification of the EMS system or emergency response team occurs automatically when the AED is removed from its storage compartment. In the hospital AEDs may be kept with other resuscitation equipment, typically on a code cart that can be wheeled to the site of an emergency.

Once the AED arrives, put it next to the victim on the side with the rescuer who will operate it. This position provides ready access to the AED controls and easier placement of electrode pads. It also allows a second rescuer to perform CPR from the opposite side of the victim without interfering with AED operation.

AEDs are available in different models. There are small differences from model to model, but all AEDs operate in basically the same way.[62,63] The 4 universal steps of AED operation are as follows:

Step 1: POWER ON the AED

The first step in operating an AED is to turn the power on. This initiates voice prompts, which guide the operator through subsequent steps. To turn the AED on, press a power switch or lift the monitor cover or screen to the "up" position.

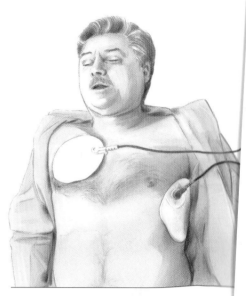

FIGURE 6. AED electrode pad placement on the victim.

Step 2: Attach Adult Electrode Pads

Quickly attach the self-adhesive electrode pads directly to the skin of the victim's chest. Be sure to choose the correct pad for the age and size (adult vs child) of the victim. Do not use child pads for adult victims. In some models the pads and cables are preconnected; in others you make the connections (see Figure 5).

Place one electrode pad on the upper-right sternal border (directly below the

Foundation Facts: Making the Connections

AEDs typically require that 4 objects be connected in a line: the **AED** is connected to the **connecting cables,** to the **AED electrode pads,** to the **victim's chest.** Remember:

1. The **AED** is joined to the
2. **connecting cables,** which are joined to the
3. **AED electrode pads,** which are attached to
4. the **victim's chest**

AED manufacturers have not yet standardized these connections. Learn the characteristics of the particular AED you will be using during the course. In newer AED models the electrode pads are preattached to the connecting cables, and the connecting cables are preattached to the AED. The only thing the operator has to do is open the electrode pad package and attach the pads to the victim's chest.

Learn exactly how much of the AED "circuit" you must put together for your AED before you need it in an emergency. If you are confronted with an unfamiliar AED system, remember that you can figure out the connections by recalling the 4 elements that must be joined: **AED, cables, electrode pads, victim** (Figure 5).

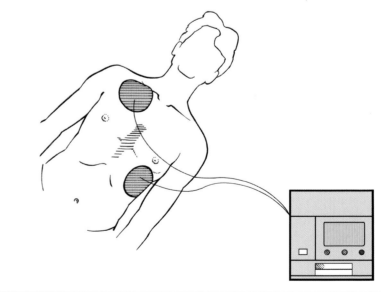

FIGURE 5. AED unit, cables, and electrode connection to patient.

After 60 seconds most devices will prompt a check for signs of circulation. If VF continues, deliver additional rounds of 3 "stacked" shocks (each will be preceded by a brief period of analysis). Provide sets of 3 stacked shocks alternating with 60 seconds of CPR until the AED gives a *"no shock indicated"* message or until ACLS is available.

The rescuer should *not* check for signs of circulation between stacked shocks, ie, after shocks 1 and 2, 4 and 5, 7 and 8, etc. Checking for signs of circulation between shocks delays rapid identification of persistent VF and also interrupts delivery of the shock. Studies have shown that rapid sequential shocks modestly reduce transthoracic impedance for each subsequent shock, so that increased energy is actually delivered to the heart with each successive shock.

"No Shock Indicated" Message: Signs of Circulation Absent

When the AED gives a *"no shock indicated"* message, check for signs of circulation. If there are no signs of circulation, resume CPR. If the victim has no signs of circulation despite CPR and 3 analyses produce 3 *"no shock indicated"* messages, there is a low probability that the rhythm is shockable (asystole is likely to be present). Therefore, rhythm analysis should be repeated only after 1- to 2-minute intervals of CPR. The outcome for these victims is poor, and consideration should be given to discontinuing CPR, particularly if no special resuscitation situations are present that suggest the likelihood of survival despite a prolonged arrest.

"No Shock Indicated" Message: Signs of Circulation Present

If signs of circulation are present, check breathing. If the victim is not breathing normally, provide rescue breathing at a rate of 10 to 12 breaths per minute. If the victim is breathing adequately, place him or her in a recovery position. The AED should always remain attached until the arrival of

---

Critical Concepts: "Shock/No Shock Indicated" Messages and Related Actions

- If the AED displays a *"shock indicated"* or *"shock advised"* message, clear the victim and then press the SHOCK button.

- If the AED indicates *"no shock indicated,"* check for signs of circulation.

- If there are no signs of circulation, resume CPR for approximately 1 minute. Then check for signs of circulation again.

- If no signs of circulation are found, analyze the victim's rhythm again.

- After 3 *"no shock indicated"* messages, perform 1 to 2 minutes of CPR.

- Repeat the analyze period every 1 to 2 minutes as you continue to do CPR.

EMS personnel. If VT/VF recurs, most AEDs will prompt the rescuer to check for signs of circulation. The device will then charge automatically and advise the rescuer to deliver an additional shock.

AEDs in a Moving Ambulance

AEDs can be left in place during transport of the patient in a moving vehicle. But never push the ANALYZE button in a moving ambulance — the movement of the vehicle can interfere with rhythm assessment, and artifact can simulate VF.[12,56] Some devices continuously analyze the patient. If a patient requires rhythm analysis during transport or if the AED prompts the rescuer to check the patient or recommends a shock, bring the vehicle to a complete stop, then reanalyze.

Integration of CPR and AED Use

When arriving at the scene of a suspected cardiac arrest, rescuers must rapidly integrate CPR with use of the AED. In most settings healthcare providers will have the benefit of having 1 or more persons to assist and perform the multiple actions needed to resuscitate a victim of sudden cardiac death. In general, 3 actions must occur simultaneously at the scene of a cardiac arrest:

1. Activation of the emergency response system (eg, hospital code team for inpatient resuscitation)

2. CPR

3. Operation of the AED

When 2 or more rescuers are present at the scene, these functions can be initiated simultaneously. AED operators should be trained in scene leadership and team management to ensure timely and effective actions by multiple rescuers.[109]

One Rescuer With an AED

In some situations 1 rescuer with immediate access to an AED may respond to a cardiac arrest. The rescuer should quickly activate the EMS system or call a code (in hospital) to summon ACLS providers. The recommended rescue sequence for 1 rescuer with an AED is as follows:

1. Verify unresponsiveness

2. Activate the emergency response system (call a code in hospital)

3. Open the airway, check breathing

4. If the victim is not breathing effectively, give 2 ventilations

5. Check for signs of circulation. If there are no signs of circulation, attach the AED and proceed with the AED treatment algorithm. The AED operator should take the following actions:

FIGURE 7. Second rescuer places AED beside victim's left ear.

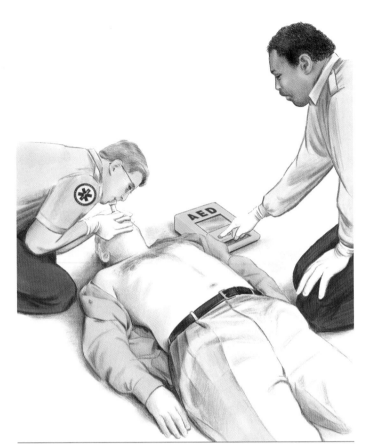

FIGURE 8. Operator turns AED on.

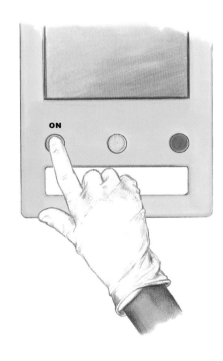

- **POWER ON** the AED and follow voice prompts. Some devices will turn on when the AED lid or carrying case is opened.

- **ATTACH** the AED.
  - Select the correct pads for victim's size and age (adult vs child).
  - Peel the backing from the pads.
  - ATTACH the adhesive pads to the victim's bare chest.
  - Attach the electrode cable to the AED (if not preconnected).

- Allow the AED to **ANALYZE** the victim's rhythm ("clear" victim during analysis).

- **Deliver a SHOCK if needed** ("clear" victim before shock).

Reasonable variations in this sequence are acceptable.

Two-Rescuer AED Sequence of Action

1. **Verify unresponsiveness:** if victim is unresponsive:
   - Call 911 (or other emergency response number).
   - Get the AED located next to the telephone:
     - The person who calls 911 gets the AED.
     - The person who will use the AED stays with the victim and performs CPR until the AED arrives. (In many circumstances these roles may be reversed.)

2. **Open airway:** head tilt–chin lift (or jaw thrust if trauma is suspected)

3. **Check for effective breathing:** provide breathing if needed:
   - Check for breathing *(look, listen, and feel).*
   - If not breathing, give 2 slow breaths:
     - A face shield is more likely to be available to the first rescuer outside the hospital.
     - A mouth-to-mask device should be available in the AED carrying case.
     - A bag-mask device is often available in the healthcare setting.

4. **Check for signs of circulation:** if no signs of circulation are present:
   - Perform chest compressions and prepare to attach the AED:
     - If there is any doubt that the signs of circulation are present, the first rescuer initiates chest compressions while the second rescuer prepares to use the AED.
     - Remove clothing covering the victim's chest to provide chest compressions and apply the AED electrode pads.

5. **Attempt defibrillation with the AED:** if no signs of circulation are present:
   - When the AED arrives, place it near the rescuer who will be operating it. The AED is usually placed on the side of the victim opposite the rescuer who is performing CPR (Figure 7).
   - The caller begins performing CPR while the rescuer who was performing CPR prepares to operate the AED. (It is acceptable to reverse these roles.)

Figure 9. Electrodes are attached to victim and then to AED.

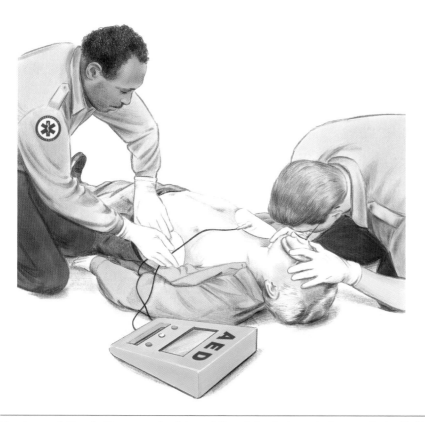

The AED operator takes the following actions:

- **POWER ON** the AED first (some devices will turn on automatically when the AED lid or carrying case is opened) (Figure 8).

- **ATTACH** the AED to the victim (Figure 9):
  — Select correct pads for the victim's size and age.
  — Peel the backing from the pads.
  — Ask the rescuer performing CPR to stop chest compressions. ATTACH adhesive electrode pads to the victim's bare chest.
  — Attach the AED connecting cables to the AED (if not preconnected).

- **ANALYZE** rhythm:
  — Clear the victim before and during analysis (Figure 10A).
  — Check that no one is touching the victim.
  — Press the ANALYZE button (Figure 10B) to start rhythm analysis (some brands of AEDs do not require this step).

Figure 10. **A.** The operator "clears" the victim before rhythm analysis. **B.** If needed, the operator then activates the "ANALYZE" feature of the AED.

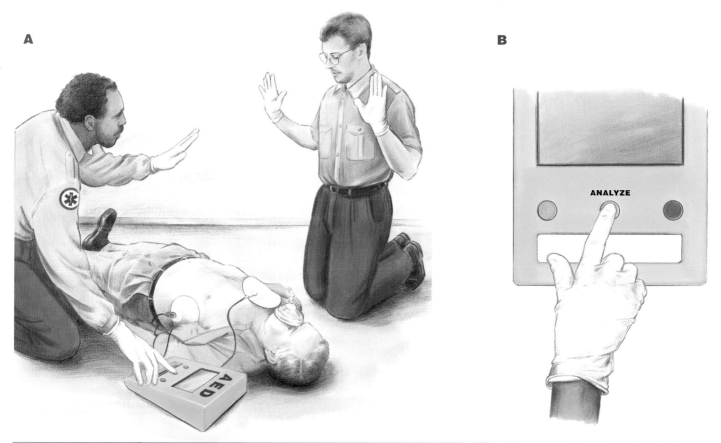

A

B

FIGURE 11. **A.** The operator "clears" the victim before delivering a shock. **B.** When everyone is "clear" of the victim, the operator presses the SHOCK button.

A

B

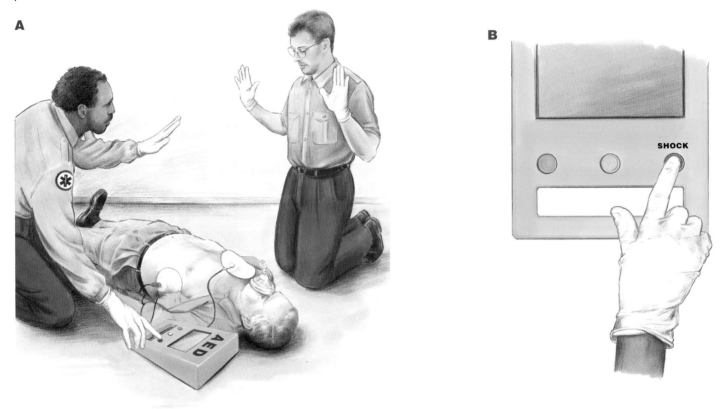

FIGURE 12. If no shock is indicated, the rescuer checks for signs of circulation, including a pulse.

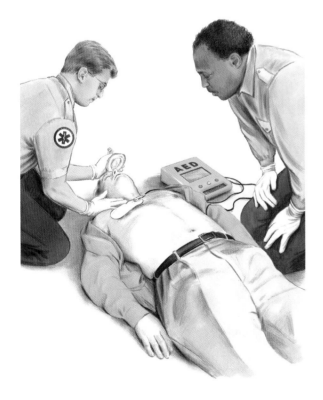

- ■ *"Shock Indicated"* **message:**

  — Clear the victim once more before pushing the SHOCK button (*"I'm clear, you're clear, oxygen's clear, everybody's clear"*) (Figure 11A).

  — Check that no one is touching the victim.

  — Press the SHOCK button (victim may display muscle contractions) (Figure 11B).

  — Press the ANALYZE and SHOCK buttons up to 2 more times if the AED signals *"shock advised"* or *"shock indicated."* (Clear the victim before each analysis and shock.)

- ■ *"No Shock Indicated"* **message:**

  — Check for signs of circulation (including a pulse) (Figure 12). If signs of circulation are present, check breathing:

    ■ If breathing is inadequate, assist breathing.

    ■ If breathing is adequate, place the victim in the recovery position, with the AED attached.

  — If no signs of circulation are present, resume CPR for 1 minute, then recheck for signs of circulation.

    ■ If there are still no signs of circulation, analyze rhythm, then follow the *"shock indicated"* or *"no shock indicated"* steps as appropriate.

Care After Successful Conversion

When signs of adequate circulation and breathing return, place the patient in the recovery position and leave the AED attached. Continue to assess the victim. Many AEDs continuously monitor the rhythm and advise the operator (*"check patient"* or *"check for signs of circulation"*) if VT/VF recurs. It is important to check breathing and signs of circulation frequently to monitor the victim's status.

PAD programs in the out-of-hospital setting should coordinate with the local EMS system to ensure seamless transfer of care after arrival of BLS or ACLS healthcare providers. When AEDs are used in the hospital, the AED can remain attached to the patient during transfer or transport to an ICU bed.

The algorithm in Figure 13 summarizes the approach to the cardiac arrest victim when an AED is used out-of-hospital.

Device Maintenance and Quality Assurance

Appropriate maintenance of the AED is vital for proper operation.[110,111] Checklists have been developed to ensure that the AED functions properly and to identify and prevent deficiencies by providing uniform device testing and increasing user familiarity with the equipment.[112] Newer AED models require almost no maintenance. These devices conduct a self-check of operation and readiness. Nonetheless, operators trained to use an AED must still make sure the AED is ready to use at any time.

AED manufacturers provide specific recommendations for maintenance and readiness, which should be followed carefully. Checklists can be obtained from manufacturers so that healthcare providers can sign off on AED readiness for use daily. If such a checklist is unavailable for any reason, healthcare providers can use the general checklist provided in Table 1.

Medical Direction

Within the constraints of state laws, ambulance providers, nurses, technicians, physician's assistants, and lay rescuers can perform some medical procedures in emergencies with a physician's medical authorization.[113] The authorizing physician assumes medical direction and takes legal responsibility for lay rescuer AED programs, BLS ambulance providers who use AEDs, and AEDs used in hospitals under protocol. The authorizing physician oversees implementation of the program, issues standing orders, and monitors the system to ensure continuous quality improvement. The rescuer must operate the AED under either the authority of the medical director or enabling administrative codes of the state or commonwealth.[113]

Case-by-Case Review

Ideally every event for which an AED is used (or could have been used) should be reviewed by the medical director or designated representative. This means that every incident in which CPR was performed or an AED was used should undergo medical review to establish whether the patient was treated according to professional standards and local standing orders. The medical review should determine whether VF and other rhythms were treated appropriately with defibrillation and BLS. Other performance dimensions that can be evaluated include command of the scene, safety, efficiency, speed, professionalism, ability to troubleshoot, completeness of patient care, and interactions with other professionals and bystanders.[114]

Quality Assurance Monitoring

Organized collection and review of patient data can identify systemwide problems and allow assessment of each link in the Chain of Survival for the adult victim of sudden cardiac death. The Utstein criteria for reporting out-of-hospital resuscitation should be used when reporting out-of-hospital arrest and resuscitation.[115] The template for use in

reporting out-of-hospital resuscitation is depicted in the *ECC Guidelines 2000*, page 363, Figure 2. Minimum data collection for reporting outcome of in-hospital resuscitation is depicted in Figure 14 of this chapter.[116] Data collection and review are quality assurance activities and as such should not expose clinical providers or organizations to increased risk of liability.

Adult victims of *witnessed* cardiac arrest of presumed cardiac etiology caused by

---

Critical Concepts: AED Maintenance

- Become familiar with your AED and how it operates.

- Check the AED for any visible problems, such as a damaged case.

- Check the *"ready-for-use"* indicator on your AED (if equipped) daily.

- Perform any other user-based maintenance according to the manufacturer's recommendations.

- Check to see that the AED carrying case contains the following accessories:

  — 2 sets of spare defibrillator electrode pads (a total of 3)

  — 2 pocket face masks

  — 1 extra battery (if appropriate for your AED; some AEDs have batteries that last for several years)

  — 2 prep razors (supplied by manufacturers)

  — 5 sterile gauze pads (4 × 4 inches), individually wrapped

  — 1 absorbent cloth towel

Remember: AED malfunctions are extremely rare. Most reported problems have been caused by the user's failure to perform maintenance on the AED.

FIGURE 13. AED algorithm for out-of-hospital use of AEDs until EMS personnel arrive.

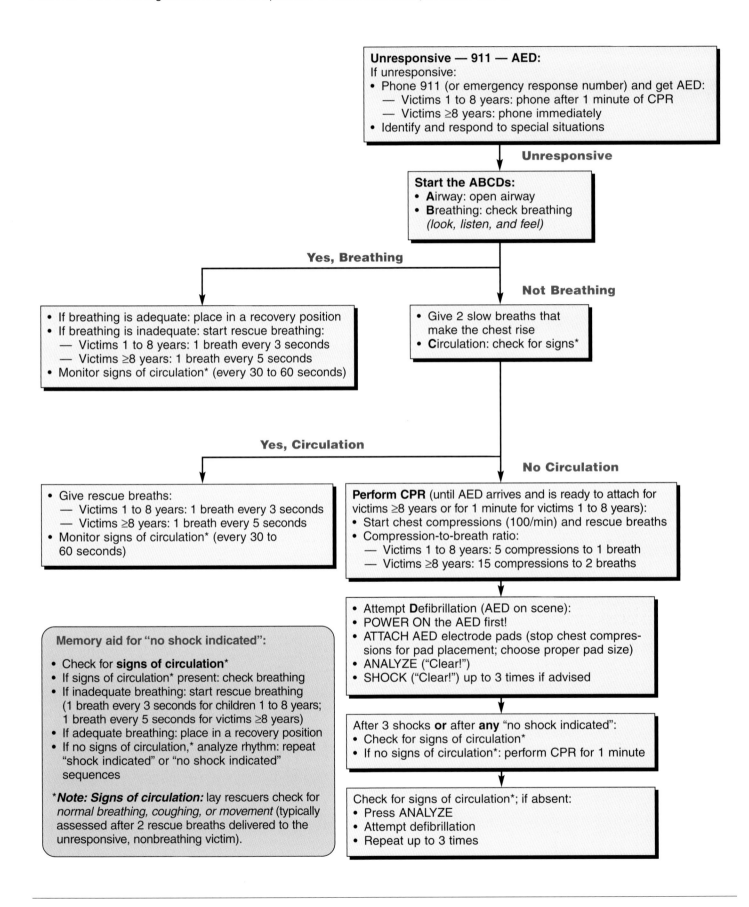

Unresponsive — 911 — AED:
If unresponsive:
• Phone 911 (or emergency response number) and get AED:
— Victims 1 to 8 years: phone after 1 minute of CPR
— Victims ≥8 years: phone immediately
• Identify and respond to special situations

Unresponsive

Start the ABCDs:
• **A**irway: open airway
• **B**reathing: check breathing
(look, listen, and feel)

Yes, Breathing

Not Breathing

• If breathing is adequate: place in a recovery position
• If breathing is inadequate: start rescue breathing:
— Victims 1 to 8 years: 1 breath every 3 seconds
— Victims ≥8 years: 1 breath every 5 seconds
• Monitor signs of circulation* (every 30 to 60 seconds)

• Give 2 slow breaths that make the chest rise
• **C**irculation: check for signs*

Yes, Circulation

No Circulation

• Give rescue breaths:
— Victims 1 to 8 years: 1 breath every 3 seconds
— Victims ≥8 years: 1 breath every 5 seconds
• Monitor signs of circulation* (every 30 to 60 seconds)

Perform CPR (until AED arrives and is ready to attach for victims ≥8 years or for 1 minute for victims 1 to 8 years):
• Start chest compressions (100/min) and rescue breaths
• Compression-to-breath ratio:
— Victims 1 to 8 years: 5 compressions to 1 breath
— Victims ≥8 years: 15 compressions to 2 breaths

Memory aid for "no shock indicated":

• Check for **signs of circulation***
• If signs of circulation* present: check breathing
• If inadequate breathing: start rescue breathing (1 breath every 3 seconds for children 1 to 8 years; 1 breath every 5 seconds for victims ≥8 years)
• If adequate breathing: place in a recovery position
• If no signs of circulation,* analyze rhythm: repeat "shock indicated" or "no shock indicated" sequences

*__Note: Signs of circulation:__ lay rescuers check for *normal breathing, coughing, or movement* (typically assessed after 2 rescue breaths delivered to the unresponsive, nonbreathing victim).

• Attempt **D**efibrillation (AED on scene):
• POWER ON the AED first!
• ATTACH AED electrode pads (stop chest compressions for pad placement; choose proper pad size)
• ANALYZE ("Clear!")
• SHOCK ("Clear!") up to 3 times if advised

After 3 shocks **or** after **any** "no shock indicated":
• Check for signs of circulation*
• If no signs of circulation*: perform CPR for 1 minute

Check for signs of circulation*; if absent:
• Press ANALYZE
• Attempt defibrillation
• Repeat up to 3 times

FIGURE 14. Utstein criteria for reporting outcomes of in-hospital resuscitation.

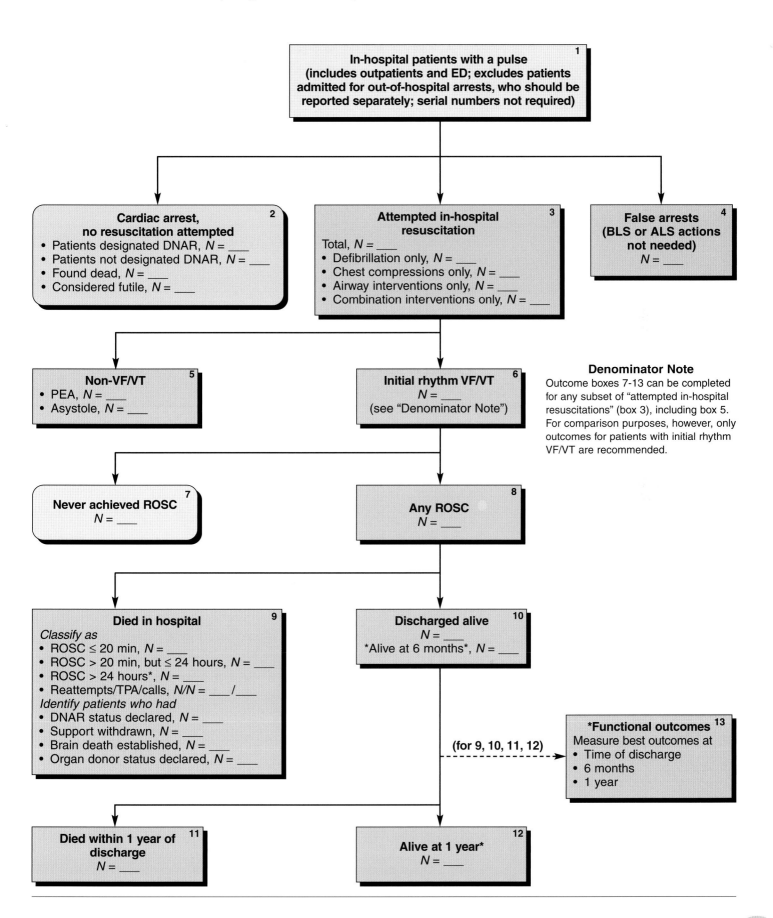

Table 1.

Readiness-for-Use Checklist: Automated External Defibrillators for Healthcare Providers: Daily/Weekly Checklist

Organization Name/Identifier _____ **Mfr/Model No.** _____ **Serial/ID No.** _____

Date ____ **Covering Period** ____ **to** ____

At the beginning of each shift or at the scheduled time, inspect the device using the checklist below. Note any inconsistencies, deficiencies, and corrective actions taken. If the device is not ready for use or is out of service, write OOS on the "day of month" line and note deficiencies in the corrective action log.

Day of Month/Signature/Unit No.

1. _____
2. _____
3. _____
4. _____
5. _____
6. _____
7. _____
8. _____
9. _____
10. _____
11. _____
12. _____
13. _____
14. _____
15. _____
16. _____
17. _____
18. _____
19. _____
20. _____
21. _____
22. _____
23. _____
24. _____
25. _____
26. _____
27. _____
28. _____
29. _____
30. _____
31. _____

Corrective Action Log

Example: 5. John Jones (signature)/Aid 2 checked Aid 2's device on the 5th day of this month and found it ready for use.

1. Defibrillator unit
a. Clean, no spills, unobstructed
b. Casing intact

2. Defibrillation cables and connectors
a. Inspect for cracks, broken wires, or damage
b. Connectors engage securely

3. Supplies available
a. Two sets of unexpired hands-free defibrillator pads in sealed packages
b. PPE — gloves, barrier device, or equivalent
c. Razor and scissors
d. Hand towel
e. *Spare event documentation device
f. *ECG paper
g. *ECG monitoring electrodes
h. *ALS module/key/equivalent

4. Power supply
a. Verify fully charged battery(ies) in place
b. *Spare charged battery available
c. *Rotate batteries per manufacturer's specifications
d. *AC power plugged into live outlet

5. Indicators and screen display
a. *POWER ON display and self-test OK
b. *ECG monitor display functional
c. *No error or service required indicator/message
d. Correct time displayed/set; synchronized with dispatch center

6. ECG paper and event documentation device
a. *Event documentation device in place and functional
b. * Adequate ECG paper
c. *ECG recorder functional

7. Charge/display cycle for defibrillation
a. Test per manufacturer's recommended test procedure
b. *Identifies shockable rhythm
c. *Charges to appropriate energy level
d. *Acceptable discharge detected

8. AED returned to patient ready status

*Applicable only if the device has this capability/feature or if required by medical authorization.

VF are the best group on which to focus because they are more homogeneous than those with nonwitnessed arrest or non-VF rhythms. Data from homogeneous groups can be compared across EMS systems or hospitals. If the arrest occurs out-of-hospital, a lower-than-expected survival to hospital discharge rate may be explained by a variety of factors, including delayed activation of EMS, long EMS response intervals, infrequent witnessed arrests, rare bystander CPR, or slow on-scene times to defibrillation. If the arrest occurs in hospital, a lower-than-expected survival to hospital discharge rate may be explained by different factors, such as the severity of underlying heart disease or other comorbidities, delay to retrieval of the AED, or problems with device maintenance or operator error. Each of these problems can be addressed with a specific programwide effort. Continued systematic and uniform data collection will determine whether the new efforts succeed (see the following section for more details about outcome reporting).

ECC Systems and the AED

The ECC Systems Concept

The term *Chain of Survival*[39] provides a useful metaphor for the elements of the ECC systems concept (see Figure 15), which summarizes the elements required to maximize survival in adults after sudden cardiac arrest.[117] The 4 links in this chain are early access to the EMS system, early CPR, early defibrillation,

and early advanced cardiovascular care. Epidemiological and clinical research have established that effective emergency cardiovascular care, whether in or out of hospital, depends on strong links that are closely interconnected.[39,45,118,119] The effectiveness of early defibrillation and PAD programs also depends on a strong Chain of Survival in the community and the hospital.

Early Defibrillation

For early defibrillation to be a reality, the first person to arrive at the scene of a cardiac arrest should have a defibrillator.[56] This concept is now internationally accepted.[117,120] Healthcare providers with a duty to perform CPR should be trained, equipped, and authorized to attempt defibrillation.[117] Early defibrillation with an AED has established benefit when performed by BLS ambulance providers,[121-123] hospital-based healthcare providers,[34-38] and trained laypersons in public access defibrillation programs.[29,30,124,125]

Out-of-Hospital BLS Providers and AEDs

The BLS provider is the most common type of emergency responder in the world. BLS rescuers provide BLS but not invasive interventions such as tracheal intubation, IV access, or IV medications. In the United States a BLS-prepared emergency responder is usually called an *emergency medical technician-basic (EMT-B)*. Because BLS providers are commonly the first emergency personnel to reach the scene of an out-of-hospital

cardiac arrest, they should be trained to use an AED.[117,120]

The clinical benefits and practical superiority of the AED are well established. Several studies have established many practical advantages of AED use by BLS ambulance providers. Initial training and continuing education programs to ensure that BLS providers can operate an AED can be simple, brief, and inexpensive. AEDs can be operated more quickly than conventional defibrillators.[69,72,73] Several studies have confirmed AED accuracy,[126] shorter times to defibrillation,[127-129] faster application of subsequent ACLS interventions,[127] and comparable[130-132] or improved[12,133-138] survival rates. Taken together, these studies stand as powerful confirmation of the value of early defibrillation by out-of-hospital emergency personnel. Early defibrillation is recommended as a standard of care for EMS personnel[33,138,139] except in sparsely populated and remote settings, where the frequency of cardiac arrest is low and rescuer response times are excessively long.[140-142]

In-Hospital Use of AEDs

An approach pioneered by William Kaye and others[34-38] is now being used by many hospitals: general care nurses are being trained to use AEDs in resuscitation attempts. In-hospital records have documented long delays (5 to 10 minutes) between collapse and first shock by conventional in-hospital response teams.[143,144] Delayed defibrillation occurs infrequently in monitored beds and critical care units,

FIGURE 15. The adult Chain of Survival.

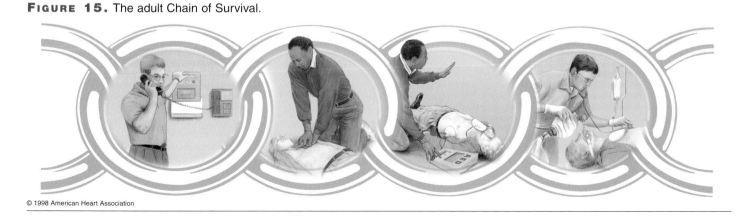

Lay rescuer AED responders are a diverse group that can be roughly categorized into 3 levels whose number and variety change daily.

Level 1: Nontraditional Responders

Nontraditional responders are persons other than healthcare personnel, such as police, firefighters, security personnel, ski patrol members, ferryboat crews, and flight attendants, whose occupations require them to respond to an emergency. Traditionally, however, they have not been asked or expected to take any action other than to perform basic CPR.

Level 2: Targeted Responders

Targeted, or *worksite*, *responders* may also be called *citizen responders*. These responders are employees of companies, corporations, or public facilities in which lay rescuer AED programs have been established. Targeted responders are located at the worksite (eg, central reception area staff) during hours when the worksite is most populated. The targeted responder is a natural choice to be the primary responder with the AED.

Level 3: Responders to Persons at High Risk

Another category of responders is *family members and friends of persons at high risk for sudden cardiac death*. They participate in early defibrillation programs and are taught CPR and use of an AED.

but it occurs more often in nonmonitored hospital beds and outpatient and diagnostic facilities, which may be occupied by hundreds of patients each day. In such areas it may be many minutes before

centralized response teams arrive with a defibrillator, attach it to the patient, and deliver shocks.[143] Resuscitation committees may inappropriately place more emphasis on *arrival* of the hospital emergency response (code) team than on *delivery of the first shock*.[34]

As with out-of-hospital care, in-hospital BLS practice must expand to include CPR *and* defibrillation.[145] Many hospitals underuse their personnel in resuscitative efforts and have not made significant attempts to ensure that early defibrillation occurs by placing AEDs in noncritical care areas.[146,147]

Several obstacles must be overcome before a quality early defibrillation program using AEDs can be successfully implemented in the hospital setting. Nurses can be trained to use an AED and retain the skills needed for its safe and effective operation.[34,148] Strategic deployment of AEDs throughout hospital areas and authorization and training of first-responding personnel in their use will be necessary to bring in-hospital use of AEDs up to the level of out-of-hospital programs.[36,37] AED training must be incorporated into BLS training for all hospital personnel expected to respond to a cardiac arrest.

Documentation of in-hospital resuscitation events is often inaccurate because each rescuer uses a different, unsynchronized time source, such as a wristwatch, wall clock, or bedside clock. As a result hospital records of resuscitation intervals are unreliable for making quantitative assessments of critical components such as time to defibrillation and other interventions during resuscitation. Recorded times must be standardized before reliable data can be collected to enable accurate assessment of resuscitation practices. In many countries AEDs can be equipped with a timing mechanism that is synchronized with governmental atomic clock satellites. The AED clock can then become the gold standard for timing resuscitation events. Accurate time-interval data must be obtained because this

information is the key to future high-quality research.

In the United States the lack of an organized systemwide resuscitation program prompted the Joint Commission for the Accreditation of Healthcare Organizations (JCAHO) to revise its standards for in-hospital resuscitation.[149] JCAHO now evaluates member hospitals on their plans to establish the following:

1. Appropriate policies, procedures, processes, or protocols governing provision of resuscitation services

2. Appropriate equipment placed strategically throughout the hospital close to areas where patients are likely to require resuscitation services

3. Ongoing review of outcomes related to resuscitation in the aggregate to identify opportunities for improvement of resuscitative efforts

4. Appropriate staff trained and competent to recognize the need for and use of designated equipment in resuscitative efforts

5. Appropriate data collection related to the process and outcomes of resuscitation, particularly the ability to track trends and changes over several years

The National Registry of Cardiopulmonary Resuscitation (NRCPR) is a national database of information on outcome of in-hospital resuscitation interventions. The AHA established the NRCPR to assist participating hospitals in systematic data collection of resuscitative efforts documenting the resuscitation performance of those hospitals over time. This information can establish the baseline performance of a participating hospital, target problem areas, and identify opportunities for improvement in its resuscitation program. Each participating hospital receives quarterly reports comparing its outcome data with that of an appropriate peer group. The NRCPR is patterned after the highly respected British Resuscitation Study (Bresus) and is based on the Utstein guidelines for collecting and reporting information from in-hospital resuscitation events.[115,116] The information collected in the NRCPR will undoubtedly be of great value to participating medical centers for quality-assurance monitoring. In addition, the registry is the largest repository of information on in-hospital cardiopulmonary arrest, so it will undoubtedly yield valuable information about large groups of inpatients with analysis within subgroups.[37] For information about subscribing to the NRCPR, contact www.info@nrcpr.org.

Modern hospitals must be capable of providing early defibrillation in patient-care areas. The goal for all hospitals should be to have first responders provide *early* defibrillation to collapsed patients in VF in all areas of the hospital and ambulatory care facilities. The time interval defined as *"early"* was discussed extensively at the International Guidelines 2000 Conference. The approach to development of early defibrillation programs should be *"the earlier the better,"* and evaluation and intervention should occur when prolonged collapse-to-shock intervals are documented. Experts at the Guidelines 2000 Conference endorsed a goal of collapse-to–first shock interval of 3±1 minutes for a high percentage of in-hospital arrests.

Lay Rescuer AED Programs

The concept of public access defibrillation (PAD) was originally developed and explored by Douglas Chamberlain in Brighton, England, and by Mickey Eisenberg in King County, Washington. Professor Chamberlain placed AEDs in train stations and commercial aircraft. Dr Eisenberg placed AEDs with families of high-risk patients. To encourage the concept of early defibrillation, the AHA Task Force on Early Defibrillation hosted 2 conferences on PAD.[32,33]

The recommendations that emerged from the 2 conferences included the recognition that automated external defibrillation is the most promising method for achieving rapid defibrillation and that AEDs and training in AED use should be available to the community.[32,33] Placement of AEDs in selected locations for immediate use by trained laypersons may be the key intervention to significantly increase survival from out-of-hospital cardiac arrest. The demonstrated safety and effectiveness of the AED makes it an ideal source of early defibrillation by trained laypersons.[56,67] Conceptually the AED is like a sharp diagnostic and therapeutic probe searching for just one phenomenon — shockable rhythm (VT/VF) — and providing a potentially lifesaving therapy over just a few milliseconds. AEDs are of no value for non-VT/VF arrests and provide no benefit after VT/VF has been terminated. Therefore, it is critical that rescuers be capable of opening the airway and providing effective ventilation and chest compressions. All persons who operate an AED must still be trained to provide effective CPR.

AED Lay Rescuers

Lay rescuer AED programs imply expanded use of AEDs in the community to the broadest possible number of rescuers while maintaining safety and effectiveness.[32,33,150] At the start of the new millennium an ever-increasing range of laypersons and healthcare professionals are learning the combined skills of CPR and AED use.

Development of Lay Rescuer AED Programs

The first step in initial planning for a lay rescuer AED program requires that the program director determine whether the population of the geographic area covered by the program will likely benefit. A variety of guidelines have been recommended to identify populations with a need for a lay rescuer AED program. Some lay rescuer AED program planners target locations with a large concentration of persons more than 50 years old, such as senior citizen centers.[151] Implementation of AED programs in places where more than 10 000 people gather has been recommended for consideration.[117]

Ideally program planners should review community-wide cardiac arrest data, identify sites with the highest incidence of cardiac arrest, and target those locations for AED placement. A few fundamental calculations are provided in the FYI box.

Location

Some data on the location and frequency of cardiac arrests in metropolitan areas is available. In Seattle and King County, Washington, for example, the incidence of cardiac arrest is greatest at the international airport, then (in decreasing order of frequency) the county correctional facilities, shopping malls, public sports venues, industrial sites, golf courses, shelters, ferries/train terminals, health clubs/gyms, and community/senior centers.[152] The site-specific incidence and proposed distribution of AEDs within those sites is likely to vary with each community. To optimize the benefit of limited healthcare resources in each community, it is essential for program planners to implement the use of AEDs in locations with the highest incidence of cardiac arrest.

Accordingly, the evidence supports the establishment of lay rescuer AED programs in sites that

1. Have a frequency of cardiac arrest events for which there is a reasonable probability of AED use (an estimated event rate of 1 sudden cardiac arrest per 1000 adult person-years)

2. Cannot reliably achieve an EMS call-to-shock interval of less than 5 minutes with conventional EMS services

3. Can reliably achieve (in more than 90% of cases) a collapse-to-shock interval of less than 5 minutes by training and equipping laypersons to function as first responders in the community so that they recognize cardiac arrest, phone 911 (or other emergency response number), initiate CPR, and attach and operate an AED

FYI: Calculations to Estimate the Frequency of Sudden Cardiac Arrest and Need for a Lay Rescuer AED Program

1. *Frequency of sudden cardiac arrest*

a. 1 sudden cardiac arrest per 1000 adult population (victim is typically more than 40 years of age) per year

b. 1000 people more than 40 years old living 365 days (24 h/d) per year is 1000 person-years (this is equivalent to 1 sudden cardiac arrest per 8.76 million person-hours)

c. To calculate the number of cardiac arrests in a stadium in which 100 000 adults are present for 5 hours at a time for a football game represents 500 000 person-hours per football game. Anticipate 1 sudden cardiac arrest every 17.5 games (1 arrest per 8.76 million person-hours divided by 500 000 person-hours per game).

2. *Calculating the need for a lay rescuer AED program*

a. A lay rescuer AED program is generally thought to be advisable if it results in 1 "defibrillation opportunity" per AED every 5 years. The 5-year range is now the average life expectancy of an AED.

b. The numbers described in the first calculation above could be converted from 1 sudden cardiac arrest per 1000 adults per year to 1 sudden cardiac arrest per 200 adults every 5 years.

c. 1 use of an AED every 5 years would be expected for every community in which there are 200 person-years (200 × 365 d/y × 24 h/d = 1.752 million person-hours or approximately 20% of the numbers in 1 above)

Coordination With EMS

Lay rescuer AED program planners coordinate AED programs with the local EMS system. Elements of coordination may include but are not limited to medical direction, assistance in planning AED deployment and AED protocols, training, continuous quality improvement, monitoring, and review of AED events. Integration with the local EMS dispatch system is important because many dispatch systems use phone-directed protocols to assist rescuers in the use of the AED if needed and will notify EMS en route that an AED is being used at the scene.[153,154] The American College of Emergency Physicians has issued a policy statement endorsing coordination with EMS systems to ensure medical direction of AED programs, including those in which bystanders use AEDs.[155]

Elements of Successful Lay Rescuer AED Programs

Objective data on the details of successful lay rescuer AED programs is lacking. Nonetheless, rational conjecture plus data extrapolated from other sources have identified many elements as keys to successful lay rescuer AED programs. There must be a strong Chain of Survival in the community. Innovative methods for training laypersons in the use of AEDs, such as those used in the AHA Heartsaver AED Course,[109] provide effective, quality education. Incorporating EMS and EMS dispatch into the lay rescuer AED program allows dispatchers to alert a caller to the nearest AED location and provide instruction by telephone if needed. It also allows the EMS system to learn to operate specific types of AEDs in advance, enabling seamless patient care.[153,154]

Performance of continuous quality improvement is vital to a successful lay rescuer AED program. The program director should carefully select AED rescuers who are motivated, available during the expected response period, and capable of performing their duties. A specific response plan should be implemented in each site, with the target being a collapse-to-defibrillation time of 4 to 5 minutes or less. Ideally AEDs are located throughout the facility so that the walk to get an AED is 1.5 minutes or less (meaning that a round trip to get the AED and return to the victim's side will require no more than 3 minutes). The AHA recommends that the lay rescuer AED program director or trainer conduct frequent unannounced practice drills and evaluation of performance and response times.

The most frequent cause of allegations of AED "malfunction" is a lack of maintenance.[110,111] The AED must be maintained according to the manufacturer's specifications[112] (see Table 2). Regular system evaluations should be conducted. Lay rescuer AED program directors are learning the value of attending to the emotional needs of lay rescuers, who are not accustomed to providing lifesaving care in an emergency.[156] Case-by-case review with laypersons and critical-incident stress debriefing provide important support for participants in lay rescuer AED programs.[156] One person should be responsible for the quality of training and medical care provided by lay responders. Finally, lay rescuer AED programs must comply with state law.

Effectiveness of Lay Rescuer AED Programs

Several studies have shown that early defibrillation not only saves lives but also is cost-effective. The cost-effectiveness of AED use by BLS ambulance providers and in lay rescuer AED programs has been compared with other medical interventions.[57,151,157,158] This data establishes the substantial survival benefits and attractive cost-effectiveness of well-designed and implemented lay rescuer AED programs.

Table 2.

Readiness-for-Use Checklist: Lay Rescuer AED Program
Date _____ Covering Period _____ to _____
*(This checklist can cover 1 month if **daily** check is used or 1 year if **monthly** check is used.)*

Organization Name/Identifier _____ **Mfr/Model No.** _____ **Serial/ID No.** _____

At the beginning of each shift or scheduled time, inspect the AED, using the checklist below. Note any inconsistencies, deficiencies, and corrective actions taken. If the device is not ready for use or out of service, write OOS on the "day of month" line and note deficiencies in the corrective action log.

Daily check:
1. Visually inspect the AED (if in "alarmed" holder):
  a. In proper location
  b. Clean, no spills
  c. No signs of tampering or inappropriate opening
  d. All readiness-for-use indicators, including battery, indicate "ready"

Monthly check (assuming no clinical uses):
2. Defibrillator cables and connectors
  a. Inspect for any outward signs of damage
  b. Engage/disengage connectors (pads to cables, cables to AED)
3. Supplies available
  a. 3 sets of unexpired hands-free defibrillator pads in sealed packages
  b. Personal protective equipment (gloves, barrier device)
  c. Razor and scissors
  d. Hand towel
  e. *Spare event documentation module ("Flash" card, PCMCIA card, magnetic storage)
4. Power supply
  a. Inspect battery-status display
  b. Verify AED signals "AED ready for use" or equivalent
  c. *AC power plugged into main if battery requires "trickle charge"
5. Indicators and screen display
  a. *POWER ON, self-test runs, display runs, verify OK
  b. *Monitor display functional
  c. *No "error" or "service required" indicator/message
  d. *Correct time displayed/set; synchronized with dispatch center/set
6. ECG event documentation module
  a. Follow manufacturer's recommendations
  b. *Event documentation module in place and functional
7. Charge/discharge cycle to simulated VF
  a. Perform charge/discharge test cycle per mfr's recommendations
  b. Input shockable rhythm (VF); use proper connection components
  c. *AED analysis identifies shockable rhythm
  d. *Charges to appropriate energy level
  e. *Acceptable discharge detected
8. AED returned to ready-for-use status

Indicates features that vary greatly among AED brands and models. Applies only to devices with this capability or feature or if required by medical authority.

Day of Month/Signature/Unit No.

1. _____
2. _____
3. _____
4. _____
5. _____
6. _____
7. _____
8. _____
9. _____
10. _____
11. _____
12. _____
13. _____
14. _____
15. _____
16. _____
17. _____
18. _____
19. _____
20. _____
21. _____
22. _____
23. _____
24. _____
25. _____
26. _____
27. _____
28. _____
29. _____
30. _____
31. _____

Example: *5. John Jones (signature)/AED 2 checked on October 5 and found ready for use.*

Corrective Action Log

_____
_____
_____
_____
_____
_____
_____
_____

Month/Signature/Unit No.

January: _____
February: _____
March: _____
April: _____
May: _____
June: _____
July: _____
August: _____
September: _____
October: _____
November: _____
December: _____

The National Heart, Lung, and Blood Institute (NHLBI), in partnership with the AHA and industry, has embarked on a multisite, controlled, prospective clinical trial to determine the efficacy and cost-effectiveness of placing AEDs in a variety of public settings. Such definitive scientific evidence is essential for decision making related to the potentially huge lay rescuer AED program initiative. Final results from the clinical trial are not expected for 3 years or longer.

Lay Rescuer AED Program Legislation

Most states have adopted legislation that has extended limited immunity (most often, Good Samaritan immunity) to lay rescuers who use AEDs. In states without provisions for such immunity, recent federal legislation signed into law provides limited immunity to lay rescuers using AEDs and owners who place AEDs on their premises. Because state legislation varies with respect to immunity coverage and training requirements, the AHA has recommended that certain elements be included in lay rescuer AED program legislation.[32,33]

Critical elements in state legislation include limited immunity for the lay rescuer who uses the AED as a Good Samaritan and the requirement that the rescuer be trained in both CPR and AED use according to nationally recognized course protocols. *Highly recommended* elements include conferring limited immunity to owners of premises in which AEDs are located, physicians who prescribe AEDs for home or other use, and instructors who teach CPR and AED use. There should be physician authorization for AED use and physician involvement in the AED program. The AED should be maintained and operated according to the manufacturer's specifications and the PAD program integrated into the existing EMS system. *Recommended* elements include case-by-case review with a physician or medical authority and specification that persons not trained in AED use can use an AED if they are acting as Good Samaritans.[32,33]

Most states have passed legislation enabling lay rescuer AED programs.[159] The laws regarding use of AEDs vary from state to state. Laypersons using AEDs should be aware of and comply with state laws when operating AEDs. In the United States the AHA 4-hour Heartsaver AED Course[109] is the model for documented effective training in the skills of CPR and AED use and has been approved by most states for training laypersons.

Education and Training

Skills Maintenance

Survey results and experience in rural communities have demonstrated that an emergency responder may go several years without treating a patient in cardiac arrest.[140-142] Therefore, every program director must determine how to ensure correct performance of BLS and use of an AED when such an event occurs. Principles of adult education suggest that frequent practice of psychomotor skills such as use of an AED in a simulated cardiac arrest offers the best skills maintenance.

Frequency of Practice

The frequency and content of these practice sessions have been established by several successful programs.[6,55,107,140] At present many programs promote practice drills every 3 to 6 months, an interval they consider satisfactory. Many EMS personnel and systems drill as often as once a month. The most successful long-term skills maintenance occurs when individual rescuers perform a quick check of the equipment frequently and regularly. This check includes a visual inspection of the defibrillator components and controls and a mental review of the steps to be followed and controls to be operated during a cardiac arrest.

The AHA ECC Committee as well as international resuscitation councils encourage routine skills review and practice sessions at least every 6 months. The required AHA renewal interval is 2 years. Resuscitation councils outside the United States recommend a renewal interval of 1 to 2 years for certification according to the certifying body.

The Future of Lay Rescuer AED Programs

The future of lay rescuer AED programs is likely to include further improvements in device design, making AEDs easier to use, lighter, and less expensive. Public access to AEDs is growing, and implementation of AEDs in a diversity of settings is increasing. Survival from VF cardiac arrest will continue to increase if AED programs are well implemented and AEDs are used within the first few minutes after cardiac arrest.

Summary of Key Concepts

- The time from collapse to defibrillation is the single greatest determinant of survival from cardiac arrest.

- Public access defibrillation expands the routine use of AEDs within the community to the broadest number of rescuers while maintaining safety and effectiveness.

- The purpose of an AED is to provide the earliest possible defibrillation to victims of VF.

- The 4 steps of AED operation are (1) **POWER ON** the AED first!, (2) **ATTACH** adhesive electrode pads to the victim's chest (stop chest compressions), (3) **ANALYZE** the victim's rhythm, and (4) charge the AED and deliver the **SHOCK** (if indicated)

- Proper AED electrode pad placement can be achieved by viewing the illustration on the AED or the surface of the electrode pads. One pad is placed in the upper right sternal border directly below the clavicle. The other pad is placed lateral to the left nipple, with the top margin of the pad a few inches below the axilla.

- The AED operator is responsible for ensuring that that no one is touching the victim during the analyze, charging, and shock modes. Touching the patient during the analyze mode interferes with the device's interpretation of the victim's rhythm. Partial transfer of the shock to bystanders is possible if someone is touching the victim during the charging and shock modes.

✓ The following situations require a change in actions when using an AED: a victim who (1) is a child less than 8 years old (use child pads if available), (2) whose chest is covered by water (move victim out of water, wipe chest), (3) has an implanted pacemaker or defibrillator (place the electrode pad away from the device), or (4) has a transdermal medication patch (remove the patch and clean the chest wall).

✓ If both adult and child pads are available, the rescuer should be sure to use adult pads for adult victims and child pads for victims less than 8 years of age.

✓ The sequence of actions following a *"no shock indicated"* AED message is

1. Check for signs of circulation

2. If signs of circulation are present, check breathing:

   ■ If breathing is inadequate, assist breathing.

   ■ If breathing is adequate, place the victim in the recovery position, but leave the AED attached to the patient.

3. If signs of circulation are not present, resume CPR for 1 minute, then recheck the pulse.

4. If no pulse, analyze the rhythm.

5. After rhythm analysis, follow the *"shock indicated"* or *"no shock indicated"* steps.

✓ The 3 clinical findings that indicate the need to begin chest compressions and attach an AED are the 3 criteria for establishing the presence of cardiac arrest:

■ Unresponsiveness

■ No effective breathing

■ No signs of circulation

✓ Rescuers who find an unresponsive adult victim should activate the emergency response system (and get the AED), perform CPR, and if cardiac arrest is present, attach and use the AED.

Review Questions

1. You find an unresponsive adult. After you activate the emergency response system and get the AED, you return to the victim. When you discover that the victim is not breathing, you open the airway and provide 2 breaths. You find no pulse and no signs of circulation, and you prepare to operate the AED. What are the 4 universal steps required to operate an AED?

   a. phone 911, begin CPR, use the AED, and provide advanced life support

   b. move the victim to a safe place, attach the electrode pads to the victim's chest, attach the cables to the electrode pads, and attach the cables to the AED

   c. check for a pulse, POWER ON, deliver a shock, and then analyze the victim's rhythm

   d. POWER ON, ATTACH the electrode pads to the victim's chest and the AED, ANALYZE the victim's rhythm, and deliver a shock if needed

2. You are assessing a 42-year-old woman and note that she has a pulse, although it is weak. But her face has turned blue and she is not breathing. Your next step is to

   a. attach the AED and start the SHOCK cycle

   b. attach the AED and press "ANALYZE"

   c. open the airway and initiate rescue breathing

   d. attach the AED and monitor the victim's rhythm

3. You see a middle-aged man clutch his chest and collapse to the ground. Which of the following groups of clinical criteria indicate the need for initiating chest compressions and use of an AED?

   a. unresponsive, weak pulse, no breathing

   b. unresponsive, no pulse, weak breathing

   c. unresponsive, weak pulse, weak breathing

   d. unresponsive, no pulse, no breathing

4. You are alone when you see an adult suddenly collapse. The correct sequence of actions to take is

   a. phone the emergency response system, verify unresponsiveness, perform ABCD

   b. phone 911, ABCD, verify unresponsiveness

   c. verify unresponsiveness, activate the emergency response system, then begin ABCD

   d. verify unresponsiveness, begin the ABCDs, activate the emergency response system

5. You attach an AED to the chest of a 43-year-old victim who is unresponsive, not breathing, and pulseless. After 3 shocks the AED advises *"no shock indicated,"* and the victim is still pulseless. What should you do?

   a. continue a second set of 3 shocks

   b. press the ANALYZE button and defibrillate if appropriate

   c. perform CPR for 1 minute, check signs of circulation, and if absent, press ANALYZE

   d. perform CPR until EMS arrives

6. You are treating a victim of cardiac arrest with an AED. You have powered on the AED, attached the AED electrode pads, and pushed the ANALYZE button. The AED has charged and gives the *"shock indicated"* message. Your next step is to

   a. push the SHOCK button

   b. clear the victim and ensure that no one is touching the patient

   c. press ANALYZE

   d. check pulse

How did you do?

Answers: **1,** d; **2,** c; **3,** d; **4,** c; **5,** c; **6,** b.

References

1. Atkins JM. Emergency medical service systems in acute cardiac care: state of the art. *Circulation.* 1986;74(suppl 6, pt 2):IV-4-IV-8.

2. Cummins RO, Eisenberg MS, Stults KR. Automatic external defibrillators: clinical issues for cardiology. *Circulation.* 1986;73: 381-385.

3. White RD. EMT-defibrillation: time for controlled implementation of effective treatment. *American Heart Association Emergency Cardiac Care National Faculty Newsletter.* 1986;8:1-3.

4. Atkins JM, Murphy D, Allison EJ Jr, Graves JR. Toward earlier defibrillation. *J Emerg Med Serv.* 1986;11:70.

5. Eisenberg MS, Cummins RO. Defibrillation performed by the emergency medical technician. *Circulation.* 1986;74(suppl 6, pt 2): IV-9-IV-12.

6. Cummins RO. EMT-defibrillation: national guidelines for implementation. *Am J Emerg Med.* 1987;5:254-257.

7. Ruskin JN. Automatic external defibrillators and sudden cardiac death. *N Engl J Med.* 1988;319:713-715.

8. Cummins RO, Eisenberg MS. EMT-defibrillation: a proven concept. *American Heart Association Emergency Cardiac Care National Faculty Newsletter.* 1984;1:1-3.

9. Cummins RO, Eisenberg MS, Moore JE, Hearne TR, Andresen E, Wendt R, Litwin PE, Graves JR, Hallstrom AP, Pierce J. Automatic external defibrillators: clinical, training, psychological, and public health issues. *Ann Emerg Med.* 1985;14:755-760.

10. Newman MM. National EMT-D study. *J Emerg Med Serv.* 1986;11:70-72.

11. Newman MM. The survival advantage: early defibrillation programs in the fire service. *J Emerg Med Serv.* 1987;12:40-46.

12. Sedgwick ML, Watson J, Dalziel K, Carrington DJ, Cobbe SM. Efficacy of out-of-hospital defibrillation by ambulance technicians using automated external defibrillators: the Heartstart Scotland Project. *Resuscitation.* 1992;24:73-87.

13. Mols P, Beaucarne E, Bruyninx J, Labruyere JP, De Myttenaere L, Naeije N, Watteeuw G, Verset D, Flamand JP. Early defibrillation by EMTs: the Brussels experience. *Resuscitation.* 1994;27:129-136.

14. Stapczynski JS, Svenson JE, Stone CK. Population density, automated external defibrillator use, and survival in rural cardiac arrest. *Acad Emerg Med.* 1997;4:552-558.

15. Cummins RO, Eisenberg MS, Bergner L, Hallstrom A, Hearne T, Murray JA. Automatic external defibrillation: evaluations of its role in the home and in emergency medical services.

Ann Emerg Med. 1984;13(suppl 9, pt 2): 798-801.

16. Jacobs L. Medical, legal, and social implications of automatic external defibrillators. *Ann Emerg Med.* 1986;15:863-864.

17. White RD, Vukov LF, Bugliosi TF. Early defibrillation by police: initial experience with measurement of critical time intervals and patient outcome. *Ann Emerg Med.* 1994;23: 1009-1013.

18. White RD, Asplin BR, Bugliosi TF, Hankins DG. High discharge survival rate after out-of-hospital ventricular fibrillation with rapid defibrillation by police and paramedics. *Ann Emerg Med.* 1996;28:480-485.

19. White RD, Hankins DG, Bugliosi TF. Seven years' experience with early defibrillation by police and paramedics in an emergency medical services system. *Resuscitation.* 1998;39: 145-151.

20. Davis EA, Mosesso VN Jr. Performance of police first responders in utilizing automated external defibrillation on victims of sudden cardiac arrest. *Prehosp Emerg Care.* 1998;2: 101-107.

21. Mosesso VN Jr, Davis EA, Auble TE, Paris PM, Yealy DM. Use of automated external defibrillators by police officers for treatment of out-of-hospital cardiac arrest. *Ann Emerg Med.* 1998;32:200-207.

22. Davis EA, McCrorry J, Mosesso VN Jr. Institution of a police automated external defibrillation program: concepts and practice. *Prehosp Emerg Care.* 1999;3:60-65.

23. O'Rourke MF, Donaldson E, Geddes JS. An airline cardiac arrest program. *Circulation.* 1997;96:2849-2853.

24. Wolbrink A, Borrillo D. Airline use of automatic external defibrillators: shocking developments. *Aviat Space Environ Med.* 1999;70: 87-88.

25. Eisenberg MS, Horwood BT, Cummins RO, Reynolds-Haertle R, Hearne TR. Cardiac arrest and resuscitation: a tale of 29 cities. *Ann Emerg Med.* 1990;19:179-186.

26. Gundry JW, Comess KA, DeRook FA, Jorgenson D, Bardy GH. Comparison of naïve sixth-grade children with trained professionals in the use of an automated external defibrillator. *Circulation.* 1999;100:1703-1707.

27. Valenzuela TD, Roe DJ, Nichol G, Clark LL, Spaite DW. Casino project: implications for public access defibrillation. *Acad Emerg Med.* 2000;7:426.

28. Eisenberg MS, Moore J, Cummins RO, Andresen E, Litwin PE, Hallstrom AP, Hearne T. Use of the automatic external defibrillator in homes of survivors of out-of-hospital ventricular fibrillation. *Am J Cardiol.* 1989;63:443-446.

29. Caffrey S, Willoughby PJ, Pepe PE, Becker LB. Public use of automated external defibrillators. *New Engl J Med.* 2002;347:1242-1247.

30. McKenas DK. On-board defibrillators. *Aviat Space Environ Med.* 1999;70:533.

31. Wassertheil J, Keane G, Fisher N, Leditschke JF. Cardiac arrest outcomes at the Melbourne Cricket Ground and Shrine of Remembrance, using a tiered response strategy: a forerunner to public access defibrillation. *Resuscitation.* 2000;44:97-104.

32. Nichol G, Hallstrom AP, Kerber R, Moss AJ, Ornato JP, Palmer D, Riegel B, Smith S Jr, Weisfeldt ML. Special report: American Heart Association report on the second public access defibrillation conference, April 17-19, 1997. *Circulation.* 1998;97:1309-1314.

33. Weisfeldt ML, Kerber RE, McGoldrick RP, Moss AJ, Nichol G, Ornato JP, Palmer DG, Riegel B, Smith SC Jr. Public access defibrillation: a statement for healthcare professionals from the American Heart Association Task Force on Automatic External Defibrillation. *Circulation.* 1995;92:2763.

34. Kaye W, Mancini ME, Giuliano KK, Richards N, Nagid DM, Marler CA, Sawyer-Silva S. Strengthening the in-hospital chain of survival with rapid defibrillation by first responders using automated external defibrillators: training and retention issues. *Ann Emerg Med.* 1995;25: 63-168.

35. Kaye W, Mancini ME, Richards N. Organizing and implementing a hospital-wide first-responder automated external defibrillation program: strengthening the in-hospital chain of survival. *Resuscitation.* 1995;30:151-156.

36. Destro A, Marzaloni M, Sermasi S, Rossi F. Automatic external defibrillators in the hospital as well? *Resuscitation.* 1996;31:39-43; discussion 43-44.

37. Kaye W, Mancini ME. Improving outcome from cardiac arrest in the hospital with a reorganized and strengthened chain of survival: an American view. *Resuscitation.* 1996;31: 181-186.

38. Mancini ME, Kaye W. In-hospital first-responder automated external defibrillation: what critical care practitioners need to know. *Am J Crit Care.* 1998;7:314-319.

39. Cummins RO, Ornato JP, Thies WH, Pepe PE. Improving survival from sudden cardiac arrest: the "chain of survival" concept: a statement for health professionals from the Advanced Cardiac Life Support Subcommittee and the Emergency Cardiac Care Committee, American Heart Association. *Circulation.* 1991;83: 1832-1847.

40. McIntyre KM. Cardiopulmonary resuscitation and the ultimate coronary care unit. *JAMA.* 1980;244:510-511.

41. Eisenberg MS, Cummins RO, Damon S, Larsen MP, Hearne TR. Survival rates from out-of-hospital cardiac arrest: recommendations for uniform definitions and data to report. *Ann Emerg Med.* 1990;19:1249-1259.

42. Eisenberg MS, Copass MK, Hallstrom A, Cobb LA, Bergner L. Management of out-of-hospital cardiac arrest: failure of basic emergency medical technician services. *JAMA.* 1980;243:1049-1051.

43. Eisenberg MS, Hallstrom AP, Copass MK, Bergner L, Short F, Pierce J. Treatment of ventricular fibrillation: emergency medical technician defibrillation and paramedic services. *JAMA.* 1984;251:1723-1726.

44. Weaver WD, Copass MK, Bufi D, Ray R, Hallstrom AP, Cobb LA. Improved neurologic recovery and survival after early defibrillation. *Circulation.* 1984;69:943-948.

45. Larsen MP, Eisenberg MS, Cummins RO, Hallstrom AP. Predicting survival from out-of-hospital cardiac arrest: a graphic model. *Ann Emerg Med.* 1993;22:1652-1658.

46. Eisenberg M, Bergner L, Hallstrom A. Paramedic programs and out-of-hospital cardiac arrest, II: impact on community mortality. *Am J Public Health.* 1979;69:39-42.

47. Fletcher GF, Cantwell JD. Ventricular fibrillation in a medically supervised cardiac exercise program: clinical, angiographic, and surgical correlations. *JAMA.* 1977;238:2627-2629.

48. Haskell WL. Cardiovascular complications during exercise training of cardiac patients. *Circulation.* 1978;57:920-924.

49. Hossack KF, Hartwig R. Cardiac arrest associated with supervised cardiac rehabilitation. *J Card Rehabil.* 1982;2:402-408.

50. Van Camp SP, Peterson RA. Cardiovascular complications of outpatient cardiac rehabilitation programs. *JAMA.* 1986;256:1160-1163.

51. Eisenberg MS, Copass MK, Hallstrom AP, Blake B, Bergner L, Short FA, Cobb LA. Treatment of out-of-hospital cardiac arrests with rapid defibrillation by emergency medical technicians. *N Engl J Med.* 1980;302:1379-1383.

52. Stults KR, Brown DD, Schug VL, Bean JA. Prehospital defibrillation performed by emergency medical technicians in rural communities. *N Engl J Med.* 1984;310:219-223.

53. Vukov LF, White RD, Bachman JW, O'Brien PC. New perspectives on rural EMT defibrillation. *Ann Emerg Med.* 1988;17:318-321.

54. Bachman JW, McDonald GS, O'Brien PC. A study of out-of-hospital cardiac arrests in northeastern Minnesota. *JAMA.* 1986;256:477-483.

55. Olson DW, LaRochelle J, Fark D, Aprahamian C, Aufderheide TP, Mateer JR, Hargarten KM, Stueven HA. EMT-defibrillation: the Wisconsin experience. *Ann Emerg Med.* 1989;18:806-811.

56. Cummins RO. From concept to standard-of-care? Review of the clinical experience with automated external defibrillators. *Ann Emerg Med.* 1989;18:1269-1275.

57. Cobb LA, Fahrenbruch CE, Walsh TR, Copass MK, Olsufka M, Breskin M, Hallstrom AP. Influence of cardiopulmonary resuscitation prior to defibrillation in patients with out-of-hospital ventricular fibrillation. *JAMA.* 1999;281:1182-1188.

58. Valenzuela TD, Roe DJ, Cretin S, Spaite DW, Larsen MP. Estimating effectiveness of cardiac arrest interventions: a logistic regression survival model. *Circulation.* 1997;96:3308-3313.

59. Holmberg M, Holmberg S, Herlitz J, Gardelov B. Survival after cardiac arrest outside hospital in Sweden. *Resuscitation.* 1998;36:29-36.

60. Valenzuela TD, Spaite DW, Meislin HW, Clark LL, Wright AL, Ewy GA. Case and survival definitions in out-of-hospital cardiac arrest: effect on survival rate calculation. *JAMA.* 1992;267:272-274.

61. Valenzuela TD, Spaite DW, Meislin HW, Clark LL, Wright AL, Ewy GA. Emergency vehicle intervals versus collapse-to-CPR and collapse-to-defibrillation intervals: monitoring emergency medical services system performance in sudden cardiac arrest. *Ann Emerg Med.* 1993;22:1678-1683.

62. Stults KR, Cummins RO. Fully automatic vs shock advisory defibrillators: what are the issues? *J Emerg Med Serv.* 1987;12:71-73.

63. Stults KR, Brown DD, Cooley F, Kerber RE. Self-adhesive monitor/defibrillation pads improve prehospital defibrillation success. *Ann Emerg Med.* 1987;16:872-877.

64. Cummins RO, Stults KR, Haggar B, Kerber RE, Schaeffer S, Brown DD. A new rhythm library for testing automatic external defibrillators: performance of three devices. *J Am Coll Cardiol.* 1988;11:597-602.

65. Diack AW, Welborn WS, Rullman RG, Walter CW, Wayne MA. An automatic cardiac resuscitator for emergency treatment of cardiac arrest. *Med Instrument.* 1979;13:78-83.

66. Jaggarao NS, Heber M, Grainger R, Vincent R, Chamberlain DA, Aronson AL. Use of an automated external defibrillator-pacemaker by ambulance staff. *Lancet.* 1982;2:73-75.

67. Cummins RO, Eisenberg M, Bergner L, Murray JA. Sensitivity, accuracy, and safety of an automatic external defibrillator. *Lancet.* 1984;2:318-320.

68. Cummins RO, Eisenberg MS, Litwin PE, Graves JR, Hearne TR, Hallstrom AP. Automatic external defibrillators used by emergency medical technicians: a controlled clinical trial. *JAMA.* 1987;257:1605-1610.

69. Stults KR, Brown DD, Kerber RE. Efficacy of an automated external defibrillator in the management of out-of-hospital cardiac arrest: validation of the diagnostic algorithm and initial clinical experience in a rural environment. *Circulation.* 1986;73:701-709.

70. Jakobsson J, Nyquist O, Rehnqvist N. Effects of early defibrillation of out-of-hospital cardiac arrest patients by ambulance personnel. *Eur Heart J.* 1987;8:1189-1194.

71. Gray AJ, Redmond AD, Martin MA. Use of the automatic external defibrillator-pacemaker by ambulance personnel: the Stockport experience. *Br Med J.* 1987;294:1133-1135.

72. Weaver WD, Hill D, Fahrenbruch CE, Copass MK, Martin JS, Cobb LA, Hallstrom AP. Use of the automatic external defibrillator in the management of out-of-hospital cardiac arrest. *N Engl J Med.* 1988;319:661-666.

73. Dickey W, Dalzell GW, Anderson JM, Adgey AA. The accuracy of decision-making of a semi-automatic defibrillator during cardiac arrest. *Eur Heart J.* 1992;13:608-615.

74. Monsieurs KG, Conraads VM, Goethals MP, Bossaert LL, Snoeck JP. Semi-automatic defibrillation and implanted cardiac pacemakers: understanding the interactions during resuscitation. *Resuscitation.* 1995;30:127-131.

75. Kerber RE, Martins JB, Kienzle MG, Constantin L, Olshansky B, Hopson R, Charbonnier F. Energy, current, and success in defibrillation and cardioversion: clinical studies using an automated impedance-based method of energy adjustment. *Circulation.* 1988;77:1038-1046.

76. Geddes LA, Tacker WA, Rosborough JP, Moore AG, Cabler PS. Electrical dose for ventricular defibrillation of large and small animals using precordial electrodes. *J Clin Invest.* 1974;53:310-319.

77. Gutgesell HP, Tacker WA, Geddes LA, Davis S, Lie JT, McNamara DG. Energy dose for ventricular defibrillation of children. *Pediatrics.* 1976;58:898-901.

78. Dahl CF, Ewy GA, Warner ED, Thomas ED. Myocardial necrosis from direct current countershock: effect of paddle electrode size and time interval between discharges. *Circulation.* 1974;50:956-961.

79. Pantridge JF, Adgey AA, Webb SW, Anderson J. Electrical requirements for ventricular defibrillation. *Br Med J.* 1975;2:313-315.

80. Weaver WD, Cobb LA, Copass MK, Hallstrom AP. Ventricular defibrillation — a comparative trial using 175-J and 320-J shocks. *N Engl J Med.* 1982;307:1101-1106.

81. Bardy GH, Gliner BE, Kudenchuk PJ, Poole JE, Dolack GL, Jones GK, Anderson J, Troutman C, Johnson G. Truncated biphasic pulses for transthoracic defibrillation. *Circulation.* 1995;91:1768-1774.

82. Bardy GH, Marchlinski FE, Sharma AD, Worley SJ, Luceri RM, Yee R, Halperin BD, Fellows CL, Ahern TS, Chilson DA, Packer DL, Wilber DJ, Mattioni TA, Reddy R, Kronmal RA, Lazzara R. Multicenter com-

parison of truncated biphasic shocks and standard damped sine wave monophasic shocks for transthoracic ventricular defibrillation. Transthoracic Investigators. *Circulation.* 1996;94:2507-2514.

83. Mittal S, Ayati S, Stein KM, Knight BP, Morady F, Schwartzman D, Cavlovich D, Platia EV, Calkins H, Tchou PJ, Miller JM, Wharton JM, Sung RJ, Slotwiner DJ, Markowitz SM, Lerman BB. Comparison of a novel rectilinear biphasic waveform with a damped sine wave monophasic waveform for transthoracic ventricular defibrillation. ZOLL Investigators. *J Am Coll Cardiol.* 1999;34:1595-1601.

84. Mittal S, Ayati S, Stein KM, Schwartzman D, Cavlovich D, Tchou PJ, Markowitz SM, Slotwiner DJ, Scheiner MA, Lerman BB. Transthoracic cardioversion of atrial fibrillation: comparison of rectilinear biphasic versus damped sine wave monophasic shocks. *Circulation.* 2000;101:1282-1287.

85. Cummins RO, Hazinski MF, Kerber RE, Kudenchuk P, Becker L, Nichol G, Malanga B, Aufderheide TP, Stapleton EM, Kern K, Ornato JP, Sanders A, Valenzuela T, Eisenberg M. Low-energy biphasic waveform defibrillation: evidence-based review applied to emergency cardiovascular care guidelines: a statement for healthcare professionals from the American Heart Association Committee on Emergency Cardiovascular Care and the Subcommittees on Basic Life Support, Advanced Cardiac Life Support, and Pediatric Resuscitation. *Circulation.* 1998;97:1654-1667.

86. Eisenberg M, Bergner L, Hallstrom A. Epidemiology of cardiac arrest and resuscitation in children. *Ann Emerg Med.* 1983;12:672-674.

87. Kuisma M, Suominen P, Korpela R. Paediatric out-of-hospital cardiac arrests — epidemiology and outcome. *Resuscitation.* 1995;30:141-150.

88. Hickey RW, Cohen DM, Strausbaugh S, Dietrich AM. Pediatric patients requiring CPR in the prehospital setting. *Ann Emerg Med.* 1995;25:495-501.

89. Sirbaugh PE, Pepe PE, Shook JE, Kimball KT, Goldman MJ, Ward MA, Mann DM. A prospective, population-based study of the demographics, epidemiology, management, and outcome of out-of-hospital pediatric cardiopulmonary arrest. *Ann Emerg Med.* 1999;33:174-184.

90. Fingerhut LA, Cox CS, Warner M. International comparative analysis of injury mortality: findings from the ICE on injury statistics. International Collaborative Effort on Injury Statistics. *Adv Data.* October 7, 1998; Number 303:1-20.

91. Peters KD, Kochanek KD, Murphy SL. Deaths: final data for 1996. *Natl Vital Stats Rep.* 1998;47:1-100.

92. Mogayzel C, Quan L, Graves JR, Tiedeman D, Fahrenbruch C, Herndon P. Out-of-hospital ventricular fibrillation in children and adolescents: causes and outcome. *Ann Emerg Med.* 1995;25:484-491.

93. Appleton GO, Cummins RO, Larson MP, Graves JR. CPR and the single rescuer: at what age should you "call first" rather than "call fast"? *Ann Emerg Med.* 1995;25:492-494.

94. Ronco R, King W, Donley DK, Tilden SJ. Outcome and cost at a children's hospital following resuscitation for out-of-hospital cardiopulmonary arrest. *Arch Pediatr Adolesc Med.* 1995;149:210-214.

95. Walsh CK, Krongard E. Terminal cardiac electrical activity in pediatric patients. *Am J Cardiol.* 1983;51:559-561.

96. Safranek DJ, Eisenberg MS, Larsen MP. The epidemiology of cardiac arrest in young adults. *Ann Emerg Med.* 1992;21:1102-1106.

97. Losek JD, Hennes H, Glaeser P, Hendley G, Nelson DB. Prehospital care of the pulseless, nonbreathing pediatric patient. *Am J Emerg Med.* 1987;5:370-374.

98. Cecchin F, Jorgenson DB, Berul CI, Perry JC, Zimmerman AA, Duncan BW, Lupinetti FM, Snyder D, Lyster TD, Rosenthal GL, Cross B, Atkins DL. Is arrhythmia detection by automatic external defibrillator accurate for children? Sensitivity and specificity of an automatic external defibrillator algorithm in 696 pediatric arrhythmias. *Circulation.* 2001;103:2483-2488.

99. Atkinson E, Mikysa B, Conway JA, Parker M, Christian K, Deshpande J, Knilans TK, Smith J, Walker C, Stickney RE, Hampton DR, Hazinski MF. Specificity and sensitivity of automated external defibrillator rhythm analysis in infants and children. *Ann Emerg Med.* In press.

100. Samson RA, Berg RA, Bingham R, Biarent D, Coovadia A, Hazinski MF, Hickey RW, Nadkarni V, Nichol G, Tibballs J, Reis AG, Tse S, Zideman D, Potts J, Uzark K, Atkins D. Use of automated external defibrillators for children: an update: an advisory statement from the Pediatric Advanced Life Support Task Force, International Liaison Committee on Resuscitation. *Circulation.* 2003;107:3250-3255.

101. Clark CB, Davies LR, Kerber RE. Pediatric defibrillation: biphasic vs. monophasic waveforms in an experimental model. *Circulation.* 1999;200:I-90.

102. Tang W, Weil MH, Sun S, Yamaguchi H, Povoas HP, Pernat AM, Bisera J. The effects of biphasic and conventional monophasic defibrillation on postresuscitation myocardial function. *J Am Coll Cardiol.* 1999;34:815-822.

103. Babbs CF, Tacker WA, VanVleet JF, Bourland JD, Geddes LA. Therapeutic indices for transchest defibrillator shocks: effective, damaging, and lethal electrical doses. *Am Heart J.* 1980;99:734-738.

104. Lubitz DS, Seidel JS, Chameides L, Luten RC, Zaritsky AL, Campbell FW. A rapid method for estimating weight and resuscitation drug dosages from length in the pediatric age group. *Ann Emerg Med.* 1988;17:576-581.

105. Calle PA, Buylaert W. When an AED meets an ICD ... automated external defibrillator: implantable cardioverter defibrillator. *Resuscitation.* 1998;38:177-183.

106. Panacek EA, Munger MA, Rutherford WF, Gardner SF. Report of nitropatch explosions complicating defibrillation. *Am J Emerg Med.* 1992;10:128-129.

107. Bissing JW, Kerber RE. Effect of shaving the chest of hirsute subjects on transthoracic impedance to self-adhesive defibrillation electrode pads. *Am J Cardiol.* 2000;86:587-589.

108. Gibbs W, Eisenberg M, Damon SK. Dangers of defibrillation: injuries to emergency personnel during patient resuscitation. *Am J Emerg Med.* 1990;8:101-104.

109. Aufderheide T, Stapleton ER, Hazinski MF, Cummins RO. *Heartsaver AED for the Lay Rescuer and First Responder.* Dallas, Tex: American Heart Association; 1999.

110. Emergency Care Research Institute. Hazard: user error and defibrillator discharge failures. *Health Devices.* 1986;15:340-343.

111. Cummins RO, Chesemore K, White RD. Defibrillator failures: causes of problems and recommendations for improvement. Defibrillator Working Group. *JAMA.* 1990;64:1019-1025.

112. White RD. Maintenance of defibrillators in a state of readiness. *Ann Emerg Med.* 1993;22(2 pt 2):302-306.

113. White RD. AED (automated external defibrillator): a physician's responsibility. *J Emerg Med Serv.* 1992;17:8-9.

114. Cummins RO, Austin D Jr, Graves JR, Hambly C. An innovative approach to medical control: semiautomatic defibrillators with solid-state memory modules for recording cardiac arrest events. *Ann Emerg Med.* 1988;17:818-824.

115. Cummins RO, Chamberlain DA, Abramson NS, Allen M, Baskett P, Becker L, Bossaert L, Delooz H, Dick W, Eisenberg M, et al. Recommended guidelines for uniform reporting of data from out-of-hospital cardiac arrest: the Utstein Style. *Ann Emerg Med.* 1991;20:861-874.

116. Cummins RO, Chamberlain D, Hazinski MF, Nadkarni V, Kloeck W, Kramer E, Becker L, Robertson C, Koster R, Zaritsky A, Bossaert L, Ornato JP, Callanan V, Allen M, Steen P,

Connolly B, Sanders A, Idris A, Cobbe S. Recommended guidelines for reviewing, reporting, and conducting research on in-hospital resuscitation: the in-hospital "Utstein style." A statement for healthcare professionals from the American Heart Association, the European Resuscitation Council, the Heart and Stroke Foundation of Canada, the Australian Resuscitation Council, and the Resuscitation Councils of Southern Africa. *Resuscitation.* 1997;34:151-183.

117. American Heart Association, International Liaison Committee on Resuscitation (ILCOR). Guidelines 2000 for cardiopulmonary resuscitation and emergency cardiovascular care. International Consensus on Science. *Circulation.* 2000;102(suppl I):I-1-I-384.

118. Murphy DM. Rapid defibrillation: fire service to lead the way. *J Emerg Med Serv.* 1987;12: 67-71.

119. Newman MM. Chain of Survival concept takes hold. *J Emerg Med Serv.* 1989;14:11-13.

120. Bossaert L, Handley A, Marsden A, Arntz R, Chamberlain D, Ekstrom L, Evans T, Monsieurs K, Robertson C, Steen P. European Resuscitation Council guidelines for the use of automated external defibrillators by EMS providers and first responders: a statement from the Early Defibrillation Task Force, with contributions from the Working Groups on Basic and Advanced Life Support, and approved by the Executive Committee. *Resuscitation.* 1998;37:91-94.

121. Walters G, Glucksman E, Evans TR. Training St. John Ambulance volunteers to use an automated external defibrillator. *Resuscitation.* 1994;27:39-45.

122. Weaver WD, Sutherland K, Wirkus MJ, Bachman R. Emergency medical care requirements for large public assemblies and a new strategy for managing cardiac arrest in this setting. *Ann Emerg Med.* 1989;18: 155-160.

123. Watts DD. Defibrillation by basic emergency medical technicians: effect on survival. *Ann Emerg Med.* 1995;26:635-639.

124. Fenner P, Leahy S. Successful defibrillation on a beach by volunteer surf lifesavers. *Med J Aust.* 1998;168:169.

125. Riegel B. Training nontraditional responders to use automated external defibrillators. *Am J Crit Care.* 1998;7:402-410.

126. Herlitz J, Bang A, Axelsson A, Graves JR, Lindqvist J. Experience with the use of automated external defibrillators in out-of-hospital cardiac arrest. *Resuscitation.* 1998;37:3-7.

127. Hoekstra JW, Banks JR, Martin DR, Cummins RO, Pepe PE, Stueven HA, Jastremski M, Gonzalez E, Brown CG. Effect of first-responder automated defibrillation on time to therapeutic interventions during out-of-hospital cardiac arrest: the Multicenter High Dose Epinephrine Study Group. *Ann Emerg Med.* 1993;22:1247-1253.

128. Shuster M, Keller JL. Effect of fire department first-responder automated defibrillation. *Ann Emerg Med.* 1993;22:721-727.

129. Calle P, Van Acker P, Buylaert W, Quets A, Corne L, Delooz H, Bossaert L, Martens P, Mullie A. Should semi-automatic defibrillators be used by emergency medical technicians in Belgium? The Belgian Cerebral Resuscitation Study Group. *Acta Clin Belg.* 1992;47:6-14.

130. Calle PA, Verbeke A, Vanhaute O, Van Acker P, Martens P, Buylaert W. The effect of semi-automatic external defibrillation by emergency medical technicians on survival after out-of-hospital cardiac arrest: an observational study in urban and rural areas in Belgium. *Acta Clin Belg.* 1997;52:72-83.

131. Martens P, Calle P, Mullie A. Do we know enough to introduce semi-automatic defibrillation by ambulancemen in Belgium? *Eur J Med.* 1993;2:430-434.

132. Richless LK, Schrading WA, Polana J, Hess DR, Ogden CS. Early defibrillation program: problems encountered in a rural/suburban EMS system. *J Emerg Med.* 1993;11:127-134.

133. Auble TE, Menegazzi JJ, Paris PM. Effect of out-of-hospital defibrillation by basic life support providers on cardiac arrest mortality: a meta-analysis. *Ann Emerg Med.* 1995;25: 642-648.

134. Ho J, Held T, Heegaard W, Crimmins T. Automatic external defibrillation and its effects on neurologic outcome in cardiac arrest patients in an urban, two-tiered EMS system. *Prehosp Disaster Med.* 1997;12: 284-287.

135. Herlitz J, Bang A, Holmberg M, Axelsson A, Lindkvist J, Holmberg S. Rhythm changes during resuscitation from ventricular fibrillation in relation to delay until defibrillation, number of shocks delivered and survival. *Resuscitation.* 1997;34:17-22.

136. Hamer DW, Gordon MW, Cusack S, Robertson CE. Survival from cardiac arrest in an accident and emergency department: the impact of out-of-hospital advisory defibrillation. *Resuscitation.* 1993;26:31-37.

137. Arntz HR, Oeff M, Willich SN, Storch WH, Schroder R. Establishment and results of an EMT-D program in a two-tiered physician-escorted rescue system: the experience in Berlin, Germany. *Resuscitation.* 1993;26: 39-46.

138. National Heart Attack Alert Program Coordinating Committee Access to Care Subcommittee. Staffing and equipping emergency medical services systems: rapid identification and treatment of acute myocardial infarction. *Am J Emerg Med.* 1995;13:58-66.

139. Kloeck W, Cummins RO, Chamberlain D, Bossaert L, Callanan V, Carli P, Christenson J, Connolly B, Ornato JP, Sanders A, Steen P. Early defibrillation: an advisory statement from the Advanced Life Support Working Group of the International Liaison Committee on Resuscitation. *Circulation.* 1997;95:2183-2184.

140. Stults KR, Brown DD. Special considerations for defibrillation performed by emergency medical technicians in small communities. *Circulation.* 1986;74(suppl 6, pt 2):IV-13-IV-17.

141. Ornato JP, McNeill SE, Craren EJ, Nelson NM. Limitation on effectiveness of rapid defibrillation by emergency medical technicians in a rural setting. *Ann Emerg Med.* 1984;13:1096-1099.

142. Cummins RO, Eisenberg MS, Graves JR, Damon SK. EMT-defibrillation: is it right for you? *J Emerg Med Serv.* 1985;10:60-64.

143. Lazzam C, McCans JL. Predictors of survival of in-hospital cardiac arrest. *Can J Cardiol.* 1991;7:113-116.

144. Dickey W, Adgey AA. Mortality within hospital after resuscitation from ventricular fibrillation outside hospital. *Br Heart J.* 1992;67: 334-338.

145. Cummins RO, Sanders A, Mancini E, Hazinski MF. In-hospital resuscitation: a statement for healthcare professionals from the American Heart Association Emergency Cardiac Care Committee and the Advanced Cardiac Life Support, Basic Life Support, Pediatric Resuscitation, and Program Administration Subcommittees. *Circulation.* 1997; 95:2211-2212.

146. Nelson ME, Zenas CS. Losing the race to resuscitate. *Nurs Manage.* 1998;29:36D-36E, 36G.

147. Mancini ME, Kaye W. AEDs: changing the way you respond to cardiac arrest. *Am J Nurs.* 1999;99:26-31.

148. Warwick JP, Mackie K, Spencer I. Towards early defibrillation: a nurse training programme in the use of automated external defibrillators. *Resuscitation.* 1995;30:231-235.

149. Joint Commission on Accreditation of Healthcare Organizations. In-hospital resuscitation requirements reinstated for hospitals. *Joint Comm Perspect.* 1998;18:5.

150. Stoddard FG. Public access defibrillation comes of age. *Currents in Emergency Cardiovascular Care.* Winter 1996;7:1-3.

151. Nichol G, Hallstrom AP, Ornato JP, Riegel B, Stiell IG, Valenzuela T, Wells GA, White RD, Weisfeldt ML. Potential cost-effectiveness of public access defibrillation in the United States. *Circulation.* 1998;97:1315-1320.

152. Becker L, Eisenberg M, Fahrenbruch C, Cobb L. Public locations of cardiac arrest: implications for public access defibrillation. *Circulation.* 1998;97:2106-2109.

153. Zachariah BS, Pepe PE. The development of emergency medical dispatch in the USA: a historical perspective. *Eur J Emerg Med.* 1995;2:109-112.

154. Rossi R. The role of the dispatch centre in preclinical emergency medicine. *Eur J Emerg Med.* 1994;1:27-30.

155. Axelsson A, Herlitz J, Karlsson T, Lindqvist J, Reid Graves J, Ekstrom L, Holmberg S. Factors surrounding cardiopulmonary resuscitation influencing bystanders' psychological reactions. *Resuscitation.* 1998;37:13-20.

156. American College of Emergency Physicians. Early defibrillation programs. *Ann Emerg Med.* 1999;33:371.

157. Ornato JP, Craren EJ, Gonzalez ER, Garnett AR, McClung BK, Newman MM. Cost-effectiveness of defibrillation by emergency medical technicians. *Am J Emerg Med.* 1988;6:108-112.

158. Steill IG, Wells GA, Field BJ, Spaite DW, De Maio VJ, Ward R, Munkley DP, Lyver MB, Luinstra LG, Campeau T, Maloney J, Dagnone E. Improved out-of-hospital cardiac arrest survival through the inexpensive optimization of an existing defibrillation program: OPALS study phase II. Ontario Prehospital Advanced Life Support. *JAMA.* 1999;281:1175-1181.

159. SoRelle R. States set to pass laws limiting liability for lay users of automated external defibrillators. *Circulation.* 1999;99:2606-2607.

You are a medical resident. You are talking with a 42-year-old patient in his hospital room. The man is eating lunch and starts to laugh at a comment you made. Suddenly he clutches his throat and appears to be in distress. You ask, "Are you choking?" The patient nods. You ask, "Can you speak?" He shakes his head no and makes no sound. You tell him you are going to help him. You ask if he can get out of bed. He nods and stands at the side of the bed, still clutching his throat, attempting to cough.

You stand behind the patient and wrap your arms around him. You place your closed fist just above his navel and well below the xiphoid process and grab your fist with your other hand. You provide 3 upward abdominal thrusts. A piece of meat flies out of the patient's mouth. The patient recovers quickly. You carefully evaluate him to make sure that there are no complications related to the incident and remind him (and yourself) that eating and laughing is a potentially lethal combination.

Adult Foreign-Body Airway Obstruction

Overview

Severe or complete airway obstruction is an emergency that will result in death within minutes if not treated. An unresponsive victim can develop airway obstruction from intrinsic (tongue) and extrinsic (foreign body) causes. The most common cause of upper airway obstruction in the unresponsive victim is (intrinsic) obstruction by the tongue during loss of consciousness and cardiopulmonary arrest. When the unresponsive victim lies on his or her back, the tongue falls back into the pharynx, obstructing the upper airway. The epiglottis can block the entrance of the airway in unconscious victims.

Bleeding from head and facial injuries or regurgitation of stomach contents may produce upper airway obstruction, particularly if the patient is unconscious and has depressed cough and gag reflexes. In the healthcare setting these causes of airway obstruction are often successfully relieved by suctioning the pharynx.

FBAO (choking) is a relatively uncommon and preventable cause of cardiac arrest. FBAO accounts for approximately 3000 deaths annually.[1] There are 1.2 choking deaths per 100 000 population compared with 1.7 deaths for drowning, 16.5 for motor vehicle crashes, and 198 for coronary heart disease.[1-6]

FBAO is not a common problem among submersion/near-drowning victims.[7] Water does not act as a solid foreign

Learning Objectives

After reading this chapter and participating in the video segments and skills practice sessions, you should be able to

1. List the most common causes of adult foreign-body airway obstruction (FBAO)

2. List the precautions that can be implemented to prevent adult FBAO

3. Recognize the signs of severe or complete FBAO in the responsive adult

4. Describe how to perform a tongue-jaw lift and finger sweep

5. Describe the sequence of action for management of adult FBAO in

   ■ The responsive victim

   ■ The unresponsive victim

   ■ The responsive pregnant or obese victim

   ■ The unresponsive pregnant or obese victim

   ■ The self-administered Heimlich maneuver

6. Describe the sequence of action for management of the adult victim after relief of FBAO

body and does not obstruct the airway.[8] Although foreign material such as sand and seaweed has been observed in the mouth and pharynx of near-drowning victims, there is no evidence that this material acts as an obstructing foreign body.[7] Many submersion victims do not aspirate water at all, and any aspirated water will be absorbed in the upper airway and trachea. Near-drowning victims require immediate provision of CPR, particularly rescue breathing, to correct hypoxia. Therefore, efforts to relieve FBAO are not recommended for victims of near-drowning. Such efforts may produce complications and will delay CPR, the most important treatment for the submersion victim.[8]

Causes and Prevention of Adult FBAO

FBAO should be suspected when a person suddenly develops difficulty breathing and becomes cyanotic and unconscious for no apparent reason.

FBAO in adults usually occurs during eating,[9,10] and meat is the most common cause of obstruction. A variety of other foods and foreign bodies have been the cause of choking in children and some adults.[11-16] Common factors associated with choking on food include attempts to swallow large, poorly chewed pieces of food, elevated blood alcohol levels, and dentures.[11-17] Elderly patients with dysphagia are also at risk for FBAO and should be careful when drinking and eating. In restaurants choking emergencies have been mistaken for a heart attack, giving rise to the term "café coronary."[9,10]

The following precautions may help modify the risks and prevent FBAO:

- Cut food into small pieces and chew slowly and thoroughly, especially if wearing dentures.

- Avoid laughing and talking during chewing and swallowing.

- Avoid excessive intake of alcohol, particularly during meals.

Recognition of FBAO in the Responsive Adult

Because early recognition of airway obstruction is the key to successful outcome, it is important to distinguish this emergency from fainting, stroke, heart attack, epilepsy, drug overdose, or other conditions that cause sudden respiratory failure but require different treatment. Signs of FBAO are often obvious to the trained observer.

FIGURE 1. Universal choking sign.

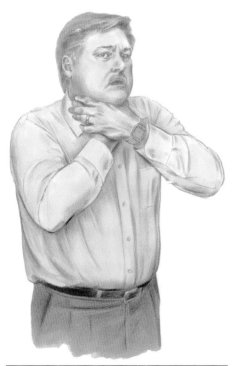

Foreign bodies may cause either *partial* or *complete* airway obstruction. With partial airway obstruction, the victim may be capable of either good or poor air exchange. With good air exchange, the victim is responsive and can cough forcefully, although wheezing may be heard between coughs.

As long as good air exchange continues, encourage the victim to continue spontaneous coughing and breathing efforts. At this point do not interfere with the victim's own attempts to expel the foreign body, but stay with the victim and monitor his or her condition. If partial airway obstruction persists, activate EMS or another emergency response system.

The victim with severe FBAO may immediately demonstrate poor air exchange or may initially demonstrate good air exchange that deteriorates to poor air exchange. Signs of poor air exchange include a weak, ineffective cough, a high-pitched noise while inhaling, increased respiratory difficulty, and possibly cyanosis. A partial obstruction with poor air exchange is treated in the same way as a complete airway obstruction.

With severe or complete airway obstruction, victims are unable to speak, breathe, or cough forcefully and may clutch their neck with the thumb and fingers, making the universal choking sign (see Critical Concepts box). Movement of air is absent.

The public should be encouraged to use the universal choking sign to indicate the need for help when choking (Figure 1).

Ask the victim if he or she is choking. If the victim nods, ask if he or she can speak. If the victim indicates no, severe or complete airway obstruction is present and you must act.

If severe or complete airway obstruction is not relieved, the victim's blood oxygen saturation will fall rapidly because the obstructed airway prevents entry of air into the lungs. If you do not act, the victim will become unresponsive and death will soon follow.

Relief of FBAO

The Heimlich maneuver is recommended for relief of FBAO in adults and children 1 to 8 years of age. It is *not* recommended for relief of FBAO in infants.[17] The terms *subdiaphragmatic abdominal thrusts* and *abdominal thrusts* have been used synonymously with the term *Heimlich maneuver* since 1976.[10]

Critical Concepts:
Signs of Severe or Complete Airway Obstruction

In a conscious, choking person the following are signs of severe or complete airway obstruction that require immediate action:

- **Universal choking sign:** the victim clutches his neck with the thumb and index finger (Figure 1)

- Inability to speak

  — Ask the victim "Are you choking?"

  — If the victim indicates yes, ask "Can you speak?"

  — If the victim is unable to speak, severe or complete airway obstruction is present and you must act.

- Weak, ineffective coughs

- High-pitched sounds or no sounds while inhaling

- Increased difficulty breathing

- Bluish skin color (cyanosis)

Note: You do *not* need to act if the victim can cough forcefully and speak. Do not interfere at this point because a strong cough is the most effective way to remove a foreign body. Stay with the victim and monitor his or her condition. If the partial obstruction persists, activate EMS or other emergency response system.

Foundation Facts:
Causes of Airway Obstruction

There are 3 common ways in which an adult's airway may become obstructed. Each is treated differently.

1. **Foreign body.** A foreign body (eg, food) may become lodged in the airway, blocking it. If the victim develops signs of severe or complete airway obstruction, perform abdominal thrusts (Heimlich maneuver) until the object is expelled or the victim becomes unresponsive. The *healthcare provider* then performs a tongue-jaw lift, removes the object if seen, attempts ventilation, and if the airway remains obstructed, performs abdominal thrusts. If the victim is pregnant or obese, perform chest thrusts instead of abdominal thrusts.

2. **Relaxed tongue.** In an unresponsive/unconscious victim (eg, after a stroke or head injury or in cardiac arrest), the tongue may fall back against the throat, blocking the airway. Use either the head tilt–chin lift or the jaw-thrust maneuver to lift the tongue away from the back of the throat (see Figure 2).

3. **Swollen air passages.** This condition is a medical problem rather than a mechanical problem, and it will *not* be eliminated by the Heimlich maneuver or by simply opening the patient's airway. Swelling and blockage of the upper or lower airways can be caused by conditions such as asthma, infection, or allergy. Positioning of the head or neck and use of the Heimlich maneuver will *not* eliminate this form of airway obstruction. Critical narrowing of the airway is a life-threatening condition. This condition cannot be resolved without the use of medications, such as epinephrine, or surgery. If the victim stops breathing, give rescue breaths.

FIGURE 2. Obstruction of the airway in the unresponsive victim is relieved by head tilt–chin lift. **A,** Obstruction by the tongue and epiglottis. When a victim is unresponsive, the tongue and epiglottis can block the upper airway. **B,** The head tilt–chin lift maneuver lifts the tongue, relieving airway obstruction.

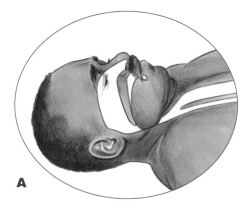

A

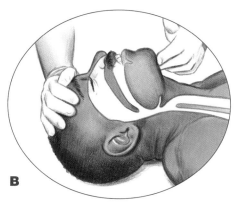

B

By elevating the diaphragm, a subdiaphragmatic abdominal thrust can force air from the lungs. This may be sufficient to create an artificial cough and expel a foreign body from the airway.[18-22] Each individual thrust should be given with the intent of relieving the obstruction. It may be necessary to repeat the thrust several times to clear the airway.[23]

Abdominal thrusts may cause complications, such as ruptured or lacerated abdominal or thoracic viscera or damage to internal organs.[23-32] After the Heimlich maneuver has been performed, the patient should be examined by his or her physician to rule out any life-threatening complications.[26]

To minimize the possibility of complications, do not place your fist on the xiphoid process or the lower margins of the rib cage. The fist should be placed well below this area but just above the navel and in the midline. Regurgitation may occur as a result of abdominal thrusts and may be associated with aspiration.[29] Under no circumstances should students practice subdiaphragmatic abdominal thrusts (the Heimlich maneuver) on each other during CPR training.

An infant's liver is relatively unprotected by the ribs. Injuries to the abdomen have been reported after performance of the Heimlich maneuver in children and

adults.[26-32] Injuries to the liver have been reported in infants after blows to the abdomen. For this reason abdominal thrusts are not recommended for relief of FBAO in the infant. Instead, alternating back blows and chest thrusts are recommended (see Chapter 9, "Pediatric Basic Life Support").

Heimlich Maneuver With Victim Standing or Sitting

Stand behind the victim, wrap your arms around the victim's waist, and continue as follows (Figure 3):

FIGURE 3. Heimlich maneuver with victim standing.

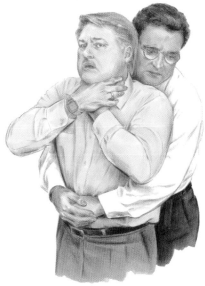

Chapter 8

1. Make a fist with one hand.

2. Place the thumb side of your fist against the victim's abdomen, in the midline, slightly above the navel and well below the tip of the xiphoid process.

3. Grasp your fist with your other hand and press your fist into the victim's abdomen with a quick upward thrust.

4. Repeat thrusts until the object is expelled from the airway or the victim becomes unresponsive.

5. Each new thrust should be a separate, distinct movement given with the intent of relieving the obstruction.[9,21,32]

If a rescuer is too short to reach around the waist of a responsive victim, the Heimlich maneuver may be performed with the victim lying down (see below).

Heimlich Maneuver With Responsive Victim Lying Down

Place the victim in the supine position (face up). Kneel astride the victim's thighs and place the heel of one hand against the victim's abdomen, in the midline, slightly above the navel and well below the tip of the xiphoid process. Place your other hand directly on top of the first. Press both hands into the abdomen with quick, upward thrusts (Figure 4). If you are in the correct position, you will be positioned over the mid-abdomen, unlikely to direct the thrust to the right or left. You can use your body weight to perform the maneuver. This maneuver is identical with the abdominal thrusts a healthcare provider performs for the unresponsive choking victim.

The Self-Administered Heimlich Maneuver

To treat your own complete FBAO, make a fist with one hand, place the thumb side on the abdomen above the navel and below the xiphoid process, grasp your fist with your other hand, and then press inward and upward toward the diaphragm with a quick motion. If this is unsuccessful, press the upper abdomen quickly over any firm surface, such as the back of a chair, side of a table, or porch railing. Several thrusts may be needed to clear the airway.

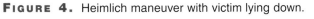

FIGURE 4. Heimlich maneuver with victim lying down.

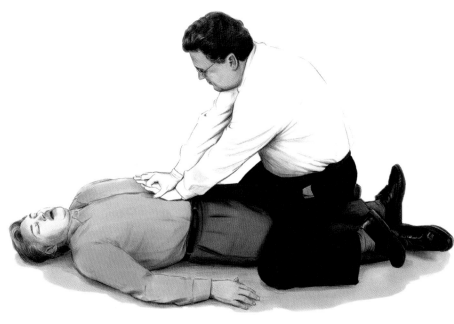

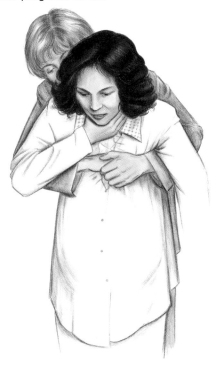

FIGURE 5. Chest thrusts for responsive pregnant victim.

Chest Thrusts With Victim Standing or Sitting

Several studies have suggested that chest compressions may generate a sufficient increase in intrathoracic pressure to relieve FBAO.[23,33,34] In fact, a recent study involving the use of cadavers has shown that chest compressions may create a peak airway pressure that is equal or superior to that created by abdominal thrusts.[33]

Chest thrusts may be used as an alternative to the Heimlich maneuver when the victim is in the late stages of pregnancy or is markedly obese. Stand behind the victim, with your arms directly under the victim's armpits, and encircle the victim's chest. Place the thumb side of one fist on the middle of the victim's breastbone, taking care to avoid the xiphoid process and the margins of the rib cage. Grab your fist with your other hand and perform backward thrusts until the foreign body is expelled or the victim becomes unresponsive (Figure 5).

Chest Thrusts With Victim Lying Down

Sometimes the Heimlich maneuver is more effective if it is performed with the victim lying down. This maneuver may be used for the victim in the late stages of pregnancy or the victim who is unresponsive and markedly obese. To perform the Heimlich maneuver with the victim lying down, place the victim on his or her back and kneel close to the victim's side. The hand position and technique for chest thrusts is the same as that for chest compressions during CPR. In the adult, for example, place the heel of your hand on the lower half of the victim's sternum. Deliver each thrust with the intent of relieving the obstruction.

Healthcare Provider Actions to Relieve FBAO in the Unresponsive Victim

Victims of FBAO initially may be responsive and then may become unresponsive. In this circumstance you know that an FBAO is the cause of the victim's symptoms, and you know to look for a foreign object in the pharynx.

The victim of FBAO may be unresponsive when you first encounter him or her. In this circumstance you probably will not know that an FBAO exists until your repeated attempts at rescue breathing are unsuccessful.

Regardless of whether the victim is responsive or unresponsive when first encountered, whenever you suspect FBAO in the unresponsive victim, you perform a sequence of actions. You open the airway with a tongue-jaw lift, look in the airway, and try to remove the foreign object with a finger sweep. You then attempt (and, if necessary, reattempt) ventilation. If these actions are unsuccessful, you will perform abdominal thrusts with the victim supine (lying on his or her back).

You will perform a slightly different sequence of actions if the victim of FBAO is responsive rather than

unresponsive when first encountered. Both sequences are reviewed here. You should first be familiar with the tongue-jaw lift and finger sweep because this is the sequence performed by the healthcare provider for the unresponsive victim of FBAO.

Tongue-Jaw Lift and Finger Sweep

The finger sweep is used to remove a foreign body from the back of the pharynx (Figure 6). It should be used by the healthcare provider only in *unresponsive* victims with complete FBAO. The finger sweep should *not* be performed if the victim is having seizures.

Responsive Victim of FBAO Becomes Unresponsive

If you see a victim collapse and know that FBAO is the cause, the following sequence of actions is recommended:

1. If you are alone, phone 911. If another rescuer is present, send that rescuer to phone 911 or activate the emergency response system while you remain with the victim. Be sure the victim is supine.

2. Perform a tongue-jaw lift, then a finger sweep to remove the object.

3. Open the airway and try to give 2 rescue breaths. If you are unable to

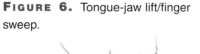

FIGURE 6. Tongue-jaw lift/finger sweep.

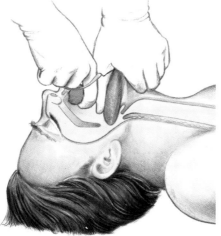

make the victim's chest rise, reposition the victim's head, reopen the airway, and try again to ventilate.

4. If you cannot deliver effective breaths (the chest does not rise) even after attempts to reposition the airway, straddle the victim's thighs and perform the Heimlich maneuver (or chest thrust for pregnant and obese patients) up to 5 times.

5. Repeat the sequence of tongue-jaw lift, finger sweep, attempt (and reattempt) to ventilate, and Heimlich maneuver — or chest thrusts — (steps 2 through 4) until the obstruction is cleared and the chest rises with ventilation or until advanced procedures are available (ie, Kelly clamp,

Magill forceps, cricothyrotomy, or needle cricothyrotomy) to establish a patent airway.

Use forceps only if you see the foreign object. Either a laryngoscope or tongue blade and flashlight can be used for direct visualization. Two types of conventional forceps are acceptable for removal of an FBAO: the Kelly clamp and the Magill forceps. Use of these devices by untrained or inexperienced persons is unacceptable. Cricothyrotomy should be performed only by healthcare providers who are trained and authorized to perform this surgical procedure.

Relief of FBAO in Victim Found Unresponsive

If a victim is found to be unresponsive and the cause is unknown, the following sequence of actions is recommended:

1. If you are alone, phone 911 or other emergency response system. If a second rescuer is present, send that rescuer to phone 911 or activate the emergency response system while you remain with the victim.

2. Open the airway and check for breathing.

3. If there is no effective breathing, attempt to provide 2 rescue breaths. If you are unable to make the chest rise, reposition the victim's head (reopen the airway) and try again to ventilate.

4. If ventilation is still unsuccessful (the chest does not rise) even after attempts to reposition the airway, straddle the victim's thighs and perform the Heimlich maneuver (or chest thrusts) up to 5 times.

5. After 5 abdominal thrusts, open the victim's airway using a tongue-jaw lift and perform a finger sweep to remove the object.

6. Repeat the sequence of attempts (and reattempts) to ventilate, Heimlich maneuver, tongue-jaw lift, and finger sweep until the obstruction is cleared or advanced procedures are available

to establish a patent airway (eg, Kelly clamps, Magill forceps, or cricothyrotomy).

7. If the obstruction is removed and the airway is cleared, check breathing. If the victim is not breathing, provide 2 rescue breaths. Then check for signs of circulation (pulse check and evidence of breathing, coughing, or movement). If there are no signs of circulation, begin chest compressions.

Lay Rescuer Actions to Relieve FBAO in the Unresponsive Victim

The 1992 recommendations[35] for treatment of FBAO in the unresponsive victim by lay rescuers were lengthy, required considerable time to teach, and were often confusing to students.[35-38] Several studies have shown that when training programs try to teach large amounts of material, poor skills retention and poor performance result.[39-45]

Studies have shown that the use of training videos that focus on the acquisition of a small number of skills produces superior levels of skills performance compared with the results of traditional CPR courses.[39-45] This data indicates a need to simplify CPR training for laypersons and focus on a small number of core skills in CPR courses. To identify core skills, the frequency and epidemiology of common cardiovascular emergencies were examined.

Epidemiological data[1-6] on FBAO fatalities does not distinguish between deaths in which the victim was responsive when first encountered and those in which the victim was unresponsive. Anecdotal evidence, however, suggests that the lay rescuer is more likely to encounter a responsive victim of FBAO than an unresponsive victim.

Because death from sudden cardiac arrest is far more common than death from choking, it is far more likely that a lay rescuer will encounter a victim of sudden cardiac arrest than a victim of cardiopulmonary arrest due to FBAO.[1-4] Adult cardiac arrest victims are more likely to

be resuscitated if the lay rescuer performs CPR and uses an AED.[34,46] This suggests that the core skills of an adult BLS course for lay rescuers should include CPR and relief of FBAO in conscious, responsive victims. Skills taught in CPR courses for lay rescuers should not include infrequently used and complex skills that are likely to distract the student from learning core skills.

On the basis of these observations, the experts at the Evidence Evaluation Conference and the Guidelines 2000 Conference recommended that the complex sequence for managing an FBAO in the unresponsive victim be eliminated from training courses for lay rescuers. Instead lay rescuers should be instructed to attempt CPR if a choking victim becomes unresponsive or if FBAO is suspected during CPR. There is one change in the CPR sequence performed by the lay rescuer: every time a rescue breath is given, open the victim's mouth widely to look for a foreign object. If you see it, try to remove it. This recommendation is designed to simplify CPR training for laypersons and ensure the acquisition of the core skills of rescue breathing and CPR while still providing effective treatment to the unresponsive victim of FBAO.

Sequence of Actions After Relief of FBAO

In the unresponsive patient the rescuer should recognize successful removal of airway obstruction by noting air movement and watching the chest rise during attempted ventilation. Relief of FBAO may also be obvious if the rescuer sees and removes a foreign body from the victim's pharynx.

After relief of FBAO the rescuer should

- Provide 2 slow rescue breaths

- Check for signs of circulation (pulse, normal breathing, coughing, and movement); if no signs of circulation are present, perform chest compressions and attach the AED

- If signs of circulation are present but the victim is not breathing, continue rescue breathing and check for signs of circulation every 30 to 60 seconds

- If signs of circulation are present and the victim is breathing adequately, place the victim in the recovery position and continue monitoring her or him until EMS personnel arrive

If an FBAO is successfully relieved with abdominal thrusts, encourage the victim to seek immediate medical attention to ensure that pulmonary aspiration or a complication of the Heimlich maneuver has not occurred.

Summary of Relief of FBAO

Anecdotal reports have documented that the techniques for relief of FBAO in a responsive victim are effective and save lives. Recognition of severe or complete FBAO is crucial to enable prompt and successful intervention. Of course, the best scenario for treatment of FBAO is prevention through public education.

Summary of Key Concepts

- In the unresponsive victim the tongue and epiglottis are the structures that most often obstruct the upper airway.

- The purpose of the head tilt–chin lift and jaw thrust is to relieve obstruction of the tongue and epiglottis.

- Signs of severe or complete airway obstruction in a responsive victim include the following:

  — The universal choking sign

  — Inability to speak. Ask the victim "Are you choking?" If the victim indicates yes, ask "Can you speak?" If the victim is unable to speak, severe or complete airway obstruction is present and you must act.

  — Weak, ineffective coughs

  — High-pitched sounds or no sound while inhaling

  — Increased difficulty breathing

  — Cyanosis

- The Heimlich maneuver should be used if the adult victim is responsive (but not speaking) and standing or sitting.

- Management of FBAO in the responsive victim includes attempts to relieve the obstruction immediately, using the Heimlich maneuver. Activate the EMS system and attach the AED only if the patient loses consciousness.

- Management of FBAO by a healthcare provider in an adult *who becomes unresponsive* includes opening the airway with the tongue-jaw lift, performing a finger sweep to remove any foreign object that is seen, attempting (and reattempting) ventilation, and performing abdominal or chest thrusts (which should be repeated until the object is removed or ventilation is successful).

- The finger sweep should be used only in the unresponsive victim. It should never be used in a seizure victim.

- For pregnant or obese victims, whether responsive or unresponsive, use chest thrusts instead of abdominal thrusts.

- It may be possible to treat one's own complete FBAO with a self-administered Heimlich maneuver.

- Lay rescuers are not taught a unique sequence for management of FBAO in the unresponsive victim: instead they are taught to perform CPR and look for an obstructing object each time they open the airway to give rescue breaths.

Review Questions

1. A 20-year-old responsive man is clutching his throat and cannot speak, breathe, or cough. You ask if he is choking, and he nods yes. You ask if he can speak and he shakes his head no. What should you do immediately?

   a. give back blows

   b. phone 911

   c. give abdominal thrusts

   d. open his airway with a tongue-jaw lift

2. A 55-year-old woman sitting at the table next to yours at a restaurant suddenly begins to cough forcefully, has very noisy breath sounds, and tells you in between fits of coughing and gasping that she is OK. You should

   a. phone 911

   b. perform the Heimlich maneuver

   c. open the airway with a tongue-jaw lift

   d. not interfere but stay with her and monitor her condition

3. You are an EMS provider called to the scene of an emergency. Upon arrival you find a 65-year-old man lying unresponsive on the floor. The victim's wife says that she thinks a loose dental appliance fell back in his throat and that he couldn't speak before he became unresponsive. You perform a head tilt–chin lift, attempt a rescue breath, and note a complete inability to get the chest to rise. Your next action should be to

   a. perform a pulse check

   b. perform a finger sweep

   c. perform up to 5 abdominal thrusts

   d. reposition the head, reopen the airway, and try to ventilate again

4. A 32-year-old woman becomes unresponsive at a restaurant. Her companions say that she suddenly stopped talking, clutched her throat with both her hands, turned blue, and collapsed. Your next action should be to

   a. have someone phone 911 and get the AED

   b. check the pulse

   c. attempt ventilation

   d. perform a finger sweep

5. You are an EMS provider treating an unresponsive adult victim of a complete airway obstruction. You have attempted and reattempted rescue breathing unsuccessfully, and you have performed 5 abdominal thrusts. Your next action should be to

   a. reposition the head and try breathing again

   b. repeat 5 abdominal thrusts

   c. perform CPR and attach the AED

   d. perform a tongue-jaw lift and finger sweep to remove the foreign object

6. You are treating an unresponsive adult victim of a complete airway obstruction. After 4 minutes of attempting to relieve the obstruction, you remove a large piece of meat from the back of the victim's throat with a finger sweep. You deliver 2 slow breaths and note that the chest rises with each rescue breath. Your next action should be to

   a. continue rescue breathing

   b. check the victim's pulse

   c. attach the AED

   d. phone 911

7. You hear a call for help in a restaurant and go to the table to investigate. A 43-year-old man is sitting at the table clutching his throat. His lips are blue, and he is unable to speak. He is drooling and is barely conscious. Your next action should be to

   a. perform a head tilt–chin lift and attempt ventilation

   b. phone 911 and get the AED

   c. perform a Heimlich maneuver

   d. perform up to 5 abdominal thrusts

How did you do?

Answers: **1,** c; **2,** d; **3,** d; **4,** a; **5,** d; **6,** b; **7,** c.

References

1. National Safety Council. *Injury Facts, 1999.* Itasca, Ill: National Safety Council; 1999:9.

2. Fingerhut LA, Cox CS, Warner M. International comparative analysis of injury mortality: findings from the ICE on injury statistics. International Collaborative Effort on Injury Statistics. *Adv Data.* October 7, 1998; Number 303:1-20.

3. Vital and Health Statistics of the Centers for Disease Control and Prevention, National Center for Health Statistics. Data on odds of death due to choking. Available at: www.cdc.gov/scientific.htm#statistics. Accessed May 7, 1998.

4. National Safety Council. *Accident Facts, 1997.* Chicago, Ill: National Safety Council; 1997.

5. Canadian Hospitals Injury Reporting and Prevention Program. *Summary Statistics CHIRPP Database for the Year 1997.*

6. Haugen RK. The café coronary: sudden death in restaurants. *JAMA.* 1963;186:142-143.

7. Manolios N, Mackie I. Drowning and near-drowning on Australian beaches patrolled by life-savers: a 10-year study, 1973-1983. *Med J Aust.* 1988;148:165-167,170-171.

8. Rosen P, Stoto M, Harley J. The use of the Heimlich maneuver in near-drowning: Institute of Medicine report. *J Emerg Med.* 1995;13:397-405.

9. Heimlich HJ. A life-saving maneuver to prevent food-choking. *JAMA.* 1975;234:398-401.

10. Ekberg O, Feinberg M. Clinical and demographic data in 75 patients with near-fatal choking episodes. *Dysphagia.* 1992;7:205-208.

11. Fioritti A, Giaccotto L, Melega V. Choking incidents among psychiatric patients: retrospective analysis of thirty-one cases from the Bologna psychiatric wards. *Can J Psychiatry.* 1997;42:515-520.

12. Lan RS. Non-asphyxiating tracheobronchial foreign bodies in adults. *Eur Respir J.* 1994;7:510-514.

13. Fitzpatrick PC, Guarisco JL. Pediatric airway foreign bodies. *J La State Med Soc.* 1998;150:138-141.

14. Jacob B, Wiebrauck C, Lamprecht J, Bonte W. Laryngologic aspects of bolus asphyxiation-bolus death. *Dysphagia.* 1992;7:31-35.

15. Chen CH, Lai CL, Tsai TT, Lee YC, Perng RP. Foreign body aspirations into the lower airway in Chinese adults. *Chest.* 1997;112:129-133.

16. Jones TM, Luke LC. Life threatening airway obstruction: a hazard of concealed eating disorders. *J Accid Emerg Med.* 1998;15:332-333.

17. American Heart Association, International Liaison Committee on Resuscitation (ILCOR). Guidelines 2000 for Cardiopulmonary Resuscitation and Emergency Cardiovascular Care. International Consensus on Science. *Circulation.* 2000;102(suppl I):I-46-I-48.

18. Committee on Emergency Medical Services, Assembly of Life Sciences, National Research Council. *Report on Emergency Airway Management.* Washington, DC: National Academy of Sciences; 1976.

19. Eigen H. Treatment of choking. *Pediatrics.* 1983;71:300-301.

20. Heimlich HJ, Hoffmann KA, Canestri FR. Food-choking and drowning deaths prevented by external subdiaphragmatic compression: physiological basis. *Ann Thorac Surg.* 1975;20:188-195.

21. Heimlich HJ, Uhley MH, Netter FH. The Heimlich maneuver. *Clin Symp.* 1979;31:1-32.

22. Nowitz A, Lewer BM, Galletly DC. An interesting complication of the Heimlich manoeuvre. *Resuscitation.* 1998;39:129-131.

23. Redding JS. The choking controversy: critique of evidence on the Heimlich maneuver. *Crit Care Med.* 1979;7:475-479.

24. Majumdar A, Sedman PC. Gastric rupture secondary to successful Heimlich manoeuvre. *Postgrad Med J.* 1998;74:609-610.

25. Bintz M, Cogbill TH. Gastric rupture after the Heimlich maneuver. *J Trauma.* 1996;40:159-160.

26. Dupre MW, Silva E, Brotman S. Traumatic rupture of the stomach secondary to Heimlich maneuver. *Am J Emerg Med.* 1993;11:611-612.

27. Anderson S, Buggy D. Prolonged pharyngeal obstruction after the Heimlich manoeuvre. *Anaesthesia.* 1999;54:308-309.

28. Heimlich HJ. Pop goes the cafe coronary. *Emerg Med.* 1974;6:154-155.

29. Orlowski JP. Vomiting as a complication of the Heimlich maneuver. *JAMA.* 1987;258:512-513.

30. Fink JA, Klein RL. Complications of the Heimlich maneuver. *J Pediatr Surg.* 1989;24:486-487.

31. van der Ham AC, Lange JF. Traumatic rupture of the stomach after Heimlich maneuver. *J Emerg Med.* 1990;8:713-715.

32. Aufderheide T, Stapleton ER, Hazinski MF, Cummins RO. *Heartsaver AED for the Lay Rescuer and First Responder.* Dallas, Tex: American Heart Association; 1999.

33. Langhelle A, Sunde K, Wik L, Steen PA. Airway pressure with chest compression versus Heimlich manoeuvre in recently dead adults with complete airway obstruction. *Resuscitation.* 2000;44:105-108.

34. Skulberg A. Chest compressions: an alternative to the Heimlich manoeuver? *Resuscitation.* 1992;24:91.

35. Emergency Cardiac Care Committee and Subcommittees, American Heart Association. Guidelines for cardiopulmonary resuscitation and emergency cardiac care. *JAMA.* 1992;268:2172-2302.

36. Emergency Cardiac Care Committee, American Heart Association. *Heartsaver ABC.* Dallas, Tex: American Heart Association; 1999.

37. Emergency Cardiac Care Committee, American Heart Association. *Heartsaver CPR in Schools.* Dallas, Tex: American Heart Association; 1999.

38. Kaye W, Rallis SF, Mancini ME, Linhares KC, Angell ML, Donovan DS, Zajano NC, Finger JA. The problem of poor retention of cardiopulmonary resuscitation skills may lie with the instructor, not the learner or the curriculum. *Resuscitation.* 1991;21:67-87.

39. Brennan RT, Braslow A. Skill mastery in cardiopulmonary resuscitation training classes. *Am J Emerg Med.* 1995;13:505-508.

40. Liberman M, Lavoie A, Mulder D, Sampalis J. Cardiopulmonary resuscitation: errors made by pre-hospital emergency medical personnel. *Resuscitation* 1999;42:47-55.

41. Kaye W, Mancini ME. Retention of cardiopulmonary skills by physicians, registered nurses, and the general public. *Crit Care Med.* 1986;14:620-622.

42. Wilson E, Brooks B, Tweed WA. CPR skills retention of lay basic rescuers. *Ann Emerg Med.* 1983;12:482-484.

43. Mancini ME, Kaye W. The effect of time since training on house officers' retention of cardiopulmonary resuscitation skills. *Am J Emerg Med.* 1985;3:31-32.

44. Mandel LP, Cobb LA. Initial and long-term competency of citizens trained in CPR. *Emerg Health Serv Q.* 1982;1:49-63.

45. Van Hoeyweghen RJ, Bossaert LL, Mullie A, Calle P, Martens P, Buylaert WA, Delooz H. Quality and efficiency of bystander CPR. Belgian Cerebral Resuscitation Study Group. *Resuscitation.* 1993;26:47-52.

46. Kern KB, Hilwig RW, Berg RA, Ewy GA. Efficacy of chest compression-only BLS CPR in the presence of an occluded airway. *Resuscitation.* 1998;39:179-188.

While you are working in the Emergency Department, a mother comes running in holding a limp infant in her arms. She calls for someone to help her. You take the infant from the mother's arms and note immediately that the infant does not respond to your touch or voice. You shout for a colleague to help. You carry the infant into the pediatric triage room and lay him down on a gurney.

The mother states that the infant, named David, has had a high fever and has been fussy. She was driving to the hospital when David had a seizure and stopped breathing. The infant is limp, with dusky lips. You grab a bag and mask and turn on the oxygen. You open the infant's airway with a head tilt–chin lift, and look, listen, and feel for breathing.

The infant has only gasping respirations, so you provide 2 breaths with bag and mask (using 100% oxygen) and note excellent chest rise with each breath. After the second breath David begins coughing and moving. He has a strong pulse. Your colleagues enter the room and begin placing ECG monitor leads on the infant's chest and establish IV access.

Pediatric Basic Life Support

Overview

The actions taken during the first few minutes of an emergency are critical to survival of the infant or child with a cardiorespiratory emergency. Pediatric basic life support (PBLS) has traditionally referred to the provision of CPR with no devices.

In recent years the practice of BLS by healthcare providers has expanded to include the use of barrier devices and airway and ventilation adjuncts, such as airways, bag-mask ventilation, and oxygen. For victims of cardiopulmonary arrest 8 years of age and older, BLS for lay and professional responders has also expanded to include the use of automated external defibrillators (AEDs).

This chapter focuses on infants from birth to 1 year of age and children from 1 to 8 years of age except in discussing prevention of injury, where adolescents are included.

In this chapter PBLS actions now include the following:

- Prevention of injuries and sudden infant death syndrome (SIDS) and other common causes of respiratory and cardiac arrest

- Prompt recognition and action for respiratory and cardiovascular emergencies to prevent respiratory and circulatory arrest

- Prompt action for any infant or child who is suddenly found to be unresponsive

- Rescue breathing for victims of respiratory arrest

  — Without barrier devices

  — With barrier devices

  — With bag-mask ventilation

- Chest compressions and rescue breathing for victims of cardiopulmonary arrest

- Recognition and relief of FBAO

This chapter will address the following aspects of BLS: (1) rescue breathing for infants and children with respiratory arrest, (2) chest compressions and rescue breathing for victims of cardiopulmonary arrest, and (3) relief of FBAO in responsive and unresponsive infants and children.

CPR and life support in the pediatric age group should be part of a community-wide Chain of Survival that links the child to the best hope of survival after emergencies. The Chain of Survival integrates education in prevention of cardiopulmonary arrest, BLS, early access to emergency medical services (EMS) systems prepared for children's needs, early and effective pediatric advanced life

Learning Objectives

After reading this chapter and participating in the skills video segments and practice sessions, you should be able to

1. List the sequence of actions you should perform when you encounter an infant (from newborn to 1 year of age) or child (1 to 8 years of age) in respiratory or cardiac arrest

2. Describe and demonstrate 1- and 2-rescuer CPR for an infant and for a child

3. Describe and demonstrate the use of the following adjuncts to ventilation:

   a. Face shield (infants and children)

   b. Pocket mask (children)

   c. Bag mask

4. Describe and demonstrate the use of cricoid pressure (the Sellick maneuver) during bag-mask ventilation for the unconscious or unresponsive infant or child

5. Describe the situations when a "phone first" approach may be appropriate for a lone rescuer with an unresponsive infant or child

6. Describe the signs of severe or complete foreign-body airway obstruction (FBAO) in the infant and child and actions to relieve it

FIGURE 1. Pediatric Chain of Survival.

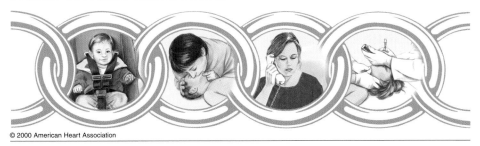

© 2000 American Heart Association

support, and pediatric postresuscitation and rehabilitative care (see Figure 1).

Sudden cardiopulmonary arrest in infants and children is much less common than sudden cardiac arrest in adults.[1] In contrast to cardiac arrest in adults, cardiac arrest in infants and children is rarely a sudden event, and noncardiac causes predominate.[1] The etiology of cardiac arrest in infants and children varies by age, setting, and the underlying health of the child. For these reasons the sequence of CPR for infants and children requires a different approach from that used for adults.

Cardiac arrest in the under-21-year-old age group occurs most commonly at either end of the age spectrum: under 1 year of age and during adolescence. In the newly born infant, respiratory failure is the most common cause of cardiopulmonary deterioration and arrest. During infancy the most common causes of arrest are sudden infant death syndrome (SIDS), respiratory diseases, airway obstruction (including foreign-body aspiration), submersion, sepsis, and neurologic disease.[2-8] Beyond 1 year of age, injuries are the leading cause of death.[9-11]

Cardiac arrest in children typically represents the terminal event of progressive shock or respiratory failure. Either shock or respiratory failure may include a compensated state from which children can rapidly deteriorate to a decompensated condition, then respiratory or cardiac arrest.

Rescuers must detect and promptly treat early signs of respiratory and circulatory failure to prevent cardiac arrest.

In children early, effective bystander CPR has been associated with successful return of spontaneous circulation and neurologically intact survival.[12,13] BLS courses should be offered to target populations such as expectant parents, child-care providers, teachers, sports supervisors, and others who regularly care for children. Parents of children with underlying conditions that predispose them to cardiopulmonary failure as well as persons who routinely care for these at-risk children should be particularly targeted for these courses.

Response to Cardiovascular Emergencies in Infants and Children

Definition of *Newly Born, Neonate, Infant, Child, and Adult*

The term *neonate* is used to describe infants in the first 28 days (month) of life.[2] The term *newly born* is used in this text to refer specifically to the neonate in the first minutes to hours after birth. This term is used to focus attention on the needs of the infant *at and immediately after birth* (including the first hours of life). The terms *newborn* or *neonate* were previously used but did not clearly refer to the first hours — rather than month — of life. The term *infant* includes the neonatal period and extends to the age of 1 year (12 months). For the purposes of this text, the term *child* refers to ages 1 to 8 years. *For the purposes of BLS only,* the term *adult* applies to victims 8 years of age through adulthood. For the purposes of pediatric *advanced* life support (PALS),

the PALS guidelines described in this text apply to infants, children, and adolescents who are cared for in pediatric facilities.

For the purposes of BLS, the term *infant* is defined by the approximate size of the young child who can receive effective chest compressions given with 2 fingers or 2 thumbs with encircling hands. Historically the use of the term *child* in the ECC guidelines has been limited to age 8 years to simplify BLS education. Cardiac compression can generally be accomplished with 1 hand for victims between the ages of 1 and 8 years. However, variability in the size of the victim or the size and strength of the rescuer can require use of the 2-finger or 2 thumb–encircling hands technique for chest compression in a small toddler or the 2-handed adult compression technique for chest compression in a large child who is 6 to 7 years of age.[14,15]

Differences in Anatomy and Physiology Affecting Cardiac Arrest and Resuscitation

Respiratory failure or arrest is a common cause of cardiac arrest during infancy and childhood. These guidelines emphasize the need for immediate provision of CPR by the lone rescuer — including opening of the airway and delivery of rescue breathing — *before* activation of the emergency response system. This emphasis on immediate support of oxygenation and ventilation is based on knowledge of the important role of respiratory failure in pediatric cardiac arrest. Optimal application of early oxygenation and ventilation requires an understanding of airway anatomy and physiology.

Airway Anatomy and Physiology

For many reasons infants and children are at risk for developing airway obstruction and respiratory failure.[16,17] The upper and lower airways of the infant and child are much smaller than the upper and lower airways of the adult. As a result, modest airway obstruction from edema, mucous plugs, or a foreign body can significantly reduce pediatric airway diameter and increase resistance to air flow and work of breathing:

1. The infant tongue is proportionally large in relation to the size of the oropharynx. As a result, posterior displacement of the tongue occurs readily and may cause severe airway obstruction in the infant.

2. In the infant and child the subglottic airway is smaller and more compliant and the supporting cartilage less developed than in the adult. As a result, this portion of the airway can easily become obstructed by mucus, blood, pus, edema, active constriction, external compression, or pressure differences created during spontaneous respiratory effort in the presence of airway obstruction. The pediatric airway is very compliant and may collapse during spontaneous respiratory effort in the face of airway obstruction.

3. The ribs and sternum normally contribute to maintenance of lung volume. In infants these ribs are very compliant and may fail to maintain lung volume, particularly when the elastic recoil of the lungs is increased or lung compliance is decreased. As a result, functional residual capacity is reduced when respiratory effort is diminished or absent. In addition, the limited support of lung volume expansion by the ribs makes the infant more dependent on diaphragm movement to generate a tidal volume. Anything that interferes with diaphragm movement (eg, gastric inflation, acute abdomen) may produce respiratory insufficiency.

4. Infants and children have limited oxygen reserve. Physiological collapse of the small airways at or below lung functional residual capacity and an interval of hypoxemia and hypercarbia preceding arrest often influence oxygen reserve and arrest metabolic conditions.[18]

Cardiac Output, Oxygen Delivery, and Oxygen Demand

Cardiac output is the product of heart rate and stroke volume. Although the pediatric heart is capable of increasing stroke volume, cardiac output during infancy and childhood is largely dependent on maintenance of an adequate heart rate. Bradycardia may be associated with a rapid fall in cardiac output, leading to rapid deterioration in systemic perfusion. In fact, bradycardia is one of the most common terminal rhythms observed in children. For this reason lay rescuers are taught to provide chest compressions when there are no observed signs of circulation. Healthcare providers are taught to provide chest compressions when there are no observed signs of circulation (including absence of a pulse) or when severe bradycardia (heart rate less than 60 beats per minute [bpm]) develops in the presence of poor systemic perfusion.

Epidemiology of Cardiopulmonary Arrest: Phone Fast (Infant/Child) Versus Phone First (Adult)

In adults most sudden, nontraumatic cardiopulmonary arrest is cardiac in origin, and the most common terminal cardiac rhythm is ventricular fibrillation (VF).[19] In research studies the gold standard for out-of-hospital adult arrest used to compare outcomes is *nontraumatic, witnessed arrest with a presenting rhythm of VF or pulseless ventricular tachycardia (VT).*[20] For these victims the time from collapse to defibrillation is the single greatest determinant of survival.[21-26] In addition, bystander CPR increases survival after sudden, witnessed adult cardiopulmonary arrest (relative odds of survival are 2.6, 95% confidence interval, 2.0 to 3.4).[27,28]

In children the incidence, precise etiology, and outcome of cardiac arrest and resuscitation are difficult to ascertain because most reports of pediatric resuscitation contain insufficient patient numbers or use exclusion criteria or definitions that are inconsistent, prohibiting broad generalization to all children.[29] The causes of

pediatric cardiopulmonary arrest are heterogeneous, including SIDS, asphyxia, near-drowning, trauma, and sepsis.[2,30-35] Therefore, there is no single gold standard for pediatric cardiac arrest for research or resuscitation outcome.[36] Reported successful outcomes from an arrest may include change in cardiac rhythm, improved hemodynamics during CPR, return of spontaneous circulation, survival to hospital admission, survival to hospital discharge, short- or long-term survival, or neurologically intact survival. Selection of the appropriate outcome variable and correlation with a single resuscitation intervention is often difficult.

If resuscitation is required in the first years of life, it is most frequently needed at birth. Approximately 5% to 10% of newly born infants require some degree of active resuscitation at birth, including stimulation to breathe,[37] and approximately 1% to 10% born in the hospital require assisted ventilation.[38] Worldwide more than 5 000 000 neonatal deaths occur annually, with asphyxia at birth the cause of approximately 19% of these deaths.[39] The implementation of relatively simple resuscitative techniques could save the lives of an estimated 1 000 000 infants per year.[40]

Throughout infancy and childhood most out-of-hospital cardiac arrest occurs in or around the home, where children are under the supervision of parents and child-care providers. In this setting conditions such as SIDS, trauma, drowning, poisoning, choking, severe asthma, and pneumonia are the most common causes of arrest. In industrialized nations trauma is the leading cause of death from the age of 6 months through young adulthood.[10]

In general, pediatric out-of-hospital arrest is characterized by a progression from hypoxia and hypercarbia to respiratory arrest and bradycardia and then asystolic cardiac arrest.[1,32,35] VT or VF has been reported in less than or equal to 15% of pediatric victims of out-of-hospital arrest[13,41,42] even when rhythm is assessed by first responders.[43,44] Survival from out-of-hospital cardiopulmonary arrest ranges from 3% to 17% in most studies,* and survivors are often neurologically devastated. Neurologically intact survival rates of 50% or greater have been reported for resuscitation of children with respiratory arrest alone,[6,51] and in some studies the presence of VT or VF is associated with a higher survival rate.[42,50]

Prompt, effective chest compressions and rescue breathing have been shown to improve return of spontaneous circulation and increase neurologically intact survival in children with cardiac arrest.[13,35] Early defibrillation can improve outcome from pediatric VT/VF (except for submersion victims[53]).[42,50]

Organized rapid delivery of out-of-hospital BLS and ALS has improved the outcome of drowning victims in cardiac arrest, perhaps the best-studied scenario of pediatric out-of-hospital cardiac arrest.[54] Because most pediatric arrests are secondary to progressive respiratory failure or shock and because VF is relatively uncommon, immediate CPR (phone fast) is recommended for lone rescuers of pediatric victims of cardiopulmonary arrest out-of-hospital rather than the adult approach (phone first). Effective BLS should be provided for infants and children as quickly as possible. The lone rescuer should provide about 1 minute of BLS before calling 911 or other emergency response number.

The need to choose between a phone first and a phone fast approach applies only if a rescuer is alone. Of course, if 2 or more rescuers are present, one rescuer should make the emergency phone call while the other begins BLS support. When several rescuers are present, the phone call should be simultaneous with provision of BLS.

In some circumstances primary arrhythmic cardiac arrest (ie, VF or pulseless VT) is more likely; in these circumstances the

*References 1, 3, 5, 6, 13, 29, 30, 35, 42, 43, 45-52

lone lay rescuer may be instructed to activate the EMS system *before* beginning CPR. Examples include the sudden collapse of children with underlying cardiac disease or a history of arrhythmia. Families of children with an *identified* risk for sudden cardiac arrest should be taught the phone first or adult sequence of CPR: if the child collapses suddenly, a lone bystander should *first* activate the local EMS or emergency medical response system and then return to the victim to begin CPR.

A *sudden* witnessed collapse in a previously healthy child or adolescent suggests cardiac arrest, and immediate activation of the EMS system may be beneficial, even if the victim is less than 8 years of age. Potential causes of sudden collapse in children with no known history of heart disease include prolonged QT syndrome, hypertrophic cardiomyopathy, and drug-induced cardiac arrest.[31,55,56] Drug-induced arrest in the adolescent age group is most likely to be related to a drug overdose.

Ideally rescuers should tailor each resuscitation sequence to the most likely cause of the victim's cardiac arrest. But this approach is impractical. Education of the lay rescuer is most effective if the message is simple and can be used in a wide variety of situations. The more complex the teaching sequence or message, the less likely that the rescuer will remember what to do and do it.[57,58] Therefore, a simple, consistent message for lone lay rescuers of most infants and children is to phone fast: provide approximately 1 minute of CPR and then activate (phone) the EMS system.

In victims 8 years and older in the out-of-hospital setting, the adult Chain of Survival and resuscitation sequence is recommended. If the victim is unresponsive, the lone rescuer should immediately activate the EMS or emergency medical response system and get the AED if available. The phone-first approach is particularly appropriate if the victim has experienced a sudden arrest.

Exceptions to the phone-first rule for unresponsive victims 8 years of age or older should be noted. These special resuscitation situations include near-drowning, trauma, drug overdose, and respiratory arrest. A victim of any age who is unresponsive from these causes will likely benefit from a phone-fast approach by the lone rescuer (provide approximately 1 minute of CPR and then activate the emergency response number). These special resuscitation situations are presented in more detail in Chapters 6 and 11.

BLS for Children With Special Needs

Children with special healthcare needs have chronic physical, developmental, behavioral, or emotional conditions and require health and related services of a type or amount not usually required by typically developing children.[59-61] These children may need emergency care for acute, life-threatening complications that are unique to their chronic conditions,[61] such as obstruction of a tracheostomy, failure of support technology (eg, ventilator failure), or progression of underlying respiratory failure or neurologic disease. Approximately half of EMS responses to children with special healthcare needs, however, are unrelated to the child's special needs and may include traditional causes of EMS calls, such as trauma,[62] which require no treatment beyond the normal EMS standard of care.

Emergency care of children with special healthcare needs can be complicated by lack of specific medical information about the child's baseline condition, medical plan of care, current medications, and any do-not-attempt-to-resuscitate orders. Certainly the best source of information about a chronically ill child is the person who cares for the child on a daily basis. If that person is unavailable or incapacitated (eg, after an automobile crash), some means is needed to access important information. A wide variety of methods have been developed to make this information immediately accessible, including the use of standard forms, containers kept in a standard place in the home (eg, the refrigerator, because most homes have one), window stickers, wallet cards, and medical alert bracelets. No single method of communicating information has proved to be superior. A standardized form, the Emergency Information Form (EIF), was developed by the American Academy of Pediatrics and the American College of Emergency Physicians[61] and is available on the Worldwide Web (http://www.pediatrics.org/cgi/content/full/104/4/e53). Parents and child-care providers should keep essential medical information at home, with the child, and at the child's school or child-care facility. Child-care providers should have access to this information and should be familiar with signs of deterioration in the child and any existing advance directives.[62,63]

If the physician, parents, and child (as appropriate) have made a decision to limit resuscitative efforts or withhold attempts at resuscitation, a physician order indicating the limits of resuscitative efforts must be written for use in the in-hospital setting; in most countries a separate order must be written for the out-of-hospital setting. Legal issues and regulations regarding requirements for these out-of-hospital no-CPR directives vary from country to country and in the United States from state to state. It is always important for families to inform the local EMS system when such directives are established for out-of-hospital care.

Whenever a child with a chronic or life-threatening condition is discharged from the hospital, parents, school nurses, and any home healthcare providers should be informed about possible complications that the child may experience, anticipated signs of deterioration, and the cause of such deterioration. Specific instructions should be given about CPR and other interventions that the child may require, as well as instructions about whom to contact and why.[63]

If the child has a tracheostomy, anyone responsible for the child's care (including parents, school nurses, and home health-care providers) should be taught to assess airway patency, clear the airway, and provide CPR with the artificial airway. If CPR is required, rescue breathing and bag-mask ventilation are performed through the tracheostomy tube. As with any form of rescue breathing, effective ventilation is judged by adequate bilateral chest expansion.

If the tracheostomy tube becomes obstructed and impossible to use even after attempts to clear the tube with suctioning, the tube should be replaced. If a clean tube is not available, provide ventilations at the tracheostomy stoma until an artificial airway can be placed. If the upper airway is patent, it may be possible to provide effective conventional bag-mask ventilation through the nose and mouth while occluding the superficial tracheal stoma site.

Out-of-Hospital (EMS) Care

EMS systems were initially created for adults in developed nations. EMS equipment, training, experience, and expertise are often less well developed to meet the needs of children. In the United States death rates are higher in children than in adults treated in the EMS system, especially in areas where tertiary pediatric care is unavailable.[64-71]

To improve pediatric out-of-hospital care, EMS personnel should be optimally trained and equipped to care for pediatric victims, medical dispatchers should use emergency protocols appropriate for children, and Emergency Departments caring for children should be appropriately staffed and equipped. Emergency Departments that care for acutely ill or injured children should have an ongoing agreement with a pediatric tertiary service through which patients can receive postresuscitation care in a pediatric intensive care unit under the supervision of trained personnel.

Prevention of Cardiopulmonary Arrest in Infants and Children

Healthcare providers are often able to educate parents and children about risk factors for injury and cardiorespiratory arrest. This section provides information about prevention of SIDS and injury, the leading causes of death in infants and children, respectively. Information provided to new or prospective parents or primary caretakers during healthcare encounters may provide them with the information they need to reduce the risk of SIDS or injury.

Reducing the Risk of Sudden Infant Death Syndrome

SIDS is the sudden death of an infant, typically between the ages of 1 month and 1 year, that is unexpected based on the infant's medical history and unexplained by other causes when a postmortem examination is performed. SIDS probably represents a variety of conditions caused by several mechanisms, including rebreathing asphyxia, with a decreased arousal and possible blunted response to hypoxemia or hypercarbia.[72-78]

The peak incidence of SIDS occurs in infants 2 to 4 months of age. From 70% to 90% of SIDS deaths are reported in the first 6 months of life.[72-78] Many characteristics are associated with increased risk of SIDS, including the prone (on the stomach) sleeping position, the winter months, lower family income, males, siblings of SIDS victims, infants whose mothers smoke cigarettes, infants who have survived severe, apparently life-threatening events, infants whose mothers are drug addicts, and infants of low birthweight.

The risk of SIDS is associated with the prone (on the stomach) sleeping position. *Infants who sleep prone have a much higher frequency of SIDS than infants who sleep supine (on the back) or on their side.*[79-81] The prone position, particularly on a soft surface, is thought to contribute to rebreathing asphyxia.[72-78] Australia, New Zealand, and several European countries have documented a significant reduction in the incidence of SIDS when parents and child-care providers are taught to place healthy infants to sleep supine or on their side.[82] This "Back to Sleep" public education campaign was introduced in the United States in 1992, when approximately 7000 infants died of SIDS. By 1997 the US SIDS death rate had been reduced to 2991.[2]

Recent reports from New Zealand[82] and England[83] have documented a slightly greater risk of SIDS when infants are placed on their side than when they are placed supine for sleep. Either side or supine position, however, continues to be associated with a much lower risk of SIDS than the prone position.

All parents and those responsible for the care of children (including healthcare providers) should be aware of the need to place healthy infants *supine* for sleeping. The supine sleeping position has not been associated with an increase in any significant adverse events, such as vomiting or aspiration.[79] A side position may be used as an alternative, but infants in this position should be propped and posi-

tioned to prevent them from rolling to the prone position. In addition, the infant should not sleep on soft surfaces, such as lambswool, fluffy comforters, or other objects that might trap exhaled air near the infant's face.

Injury: The Magnitude of the Problem

In the United States injury is the leading cause of death in children and adults 1 to 44 years of age and is responsible for more childhood deaths than all other causes combined.[9,11] Internationally injury death rates are highest for children 1 to 14 years of age and young adults 15 to 24, relative to other causes of death.[10,84] The term *injury* is emphasized rather than the term *accident* because the injury is often preventable, and the term *accident* implies that nothing can be done to prevent the episode.

The Science of Injury Control

Injury control attempts to prevent injury or minimize its effects on the child and

family in 3 phases: prevention, minimization of damage, and postinjury care. When planning injury prevention strategies, 3 principles deserve emphasis. First, passive injury prevention strategies are generally preferred because they are more likely to be used than active strategies, which require repeated, conscious effort. Second, specific instructions (eg, keep the water heater temperature 120°F to 130°F or 48.9°C to 54.4°C) are more likely to be followed than general advice (eg, reduce the maximum temperature of home tap hot water). Third, individual education reinforced by community-wide educational programs is more effective than isolated educational sessions or community-wide education alone.[85,86]

Epidemiology and Prevention of Common Injuries in Children and Adolescents

Injury prevention has the greatest effect by focusing on injuries that are frequent and for which effective strategies are available. The leading causes of death

FIGURE 2. International injury deaths for children 1 to 14 years of age. Reproduced from Fingerhut LA, Cox CS, Warner M. International comparative analysis of injury mortality: findings from the International Collaborative Effort (ICE) on injury statistics. Vital and Health Statistics, Centers for Disease Control and Prevention, National Center for Health Statistics, No. 303, October 7, 1998.

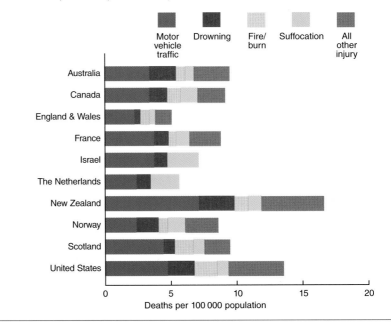

internationally in children 1 to 14 years of age are depicted in Figure 2. The 6 most common types of fatal childhood injuries amenable to injury prevention strategies are motor vehicle passenger injuries, pedestrian injuries, bicycle injuries, submersion, burns, and firearm injuries.[9,10,85,87] Prevention of these common fatal injuries would substantially reduce childhood deaths and disability internationally. For this reason information about injury prevention is included with information about infant/child resuscitation.

Motor Vehicle–Related Injuries

Motor vehicle–related trauma accounts for nearly half of all pediatric injuries and deaths in the United States and 40% of injury mortality in children 1 to 14 years of age internationally.[9,10,54] Contributing factors include failure to use proper passenger restraints, inexperienced adolescent drivers, and alcohol abuse. Each of these contributing factors should be addressed by injury prevention programs.

Proper use of child seat restraints and lap-shoulder harnesses will prevent an estimated 65% to 75% of serious injuries and fatalities to passengers 4 years of age and younger and 45% to 55% of all pediatric motor vehicle passenger injuries and deaths.[9,88] The American Academy of Pediatrics, the Centers for Disease Control and Prevention, and the National Highway Traffic Safety Administration have made the following child passenger safety recommendations:

1. Children should ride in rear-facing infant seats until they are at least 20 pounds (9 kg) *and* at least 1 year of age, with good head control. These seats should be secured in the *back* seat of the automobile.

   a. A rear-facing safety seat must *never* be placed in the front passenger seat of a car with a passenger-side airbag.

   b. Convertible seats can be used for children less than 1 year old and weighing less than 20 pounds (9 kg) if they are used in the reclined and rear-facing position.

2. A child who is 1 year old or older *and* weighs 20 to 40 pounds (9 to 18 kg) should be placed in a convertible car safety seat used in the upright and forward-facing position as long as he or she fits well in the seat. The harness straps should be positioned at or above the child's shoulders. These seats should also be placed in the *back* seat of the automobile.

3. Belt-positioning booster seats should be used for children weighing 40 to 80 pounds (18 to 36 kg) until they are at least 58 to 60 inches (4 feet, 10 inches to 5 feet or 148 cm minimum) in height. These belt-positioning seats ensure that the lap and shoulder belts restrain the child over bones rather than soft tissues.

4. Children may be restrained in automobile lap and shoulder belts when they weigh 80 pounds (36 kg) and are at least 58 inches (4 feet, 10 inches or 148 cm) tall. A properly fitting lap-shoulder belt should lie low across the child's hips while the shoulder belt lies flat across the shoulder and sternum, away from the neck and face.

5. Children approximately 12 years old and younger should not sit in the front seat of cars equipped with passenger-side air bags.[89,90]

Parents should be taught the proper use of automobile safety restraints. Children should also learn about the importance of safety restraints during their early primary school education.[91] Parents should be taught to check the installation of child passenger safety seats and follow the manufacturer's instructions carefully. If the safety seat is properly installed, it should not move more than ½ inch (1 cm) front to back or side to side when pushed.

Further development of passive restraint devices, including adjustable shoulder harnesses, automatic lap and shoulder belts, and air bags, is needed. The benefits of air bags continue to far outweigh

the risks, saving approximately 2663 lives in the United States alone from 1987 to 1997. The vast majority of the 74 US children with fatal airbag-related injuries reported through April 1999 were improperly restrained for their age or not restrained at all. They included infants restrained in rear-facing infant seats placed in the front passenger seats of cars with passenger-side airbags, children less than 4 years old restrained by lap and shoulder belts, and children who were not restrained at all. To prevent airbag and most other occupant injuries, children 12 years old and younger should be properly restrained for their age and size in the back seat of cars.

When a child is old enough (more than 12 years old) and large enough to sit in the front seat of an automobile with a passenger-side airbag, the child should be properly restrained for age and size, and the automobile seat should be moved as far back and away from the airbag cover as possible. The development of "smart" airbags that adjust inflation time and force according to the weight of the passenger should further reduce injuries related to airbags.

Adolescent drivers are responsible for a disproportionate number of motor vehicle–related injuries. Surprisingly adolescent driver education classes have increased the number of adolescent drivers at risk with no improvement in safety.[92-95] Approximately 50% of motor vehicle fatalities involving adolescents also involve alcohol. In fact, a large proportion of all pediatric motor vehicle occupant deaths occur in vehicles operated by inebriated drivers.[96-99] Although intoxication rates decreased for drivers of all age groups from 1987 to 1999, drunk drivers are still responsible for a large portion of all motor vehicle crashes and pose a significant risk to children.[9,100]

Pedestrian Injuries

Pedestrian injuries are a leading cause of death among children 5 to 9 years of age in the United States.[54,85] Pedestrian injuries typically occur when a child darts out into the street, crossing between intersections.[9] Although educational programs aimed at improving children's street-related behavior hold promise, roadway interventions, including adequate lighting, construction of sidewalks, and roadway barriers, must also be pursued in areas of high pedestrian traffic.

Bicycle Injuries

Bicycle crashes are responsible for approximately 200 000 injuries and more than 600 deaths in children and adolescents in the United States every year.[54,101] Head injuries are the cause of most bicycle injury–related morbidity and mortality. In fact, bicycle-related trauma is a leading cause of severe pediatric closed-head injuries.[102] Bicycle helmets can reduce the severity of head injuries by 85% and brain injuries by 88%. Yet many parents are unaware of the need for helmets, and children may be reluctant to wear them.[102,103] A successful bicycle helmet education program includes an ongoing community-wide multidisciplinary approach that provides focused information about the protection afforded by helmets. Such programs should ensure the acceptability, accessibility, and affordability of helmets.[101,103]

Submersion/Drowning

Internationally drowning is responsible for approximately 15% of injury deaths to children 1 to 14 years of age.[10] It is a significant cause of disability and death in children less than 4 years old and is a leading cause of death in this age group in the United States.[9,54,85,104] For every death due to submersion, 6 children are hospitalized, and approximately 20% of hospitalized survivors are severely brain damaged.[54,105]

Parents should be aware of the dangers to young children posed by any body of water. Young children and children with seizure disorders should never be left unattended in bathtubs or near swimming pools, ponds, or beaches. Some drownings in swimming pools may be prevented by completely surrounding the pool with appropriate fencing, including gates with secure latching mechanisms.[104,106] The

house will not serve as an effective barrier to the pool if it has a door opening onto the pool area.

Children more than 5 years old should learn how to swim. No one should ever swim alone, and even supervised children should wear personal flotation devices when playing in rivers, streams, or lakes.

Alcohol appears to be a significant risk factor in adolescent drowning. Adolescent education, limited access to alcohol, and the use of personal flotation devices on waterways should be encouraged.

Burns

Fires, burns, and suffocation are a leading cause of injury death worldwide.[10] Approximately 80% of fire- and burn-related deaths result from house fires, with associated smoke inhalation injury.[88,107-110] Most fire-related deaths occur in private residences, usually in homes without working smoke detectors.[88,107,108,111] From 1995 to 1996 nearly 15% of total US fatalities related to home fires were children less than 5 years old.[9] Nonfatal burns and burn complications, including smoke inhalation, scalds, and contact and electrical burns are especially likely to affect children.

Socioeconomic factors such as overcrowding, single-parent families, scarce financial resources, inadequate child care/supervision, and distance from fire department all contribute to increased risk for burn injury.

Smoke detectors are one of the most effective interventions for preventing death from burns and smoke inhalation. When used correctly, they can reduce fire-related death and severe injury by 86% to 88%.[108,111] Smoke detectors should be placed on or near the ceilings outside the doors to sleeping or napping rooms and on each floor at the top of the stairway. Parents should be aware of the effectiveness of these devices and the need to change device batteries every 6 months.

Families and schools should develop and practice a fire evacuation plan. Continued

improvements in flammability standards for furniture, bedding, and house building materials should further reduce the incidence of fire-related injuries and deaths. Child-resistant ignition products are also under investigation. School-based fire-safety programs should be continued and evaluated.

Firearm Injuries

Firearms, particularly handguns, are responsible for a large number of injuries and deaths in infants, children, and adolescents. Firearm-related deaths may be labeled as unintentional, homicide, or suicide.[2] The United States has the highest firearm-related injury rate of any industrialized nation — more than twice that of any other country.[10,112]

Although firearm-related deaths have declined from 1995 to 1997 compared with previous years,[2] firearm homicide remains the leading cause of death among African-American adolescents and young adults and the second-highest cause of death among all adolescents and young adults in the United States.[10,112,113] Firearms have been used in an increasing proportion of child and adolescent suicides. Mortality from firearm injuries is highest in young children, whether the firearm injury is unintentional or related to homicide or suicide.[114]

Most guns used in unintentional childhood shootings, school shootings, and suicides are found in the home. Many firearm owners admit to storing guns loaded and in readily accessible locations.[115] Thirty-four percent of high school students surveyed reported easy access to guns, and an increasing number of children carry guns to school.[116-118]

If guns are present in homes in which children and adolescents live and visit, it is likely that the children and adolescents will find and handle the guns. The mere presence of a gun in the home is associated with an increased likelihood of adolescent suicide[119,120] as well as an increased incidence of adult suicide or homicide.[121-123] Every gun owner, potential gun purchaser, and parent must be made aware of the risks of unsecured firearms and the need to ensure that weapons in the home are inaccessible to unsupervised children and adolescents.[124-126] Guns should be stored locked and unloaded, with ammunition stored separately from the gun. The consistent use of trigger locks may not only reduce the incidence of unintentional injury and suicide among children and young adolescents but also will most likely reduce the number of gun homicides. In addition, locked guns

obtained during burglaries would be useless. "Smart" guns, which can be fired only by the gun owner, are expected to reduce the frequency of unintentional injuries and suicides among children and young adolescents and limit the usefulness of guns obtained during burglaries.[127]

The Role of the Healthcare Provider in Injury Prevention

Healthcare providers are often in contact with prospective parents, parents, childcare providers, and teachers, as well as

older children and adolescents. These contacts can provide opportunities to educate children and those responsible for their care about the best ways to reduce injuries (see the Table). CPR and injury prevention programs in elementary schools provide additional opportunities to provide injury prevention information. Young elementary school children have shown the ability to increase their own seat belt use as well as the seat belt use of their parents and siblings.[91]

TABLE. Injury Prevention Strategies for Parents, Prospective Parents, Child-Care Providers, Teachers, and Children

Common Causes of Injury and Death	Steps to Prevent Injury or Death
Motor vehicle crash	■ "Buckle up" EVERY passenger in the vehicle. ■ Children up to 4 years and 40 lb (18 kg): use child-restraint devices. Be sure they are installed correctly! ■ Children 40 to 80 lb (18 to 36 kg): use a belt-positioning booster seat. ■ Children must be at least 58 in (148 cm) and 80 lb (36 kg) to be safely restrained in lap-shoulder belts alone. ■ Children 12 years or younger should sit in the BACK seat.
Pedestrian struck by vehicle	■ Supervise children playing near traffic. ■ Teach children to stop, look, and listen before crossing the street and to use crosswalks.
Bicycle crash	■ Be sure all bike riders ALWAYS wear bicycle helmets (ANSII or Snell approved).
Drowning	■ Supervise children who are near water (including bathtubs and swimming pools) at all times. ■ Be sure that home swimming pools are completely surrounded by fences. ■ Be sure that children wear life vests when boating.
Burns and smoke inhalation	■ Use smoke alarms. Change batteries twice a year (spring and fall). ■ Keep drapes and furniture away from heaters.
Firearms	■ Store all firearms UNLOADED and LOCKED.
Sudden infant death syndrome, choking and suffocation	■ Place a healthy term infant to sleep on his back or side. Do not place an infant on his stomach to sleep. ■ Do not allow infants and small children to play with toys that are small enough to fit through a standard toilet paper roll. ■ Do not allow children to play with plastic bags.
Poisoning	■ Keep all poisons out of the reach of children. ■ Do not store poisons in containers intended for drinking (eg, soft drink bottles). ■ Post the poison control center number near the phone.
Falls	■ Place gates on all windows above the ground floor in rooms occupied by children. ■ Use gates to block stairways from infants and toddlers.

Prevention of Choking (Foreign-Body Airway Obstruction)

Every year in the United States approximately 300 infants and children die of choking. More than 90% of deaths from foreign-body aspiration in children occur in those younger than 5 years; 65% of victims are infants.

With the development of consumer product safety standards regulating the minimum size of toys and toy parts for young children,[128,129] the incidence of foreign-body aspiration has decreased significantly. However, toys, balloons, small objects, and foods (eg, hot dogs, round candies, nuts, and grapes) may still produce FBAO[130] and should be kept away from infants and small children.

Parents and child-care providers should be taught that toys small enough to fit through a standard toilet paper roll may cause choking in young children.

Critical Concepts:
Signs of a Breathing Emergency With Poor Air Exchange — Signals to Activate the Emergency Response Number

✔ Weak cry

✔ Inability to speak or a weak voice

✔ Decreasing alertness or responsiveness

✔ Blue or pale lips and tongue

✔ Very rapid breathing with evidence that the infant or child is working hard to breathe **or**

✔ Very slow, shallow breathing (infant or child is barely breathing

Signs of Breathing Emergencies and Cardiac Arrest in Infants and Children

How to Recognize Breathing Emergencies

In children breathing emergencies can lead to cardiac arrest. Breathing emergencies can be characterized by *increased* or *decreased* breathing effort. FBAO, croup (a viral infection causing a hoarse cough), asthma, serious pneumonia, or submersion (near-drowning) may cause *increased* breathing effort. A child with any of these conditions is struggling to breathe and may breathe at a very rapid rate. The rescuer will need to decide whether the child's breathing is resulting in *poor* air exchange, which requires emergency treatment, or *good* air exchange, which provides sufficient air movement and does not require emergency treatment.

Signs of *poor* air exchange include a weak cry, inability to speak or a weak voice, decreasing alertness or responsiveness, and blue or pale lips and tongue. If you observe these signs, **activate the EMS system** and make sure that the airway is open.

Children with a *decreased* breathing effort breathe at a very slow rate or very shallowly, so they cannot maintain sufficient oxygen in the blood. If not corrected this condition can lead to respiratory or cardiac arrest. Head injury, drug intoxication, and a host of serious medical conditions that can affect the breathing control center of the brain can cause decreased breathing effort. Children with decreased breathing effort require rescue breathing and emergency treatment. Children who are severely deprived of oxygen may suffer a cardiac arrest.

Signs of Severe or Complete FBAO (Choking)

Signs of severe or complete FBAO in infants and children include the *sudden* onset of signs such as weak or silent coughing, inability to speak, stridor

(a high-pitched, noisy sound or wheezing), and increasing difficulty breathing. These signs and symptoms of airway obstruction may also be caused by *infections* such as epiglottitis and croup, which produce in-airway edema. However, signs of FBAO (rather than *infectious* airway obstruction) typically develop very suddenly, with no other

Critical Concepts:
Signs of Severe or Complete Airway Obstruction

In a responsive, choking infant or child the following are signs of severe or complete airway obstruction that require immediate action:

■ **"Universal choking sign"**: the child clutches his or her neck with the thumb and index finger (the infant will not demonstrate this sign)

■ Inability to speak (the infant will be unable to make loud sounds of any kind)

■ Ask child victim "Are you choking?" If child responds yes, ask "Can you speak?" If the child is unable to speak, severe or complete airway obstruction is present and you must act.

■ Weak, ineffective coughs

■ High-pitched sounds or no sounds while inhaling

■ Increased difficulty breathing

■ Bluish skin color (cyanosis)

Note: You do *not* need to act if the victim can cough forcefully or speak. Do not interfere at this point because a strong cough is the most effective way to remove a foreign body. Stay with the victim and monitor his or her condition. If the partial obstruction persists, activate the EMS or emergency response system.

signs of illness or infection (such as fever, signs of congestion, hoarseness, drooling, lethargy, or limpness). If the child has an *infectious* cause of airway obstruction, the Heimlich maneuver and back blows and chest thrusts will *not* relieve the airway obstruction. The child must be taken immediately to an emergency facility. If you think the signs of airway obstruction are caused by a foreign body, you should perform back blows and chest thrusts for the infant and abdominal thrusts for the child (presented later in this chapter).

Signs of Respiratory Arrest in Infants and Children

Respiratory arrest is present when the infant or child is not breathing at all or when breathing is clearly inadequate to maintain effective oxygenation and ventilation. The infant or child with respiratory arrest requires immediate support — you must open the airway and provide rescue breathing to prevent cardiac arrest and hypoxic injury to the brain and other organs.

Respiratory arrest without cardiac arrest in the out-of-hospital setting can result from a number of causes, including submersion/near-drowning, FBAO, poisoning or drug overdose, smoke inhalation, respiratory infection, electrocution, suffocation, head injuries, lightning strike, and coma of any cause. In the hospital, respiratory arrest without cardiac arrest may result from drug reaction, sedation,

Critical Concepts:

Signs of Cardiac Arrest

The healthcare provider will detect the following signs of cardiac arrest:

1. No response

2. No adequate breathing

3. No signs of circulation (no adequate breathing, no coughing, no movement), including no pulse

Critical Concepts:

Causes of Cardiac Arrest — Differences Between Infants and Children and Adults

Infants and Children	Adults
Often caused by breathing emergencies	Usually caused by abnormal heart rhythm
Onset often follows illness or injury	Onset is often sudden
Primary heart rhythm problems are uncommon, especially in children less than 8 years old	Breathing emergencies less common than sudden cardiac arrest

increased intracranial pressure, or coma of any cause. When primary respiratory arrest occurs, the heart and lungs can continue to oxygenate the blood for several minutes, and oxygen will continue to circulate to the brain and other vital organs. If rescue breathing with oxygen is provided, oxygen delivery to the brain and other vital organs may be maintained and cardiac arrest may be prevented.

Signs of Cardiac Arrest

The healthcare provider will find that the infant or child with cardiac arrest will be unresponsive, with no adequate breathing and no signs of circulation (including no pulse). The healthcare provider will recognize cardiac arrest when he or she begins to provide BLS for the unresponsive infant or child. The rescuer opens the airway and looks, listens, and feels for respirations and finds that there is no breathing at all or no adequate breathing. The rescuer then provides 2 rescue breaths. After delivering 2 effective rescue breaths that make the chest rise, the rescuer checks for signs of circulation, including a pulse, and finds that there are no signs of circulation (see Critical Concepts box, Signs of Cardiac Arrest). In the healthcare setting, if electrocardiographic (ECG) monitoring is performed, that monitoring can detect or confirm the development of an arrhythmia consistent with cardiac arrest (VT or VF).

Cardiac arrest is often a sudden event in the adult, but it does not often develop suddenly in infants or children. Cardiac

arrest in infants and children most often develops as a complication of breathing difficulties or shock or injuries (see Critical Concepts box, above).

You must remember that an unresponsive child may be in cardiac arrest. An unresponsive child is a red flag for an emergency: Act immediately!

Sequence of Pediatric BLS: The ABCs of CPR

The BLS sequence (Figure 3) described below refers to both infants (neonates outside the delivery room setting to 1 year of age) and children (1 to 8 years of age) unless specified. For BLS for children 8 years and older, see Chapter 6, "Adult CPR."

Resuscitation Sequence

To maximize survival and a neurologically intact outcome after life-threatening cardiovascular emergencies, each link in the Infant/Child Chain of Survival must be strong, including prevention of arrest, early and effective bystander CPR, rapid activation of the EMS (or other emergency response) system, and early and effective ALS (including rapid stabilization and transport to definitive care and rehabilitation).

When a child develops respiratory or cardiac arrest, immediate bystander CPR is crucial to survival. In both adult[22,27,28] and pediatric[12,13,35] studies, bystander *and older and the phone-fast sequence of resuscitation for children less than 8 years of age.*

The AHA Subcommittees on Pediatric Resuscitation and BLS and a panel addressing the citizen's response in the Chain of Survival debated a proposal to teach lay rescuers to tailor the CPR sequence and EMS activation to the likely cause of the victim's arrest rather than the victim's age. This proposed approach would teach lone lay rescuers to provide 1 minute of CPR before activating the EMS system if a victim of any age collapses with what is thought to be a probable breathing or respiratory problem. Lone lay rescuers would also be taught to activate the EMS system immediately if a victim of any age collapses suddenly (presumed sudden cardiac arrest). The proposal was rejected because inadequate data was available indicating that such an approach would improve survival, and it was clear that this approach would complicate the education of lay rescuers. CPR instruction must remain simple. Retention of CPR skills and knowledge is already suboptimal. The addition of complex instructions to existing CPR guidelines would most likely make them more difficult to teach, learn, remember, and perform.[136-142]

The phone-first and phone-fast sequences are applicable only when only 1 rescuer is present. When multiple rescuers are present, one rescuer remains with the victim of any age to begin CPR while another rescuer goes to activate the EMS or emergency response system. It is unknown how frequently 2 or more lay responders are present during initial evaluation of a pediatric cardiopulmonary emergency.

Healthcare providers, family members, and potential rescuers of infants and children at high risk for cardiopulmonary emergencies should be taught a sequence of rescue actions tailored to the potential victim's specific high-risk condition.[143] For example, parents and child-care providers of children with congenital heart disease who are known to be at risk

for arrhythmias should be instructed to phone first (activate the EMS system before beginning CPR) if they are alone and the child suddenly collapses.

Alternatively, there may be exceptions to the phone-first approach for victims 8 years of age and older, including adults. Parents of children 8 years and older who are at high risk for apnea or respiratory failure should be instructed to provide 1 minute of CPR before activating the EMS system if they are alone and find the child unresponsive. Additional conditions that would warrant a phone-fast approach (approximately 1 minute of CPR before phoning the EMS system) for the lone rescuer of a victim more than 8 years old include

■ Submersion (near-drowning)

■ Trauma

■ Drug overdose

■ Apparent respiratory arrest

Knowledgeable and experienced providers should use common sense and phone first for any apparent sudden cardiac arrest (eg, sudden collapse at any age) and phone fast in other circumstances in which breathing difficulties are documented or likely to be present (eg, trauma or apparent choking).

The rescuer calling the EMS system should be prepared to provide the following information:

1. Location of the emergency, including address and names of streets or landmarks

2. Telephone number from which the call is being made

3. What happened, eg, auto accident, drowning

4. Number of victims

5. Condition of victim(s)

6. Nature of aid being given

7. Any other information requested

The caller should hang up *only* when instructed to do so by the dispatcher. Then the caller should report back to the rescuer doing CPR.

Hospitals and medical facilities and many businesses and building complexes have established emergency medical response systems that provide a first response or early response on-site. Such a response system notifies rescuers of the location of an emergency and the type of response needed. If the cardiopulmonary emergency occurs in a facility with an established medical response system, that system should be notified because it can respond more quickly than EMS personnel arriving from outside the facility. For rescuers in these facilities, the emergency medical response system should replace the EMS system in the sequences below.

Airway
Position the Victim

If the child is unresponsive, move the child as a unit to the supine (face up) position, and place the child supine on a flat, hard surface, such as a sturdy table, the floor, or the ground. If head or neck trauma is present or suspected, move the child only if necessary and turn the head and torso as a unit. If the victim is an infant and no trauma is suspected, carry the child supported by your forearm (your forearm should support the long axis of the infant's torso, with the infant's legs straddling your elbow and your hand supporting the infant's head). It may be possible to carry the infant to the phone in this manner while beginning the steps of CPR.

Open the Airway

The most common cause of airway obstruction in the unresponsive pediatric victim is the tongue.[144-147] Therefore, once the child is found to be unresponsive, open the airway using a maneuver designed to lift the tongue away from the back of the pharynx, creating an open airway (Figure 4A, B).[148]

CPR is linked to improved return of spontaneous circulation and neurologically intact survival. The greatest impact of bystander CPR will probably be on children with noncardiac (respiratory) causes of out-of-hospital arrest.[131] Two studies have reported on the outcome of series of children who were successfully resuscitated solely by bystander CPR before EMS arrival.[13,35] The true frequency of this type of resuscitation is unknown, but it is likely to be underestimated, because victims successfully resuscitated by bystanders are often excluded from studies of out-of-hospital cardiac arrest. Unfortunately bystander CPR is provided for only approximately 30% of out-of-hospital pediatric arrests.[1,35]

Pediatric BLS guidelines delineate a series of skills performed sequentially to assess and support or restore effective ventilation and circulation to the infant or child with respiratory or cardiorespiratory arrest. Pediatric resuscitation requires a process of observation, evaluation, interventions, and assessments that is difficult to capture in a sequential description of CPR. You should initially assess the victim's responsiveness and then continuously monitor the victim's response (appearance, movement, breathing, etc) to intervention. Evaluation and intervention are often simultaneous processes, especially when more than 1 trained provider is present. Although this process is taught as a *sequence* of distinct steps to enhance skills retention, several actions may be accomplished *simultaneously* (eg, begin CPR and phone EMS) if multiple rescuers are present. The appropriate BLS actions also depend on the interval since the arrest or collapse, how the victim responded to previous resuscitative interventions, and whether special resuscitation circumstances exist (see Chapter 11).

Ensure the Safety of Rescuer and Victim

When CPR is provided out-of-hospital, first verify the safety of the scene. If resuscitation is needed near a burning building, in water, or close to electrical wires, first ensure that both the victim and rescuer are in a safe location. In the case of trauma the victim should not be moved unless it is necessary to ensure the victim's or rescuer's safety.

Although rescuer exposure during CPR carries a theoretical risk of infectious disease transmission, the risk is very low.[132] Most out-of-hospital cardiac arrests in infants and children occur at home. If the victim has an infectious disease, it is likely that family members have already been exposed to that disease or are aware of the disease and have appropriate barrier devices available. Surveys of family members indicate that risk of infection is not a concern that would prevent delivery of CPR to a loved one.[133]

Healthcare providers are required to treat all fluids from patients as potentially infectious, particularly in the hospital. Healthcare providers should use barrier devices during mouth-to-mouth breathing if a bag-mask device is unavailable and should wear gloves and protective shields during procedures that are likely to expose them to droplets of blood, saliva, or other body fluids. If neither bag-mask system nor barrier device is available, however, the healthcare provider should be prepared to initiate resuscitation without delay. The data regarding the low risk of infection associated with resuscitation is reviewed in Chapter 10 of this text.

Assess Responsiveness

Gently stimulate the child and ask loudly "Are you all right?" Quickly assess the presence or extent of injury and determine whether the child is *responsive*. Do not move or shake the victim who has sustained head or neck trauma because such handling may aggravate a spinal cord injury. If the child is responsive, he or she will answer your questions or move on command. If the child responds but is injured or needs medical assistance, you may leave the child in the position found to summon help (phone 911 or other emergency response sys-

tem). Return to the child as quickly as possible and recheck the child's condition frequently. Responsive children with respiratory distress will often assume a position that maintains airway patency and optimizes ventilation; they should be allowed to remain in the position that is most comfortable to them.

If the child is *unresponsive* and you are the only rescuer present, be prepared to provide BLS if necessary for approximately 1 minute before leaving the child to activate EMS or other emergency response system. As soon as you determine that the child is unresponsive, shout for help. If trauma has not occurred and the child is small, you may consider carrying the child with you to a telephone so that you can contact EMS more quickly. The child must be moved if he or she is in a dangerous location (eg, a burning building) or if CPR cannot be performed where the child was found (eg, submerged in water).

If a second rescuer is present during the initial assessment of the child, that rescuer should activate the EMS or emergency response system as soon as the emergency is recognized. If trauma is suspected, the second rescuer should activate the EMS (or emergency response) system and may then help immobilize the child's head and cervical spine, preventing movement of the neck (extension, flexion, and rotation) and torso. If the child must be positioned for resuscitation or moved for safety reasons, support the head and body and turn as a unit.

Activate EMS (or Emergency Response) System if Second Rescuer Is Available

The 1992 ECC guidelines[134] instructed the lone rescuer to provide approximately 1 minute of CPR before activating the EMS system in out-of-hospital arrest for infants and children up to the age of 8 years. *The ECC Guidelines 2000*[135] *recommend that the lone rescuer follow the phone-first sequence of resuscitation for adults and children 8 years of age and older and the phone-fast sequence of resuscitation for children less than 8 years of age.*

The AHA Subcommittees on Pediatric Resuscitation and BLS and a panel addressing the citizen's response in the Chain of Survival debated a proposal to teach lay rescuers to tailor the CPR sequence and EMS activation to the likely cause of the victim's arrest rather than the victim's age. This proposed approach would teach lone lay rescuers to provide 1 minute of CPR before activating the EMS system if a victim of any age collapses with what is thought to be a probable breathing or respiratory problem. Lone lay rescuers would also be taught to activate the EMS system immediately if a victim of any age collapses suddenly (presumed sudden cardiac arrest). The proposal was rejected because inadequate data was available indicating that such an approach would improve survival, and it was clear that this approach would complicate the education of lay rescuers. CPR instruction must remain simple. Retention of CPR skills and knowledge is already suboptimal. The addition of complex instructions to existing CPR guidelines would most likely make them more difficult to teach, learn, remember, and perform.[136-142]

The phone-first and phone-fast sequences are applicable only when only 1 rescuer is present. When multiple rescuers are present, one rescuer remains with the victim of any age to begin CPR while another rescuer goes to activate the EMS or emergency response system. It is unknown how frequently 2 or more lay responders are present during initial evaluation of a pediatric cardiopulmonary emergency.

Healthcare providers, family members, and potential rescuers of infants and children at high risk for cardiopulmonary emergencies should be taught a sequence of rescue actions tailored to the potential victim's specific high-risk condition.[143] For example, parents and child-care providers of children with congenital heart disease who are known to be at risk

for arrhythmias should be instructed to phone first (activate the EMS system before beginning CPR) if they are alone and the child suddenly collapses.

Alternatively, there may be exceptions to the phone-first approach for victims 8 years of age and older, including adults. Parents of children 8 years and older who are at high risk for apnea or respiratory failure should be instructed to provide 1 minute of CPR before activating the EMS system if they are alone and find the child unresponsive. Additional conditions that would warrant a phone-fast approach (approximately 1 minute of CPR before phoning the EMS system) for the lone rescuer of a victim more than 8 years old include

■ Submersion (near-drowning)

■ Trauma

■ Drug overdose

■ Apparent respiratory arrest

Knowledgeable and experienced providers should use common sense and phone first for any apparent sudden cardiac arrest (eg, sudden collapse at any age) and phone fast in other circumstances in which breathing difficulties are documented or likely to be present (eg, trauma or apparent choking).

The rescuer calling the EMS system should be prepared to provide the following information:

1. Location of the emergency, including address and names of streets or landmarks

2. Telephone number from which the call is being made

3. What happened, eg, auto accident, drowning

4. Number of victims

5. Condition of victim(s)

6. Nature of aid being given

7. Any other information requested

The caller should hang up *only* when instructed to do so by the dispatcher. Then the caller should report back to the rescuer doing CPR.

Hospitals and medical facilities and many businesses and building complexes have established emergency medical response systems that provide a first response or early response on-site. Such a response system notifies rescuers of the location of an emergency and the type of response needed. If the cardiopulmonary emergency occurs in a facility with an established medical response system, that system should be notified because it can respond more quickly than EMS personnel arriving from outside the facility. For rescuers in these facilities, the emergency medical response system should replace the EMS system in the sequences below.

Airway
Position the Victim

If the child is unresponsive, move the child as a unit to the supine (face up) position, and place the child supine on a flat, hard surface, such as a sturdy table, the floor, or the ground. If head or neck trauma is present or suspected, move the child only if necessary and turn the head and torso as a unit. If the victim is an infant and no trauma is suspected, carry the child supported by your forearm (your forearm should support the long axis of the infant's torso, with the infant's legs straddling your elbow and your hand supporting the infant's head). It may be possible to carry the infant to the phone in this manner while beginning the steps of CPR.

Open the Airway

The most common cause of airway obstruction in the unresponsive pediatric victim is the tongue.[144-147] Therefore, once the child is found to be unresponsive, open the airway using a maneuver designed to lift the tongue away from the back of the pharynx, creating an open airway (Figure 4A, B).[148]

signs of illness or infection (such as fever, signs of congestion, hoarseness, drooling, lethargy, or limpness). If the child has an *infectious* cause of airway obstruction, the Heimlich maneuver and back blows and chest thrusts will *not* relieve the airway obstruction. The child must be taken immediately to an emergency facility. If you think the signs of airway obstruction are caused by a foreign body, you should perform back blows and chest thrusts for the infant and abdominal thrusts for the child (presented later in this chapter).

Signs of Respiratory Arrest in Infants and Children

Respiratory arrest is present when the infant or child is not breathing at all or when breathing is clearly inadequate to maintain effective oxygenation and ventilation. The infant or child with respiratory arrest requires immediate support — you must open the airway and provide rescue breathing to prevent cardiac arrest and hypoxic injury to the brain and other organs.

Respiratory arrest without cardiac arrest in the out-of-hospital setting can result from a number of causes, including submersion/near-drowning, FBAO, poisoning or drug overdose, smoke inhalation, respiratory infection, electrocution, suffocation, head injuries, lightning strike, and coma of any cause. In the hospital, respiratory arrest without cardiac arrest may result from drug reaction, sedation,

> ### Critical Concepts:
> #### Signs of Cardiac Arrest
>
> The healthcare provider will detect the following signs of cardiac arrest:
>
> 1. No response
> 2. No adequate breathing
> 3. No signs of circulation (no adequate breathing, no coughing, no movement), including no pulse

> ### Critical Concepts:
> #### Causes of Cardiac Arrest — Differences Between Infants and Children and Adults
>
> | Infants and Children | Adults |
> | --- | --- |
> | Often caused by breathing emergencies | Usually caused by abnormal heart rhythm |
> | Onset often follows illness or injury | Onset is often sudden |
> | Primary heart rhythm problems are uncommon, especially in children less than 8 years old | Breathing emergencies less common than sudden cardiac arrest |

increased intracranial pressure, or coma of any cause. When primary respiratory arrest occurs, the heart and lungs can continue to oxygenate the blood for several minutes, and oxygen will continue to circulate to the brain and other vital organs. If rescue breathing with oxygen is provided, oxygen delivery to the brain and other vital organs may be maintained and cardiac arrest may be prevented.

Signs of Cardiac Arrest

The healthcare provider will find that the infant or child with cardiac arrest will be unresponsive, with no adequate breathing and no signs of circulation (including no pulse). The healthcare provider will recognize cardiac arrest when he or she begins to provide BLS for the unresponsive infant or child. The rescuer opens the airway and looks, listens, and feels for respirations and finds that there is no breathing at all or no adequate breathing. The rescuer then provides 2 rescue breaths. After delivering 2 effective rescue breaths that make the chest rise, the rescuer checks for signs of circulation, including a pulse, and finds that there are no signs of circulation (see Critical Concepts box, Signs of Cardiac Arrest). In the healthcare setting, if electrocardiographic (ECG) monitoring is performed, that monitoring can detect or confirm the development of an arrhythmia consistent with cardiac arrest (VT or VF).

Cardiac arrest is often a sudden event in the adult, but it does not often develop suddenly in infants or children. Cardiac

arrest in infants and children most often develops as a complication of breathing difficulties or shock or injuries (see Critical Concepts box, above).

*You must remember that an unresponsive child may be in cardiac arrest. An **unresponsive child is a red flag for an emergency: Act immediately!***

Sequence of Pediatric BLS: The ABCs of CPR

The BLS sequence (Figure 3) described below refers to both infants (neonates outside the delivery room setting to 1 year of age) and children (1 to 8 years of age) unless specified. For BLS for children 8 years and older, see Chapter 6, "Adult CPR."

Resuscitation Sequence

To maximize survival and a neurologically intact outcome after life-threatening cardiovascular emergencies, each link in the Infant/Child Chain of Survival must be strong, including prevention of arrest, early and effective bystander CPR, rapid activation of the EMS (or other emergency response) system, and early and effective ALS (including rapid stabilization and transport to definitive care and rehabilitation).

When a child develops respiratory or cardiac arrest, immediate bystander CPR is crucial to survival. In both adult[22,27,28] and pediatric[12,13,35] studies, bystander

FIGURE 3. Pediatric BLS Algorithm.

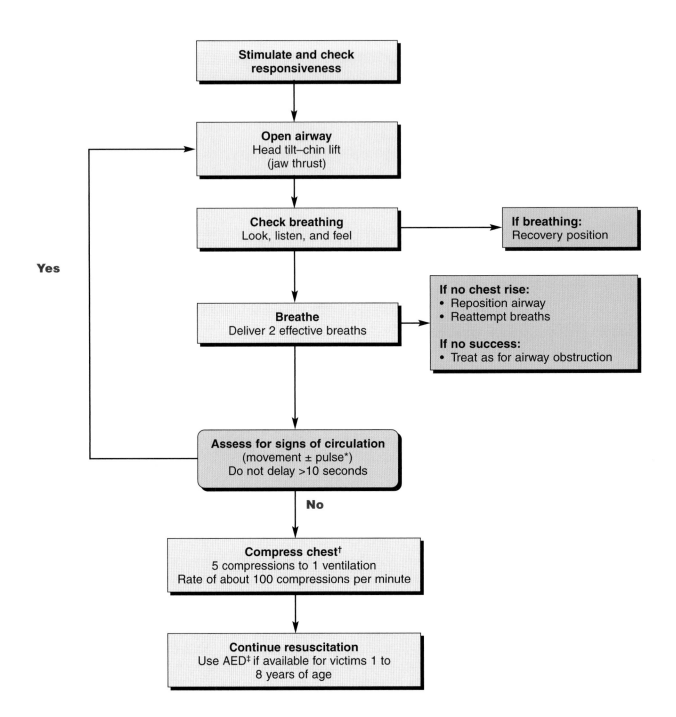

*Pulse check should be taught to healthcare providers but is not expected of laypersons.
†Continue rescue breathing and cardiopulmonary resuscitation as indicated. Activate emergency medical services as soon as possible, based on local and regional availability, training of responder, and circumstances of arrest.
‡In hospital setting, use monitor/defibrillator when available.

FIGURE 4. Relief of airway obstruction by positioning. **A,** In an unresponsive infant the prominent occiput flexes the neck. Airway obstruction can be caused by the tongue falling back into the pharynx. **B,** Maximizing airway patency by positioning the infant with the neck in a neutral position so that the tragus of the ear is level with the top (anterior) of the infant's shoulder.

A

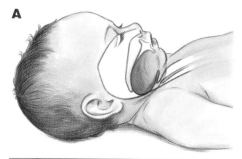

B

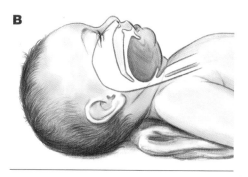

Head Tilt–Chin Lift Maneuver

If the victim is unresponsive and *trauma is not suspected,* open the child's airway by tilting the head back and lifting the chin (Figure 5A and B). Place one hand on the child's forehead and gently tilt the head back. At the same time place the fingertips of your other hand on the bony part of the child's lower jaw, near the point of the chin, and lift the chin to open the airway. Do not push on the soft tissues under the chin because this may block the airway. *If injury to the head or neck is suspected, use the jaw-thrust maneuver to open the airway; do not use the head tilt–chin lift maneuver.*

FIGURE 5. Opening of the airway with head tilt–chin lift. **A,** Infant. **B,** Child.

A

B

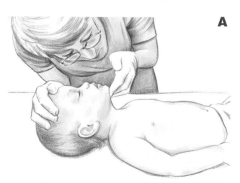

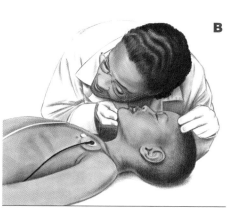

Jaw-Thrust Maneuver

If head or neck injury is suspected, use only the jaw-thrust method of opening the airway. Place 2 or 3 fingers under each side of the lower jaw at its angle and lift the jaw upward and outward (Figure 6). Your elbows may rest on the surface on which the victim is lying. If a second rescuer is present, that rescuer should immobilize the cervical spine (see "BLS for the Trauma Victim" below) after the EMS system is activated.

FIGURE 6. Jaw thrust for child victim.

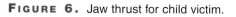
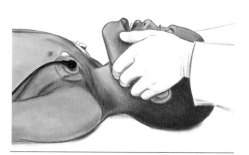

Foreign-Body Airway Obstruction

If the victim becomes unresponsive with an FBAO or if an FBAO is suspected, healthcare providers should perform a tongue-jaw lift to look for obstructing objects (see next section). Because of its complexity, however, this maneuver is not taught to lay rescuers. Instead lay rescuers are taught to perform CPR and check the victim's mouth for a foreign body each time the mouth is opened for rescue breathing.

Breathing
Assessment: Check for Breathing

Hold the victim's airway open and look for signs that the victim is breathing. *Look* for the rise and fall of the chest and abdomen, *listen* at the child's nose and mouth for exhaled breath sounds, and *feel* for air movement from the child's mouth on your cheek for no more than 10 seconds.

It may be difficult to determine whether the victim is breathing.[149,150] Healthcare providers must be able to differentiate ineffective, gasping, or obstructed breathing efforts — which require intervention — from effective breathing.[151,152] If you are not confident that respirations are adequate (effective for maintaining oxygenation and ventilation), proceed with rescue breathing.

Recovery Position

If the child is breathing spontaneously and adequately and there is no evidence of trauma, turn the child to the side in the recovery position (see Figure 7). This position should help maintain a patent airway. Although many recovery positions are used in the management of pediatric patients,[153-156] no single recovery position can be universally endorsed on the basis of scientific studies of children. There is consensus that an ideal recovery position should help maintain a patent airway and cervical spine stability, minimize risk of aspiration, limit pressure on bony prominences and peripheral nerves, enable the rescuer to see the child's respiratory effort and appearance (including color), and facilitate access to the patient for interventions.

Provide Rescue Breathing

If breathing is absent or inadequate, maintain a patent airway by head tilt–chin lift or jaw thrust. Carefully (under vision) remove any obvious airway obstruction, take a deep breath, and deliver rescue breaths. With each rescue breath, provide a volume sufficient for you to see the child's chest rise. Provide 2 slow breaths (1 to 1½ seconds per breath) to the victim, pausing after the first breath to take a breath to maximize oxygen content and minimize carbon dioxide concentration in the delivered breaths. Your exhaled air can provide oxygen to the victim, but the rescue breathing pattern you use will affect the amount of oxygen and carbon dioxide delivered to the victim.[157-159] When ventilation adjuncts and oxygen are available (eg, bag mask) to assist with ventilation, provide high-flow oxygen to all unresponsive victims or victims in respiratory distress.

Mouth-to-Mouth-and-Nose, Mouth-to-Nose, and Mouth-to-Mouth Breathing

If the victim is an infant (less than 1 year old), place your mouth over the infant's mouth and nose to create a seal (Figure 8).

Blow into the infant's nose and mouth (pausing to inhale between breaths), trying to make the chest rise with each breath. During rescue breathing attempts, maintain good head position for the infant (head tilt–chin lift to maintain a patent airway) and create an airtight seal over the airway.

A variety of alternative techniques can be used to provide rescue breathing for infants. If a rescuer with a small mouth has difficulty covering both the nose and open mouth of a large infant,[160-169] the rescuer may provide *mouth-to-nose* ventilation.[160,162] To perform mouth-to-nose ventilation, place your mouth over the infant's nose and proceed with rescue breathing. It may be necessary to close the infant's mouth during rescue breathing to prevent the rescue breaths from escaping through the infant's mouth. A chin lift will help maintain airway patency by moving the tongue forward and may help keep the mouth closed. Another alternative is to provide mouth-to-mouth breathing as you would for a child (see below).

If the victim is a large infant or a child (1 to 8 years of age), provide *mouth-to-mouth* rescue breathing. Maintain a head tilt–chin lift (to keep the airway patent) and pinch the victim's nose tightly with thumb and forefinger. Make a mouth-to-mouth seal and provide 2 rescue breaths,

FIGURE 8. Mouth-to-mouth-and-nose breathing for small infant victim.

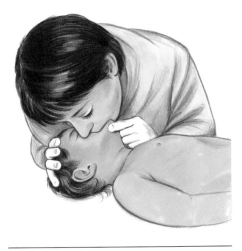

making sure that the child's chest rises visibly with each breath (see Figure 9). Inhale between rescue breaths.

Evaluate Effectiveness of Breaths Delivered

Rescue breaths provide essential support for an infant or child who is not breathing or not breathing adequately. Because children vary widely in size and lung compliance, it is impossible to make precise recommendations about the pressure or volume of breaths to be delivered during rescue breathing. Although the goal of assisted ventilation is delivery of adequate oxygen and removal of carbon dioxide with the smallest risk of iatrogenic injury, measurement of oxygen and carbon dioxide levels during pediatric BLS is often impractical. Therefore, *the volume of each rescue breath should be sufficient to cause the chest to visibly rise* without causing excessive gastric inflation.[170] *If the child's chest does not rise during rescue breathing, ventilation is inadequate.*

Because the small airway of the infant or child may provide high resistance to air flow, particularly in the presence of a large or small airway obstruction, a relatively high pressure may be required to deliver an adequate volume of air to ensure chest expansion. *The correct volume for each breath is the volume that causes the chest to rise.*

FIGURE 7. Recovery position.

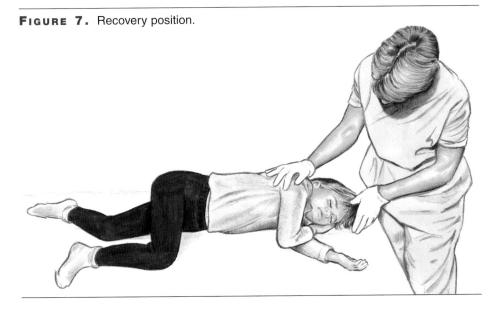

FIGURE 9. Mouth-to-mouth breathing for child victim.

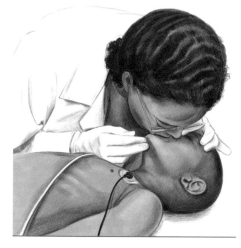

If air enters freely and the chest rises, the airway is clear. If air does not enter freely (if the chest does not rise), either the airway is obstructed or greater volume or pressure is needed to provide adequate rescue breaths. Improper opening of the airway is the most common cause of airway obstruction and inadequate ventilation during resuscitation. If air does not enter freely and the chest does not rise during initial ventilation attempts, reposition the airway and reattempt ventilation.[159] It may be necessary to move the child's head through a range of positions (only if head or neck injury is *not* suspected) to obtain optimal airway patency and effective rescue breathing.

If trauma to the head or neck is suspected, do *not* move the head to open the airway. Instead, use the jaw thrust to open the airway in these victims. If rescue breathing fails to produce chest expansion despite repeated attempts at opening the airway, FBAO may be present (see "Foreign-Body Airway Obstruction" below).

The ideal ventilation rate during CPR and low circulatory flow states is unknown. Current recommended ventilation (rescue breathing) rates are derived from normal respiratory rates for age, with some adjustments for the time needed to coordinate rescue breathing with chest compressions to ensure that ventilation is adequate.

Cricoid Pressure

Rescue breathing, especially if performed rapidly, may cause gastric inflation.[171-175] Excessive gastric inflation can interfere with rescue breathing by elevating the diaphragm and decreasing lung volume, and it may result in regurgitation of gastric contents.[170] Gastric inflation may be minimized if rescue breaths are delivered slowly during rescue breathing, because slow breaths will enable delivery of adequate tidal volume at low inspiratory pressure. Deliver rescue breaths slowly, over 1 to 1½ seconds, with a force sufficient to make the chest visibly rise.

If the victim is unconscious (unresponsive), firm but gentle pressure on the cricoid cartilage during ventilation may help compress the esophagus and decrease the amount of air transmitted to the stomach.[176,177] Healthcare providers may insert a nasogastric or orogastric tube to decompress the stomach if gastric inflation develops during resuscitation. Ideally this is done after tracheal intubation.

Ventilation With Barrier Devices

Mouth-to-mouth rescue breathing is a safe and effective technique that has saved many lives. Despite decades of experience indicating its safety for victims and rescuers alike, some potential rescuers may hesitate to perform mouth-to-mouth rescue breathing because of concerns about transmission of infectious diseases. Most children who require resuscitation outside the hospital require resuscitation at home, where the primary child-care provider is aware of the child's infectious status. Adults who work with children, particularly infants and preschool children, are exposed to pediatric infectious agents daily and often may experience the consequent illnesses. In contrast, the exposure of rescuers to victims is brief, and infections after mouth-to-mouth rescue breathing are extremely rare.[132]

Barrier devices minimize the small risk of infection. Although healthcare providers typically have access to barrier devices, in most lay rescue situations these devices

are not immediately available. If the child is unresponsive and apneic, immediate provision of mouth-to-mouth rescue breathing may be lifesaving. Rescue breathing should not be delayed while the rescuer searches for a barrier device or tries to learn how to use it.

If a barrier device for infection control is readily available, rescuers may prefer to provide rescue breathing with such a device. Barrier devices may improve aesthetics for the rescuer, but they have not been shown to reduce the risk of disease transmission.[132,178] In addition, barrier devices may increase resistance to gas flow.[179,180] Healthcare providers should be trained in the use of barrier devices and have a supply readily available in the workplace for use during any attempted resuscitation. Two broad categories of barrier devices are available: masks and face shields. Most masks have a 1-way valve, which prevents the victim's exhaled air from entering the rescuer's mouth. Face shields consist of a plastic sheet, often with a mouthpiece, to separate the victim's mouth and face from the rescuer's mouth and face. When barrier devices are used in resuscitation of infants and children, they are used in the same manner as that used in resuscitation of adults.

Mouth-to–Face Shield Ventilation

Unlike mouth-to-mask devices, face shields have only a clear plastic or silicone sheet that separates the rescuer from the victim. The mouthpiece or porous mouth seal is placed at the victim's mouth. In some models a short (1- to 2-inch) tube is part of the shield. The tube should be inserted into the mouth over the tongue. The nose is pinched closed and the rescuer seals his or her mouth around the center opening of the face shield. The patient is ventilated with slow breaths (1 to 1½ seconds) through a 1-way valve or filter in the center of the face shield, and the patient's exhaled air escapes between the shield and the victim's face when the rescuer lifts his or her mouth off the shield (see Figure 9, in Chapter 6).

The face shield should remain on the victim's face during the performance of chest compressions. If the victim begins to vomit during rescue efforts, remove the face shield and clear the airway. Because the efficacy of face shields has not been documented conclusively, healthcare professionals and those with a duty to respond should also be instructed in the use of mouth-to-mask and bag-mask devices.

The proximity of the rescuer to the victim's face and the possibility of contamination if the victim vomits are major disadvantages of face shields. Rescuers should use face shields only as a substitute for mouth-to-mouth breathing and should replace them with mouth-to-mask or bag-mask devices at the first opportunity.

Mouth-to-Mask Rescue Breathing

In mouth-to-mask breathing a transparent mask with or without a 1-way valve is used. The 1-way valve directs the rescuer's breath into the victim while diverting the victim's exhaled air away from the rescuer. Some masks have an oxygen inlet that permits administration of supplemental oxygen.

Effective use of the mask barrier device requires instruction and supervised practice. Effective mouth-to-mask ventilation can be easier to perform than mouth-to–face shield ventilation because the rescuer can use both hands to open the airway and seal the mask to the victim's face. During 2-person CPR the mask can be used in a variety of ways. The most appropriate method will depend on the experience of personnel and the equipment available. The 2 most common techniques for using the mouth-to-mask device are the lateral and cephalic techniques.

The *lateral technique* positions the rescuer at the victim's side and uses a head tilt–chin lift to open the victim's airway. It is ideal for performing 1-rescuer CPR because the rescuer can stay in the same position for both rescue breathing and chest compressions. The cephalic tech-

nique is most frequently used during 2-rescuer CPR.

Lateral Technique. Position yourself beside the victim's head in a location that will facilitate both rescue breathing and chest compressions:

- Apply the mask to the victim's face using the bridge of the nose as a guide for correct position.

- Seal the mask by placing your index finger and thumb of the hand closer to the top of the victim's head along the border of the mask and placing the thumb of your other hand along the lower margin of the mask.

- Place the remaining fingers of the hand closer to the victim's feet along the bony margin of the jaw, and lift the jaw. If spinal injury is not suspected, perform a head tilt–chin lift at the same time (Figure 10).

- Compress firmly and completely around the outside margin of the mask to provide a tight seal.

- Provide slow rescue breaths while observing for chest rise.

Cephalic Technique. Position yourself directly above the victim's head.

- Apply the mask to the victim's face, using the bridge of the nose as a guide for correct position.

- Place your thumbs and thenar eminence (portion of the palm at the base of the thumb) along the lateral edges of the mask.

- Place the index fingers of both hands under the victim's mandible and lift the jaw into the mask. Place your remaining fingers under the angle of the jaw.

- While lifting the jaw, squeeze the mask with your thumbs and thenar eminence to achieve an airtight seal (see jaw thrust).

- Provide slow rescue breaths (1 to 1½ seconds each) while observing for chest rise.

FIGURE 10. Mouth-to-mask ventilation for child victim. **A,** Lateral technique. **B,** Cephalic technique.

A

B

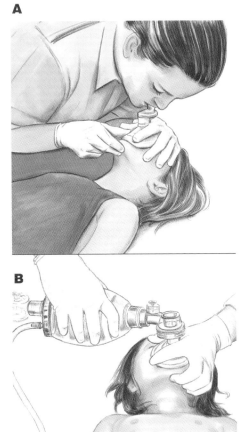

An alternative method of using the cephalic technique is to use the thumb and first finger of each hand to provide a complete seal around the edges of the mask (creating a "C" around the mouthpiece). Use the remaining fingers to lift the mandible (the 3 fingers of each hand create an "E" along the mandible). This hand placement is similar to the "E-C" clamp technique described for bag-mask ventilation in subsequent pages. If spinal injury is not suspected, tilt the head to extend the neck.

With either variation of the cephalic technique, the rescuer uses both hands to hold the mask and open the airway. In victims with suspected cervical spine injury, lift the mandible at the angles of the jaw without tilting the head.

Oral airways and cricoid pressure may be used with mouth-to-mask and any other form of rescue breathing for the unresponsive victim.

Bag-Mask Ventilation

Healthcare providers who provide BLS for infants and children should be trained to deliver effective oxygenation and ventilation with a manual resuscitator bag and mask. Ventilation with a bag-mask device requires more skill than mouth-to-mouth or mouth-to-mask ventilation and should be used only by personnel who have received proper training. Training should focus on the selection of an appropriately sized mask and bag, opening the airway and securing the mask to the face, delivering adequate ventilation, and assessing the effectiveness of ventilation. Periodic demonstration of proficiency is recommended.

Types of Ventilation Bags (Manual Resuscitators)

There are 2 basic types of manual resuscitators (ventilation bags): self-inflating and flow-inflating resuscitators. Ventilation bags used for resuscitation should be self-inflating and available in child and adult sizes suitable for the entire pediatric age range.

Flow-inflating bags (also called *anesthesia bags*) refill only with oxygen inflow, and the inflow must be individually regulated. Since flow-inflating manual resuscitators are more difficult to use, they should be used only by trained personnel.[181] Flow-inflating bags permit continuous delivery of supplemental oxygen to a spontaneously breathing victim. In contrast, self-inflating bag-mask systems that contain a fish-mouth or leaf-flap outlet valve cannot be used to provide continuous supplemental oxygen during spontaneous ventilation. When the bag is not squeezed, the child's inspiratory effort may be insufficient to open the valve. In such a case the child will receive inadequate oxygen flow (a negligible flow of oxygen escapes through the outlet valve) and will rebreathe the exhaled gases contained in the mask.

Neonatal-size (250 mL) ventilation bags may be inadequate to support the tidal volume and the longer inspiratory times required by full-term neonates and infants.[182,183] *For this reason, resuscitation bags used for ventilation of full-term newly born infants, infants, and children should have a minimum volume of 450 to 500 mL.* Studies involving infant manikins showed that effective infant ventilation can be achieved with pediatric (and larger) resuscitation bags.[169]

Regardless of the size of the manual resuscitator used, *the rescuer should use only the force and tidal volume necessary to cause the chest to rise visibly.* Excessive ventilation volumes and airway pressures may have harmful effects. They may compromise cardiac output by raising intrathoracic pressure, distending alveoli or the stomach, impeding ventilation, and increasing the risk of regurgitation and aspiration.[184] In patients with small airway obstructions (eg, asthma and bronchiolitis), excessive tidal volume and ventilation rate can result in air trapping, barotrauma, air leak, and severely compromised cardiac output. In the patient with a head injury or cardiac arrest, excessive ventilation volume and rate may result in hyperventilation, with potentially adverse effects on neurologic outcome. The goal of ventilation with a bag and mask should be to approximate normal ventilation and achieve physiological oxygen and carbon dioxide levels while minimizing risk of iatrogenic injury.

Ideally bag-mask systems used for resuscitation should either have no pressure-relief valve or have a valve with an override feature to permit use of high pressures if necessary to achieve visible chest expansion.[184] High pressures may be required during bag-mask ventilation of patients with upper- or lower-airway obstruction or poor lung compliance. In these patients a pressure-relief valve may prevent delivery of sufficient tidal volume.[185]

The self-inflating bag delivers only room air (21% oxygen) unless the bag is joined to an oxygen source. At an oxygen

inflow of 10 L/min, pediatric bag-valve devices without oxygen reservoirs deliver from 30% to 80% oxygen to the patient.[185] The actual concentration of oxygen delivered is unpredictable because a variable amount of room air is pulled into the bag to replace some of the gas mixture delivered to the patient. To deliver consistently higher oxygen concentrations (60% to 95%), all manual resuscitator devices used for resuscitation should be equipped with an oxygen reservoir. At least 10 to 15 L/min of oxygen flow is required to maintain an adequate oxygen volume in the reservoir of a pediatric manual resuscitator, and this should be considered the minimum flow rate.[185] The larger adult manual resuscitators require 15 L/min or greater oxygen flow to deliver high oxygen concentrations reliably.

Technique

To provide bag-mask ventilation, select a bag and mask of appropriate size. The mask must be able to completely cover the victim's mouth and nose without covering the eyes or overlapping the chin. Once the bag and mask are selected and connected to an oxygen supply, open the victim's airway and seal the mask to the face.

If trauma is not present, tilt the victim's head back to help open the airway. If trauma is suspected, do not move the head, but lift the jaw with a jaw thrust. The most common hand position to open the airway and seal the mask to the face is the *E-C clamp* technique. The thumb and index finger form a "C" and hold the mask on the child's face. The third, fourth, and fifth fingers form an "E" positioned under the jaw to lift the chin and jaw; this lifts the tongue away from the back of the pharynx and opens the airway. Do not put pressure on the soft tissues under the jaw because this may compress the airway. This technique should create a tight seal between the mask and the face (Figure 11A, B). Once you successfully apply the mask with one hand, compress the ventilation bag with the other hand until the chest visibly rises.

Superior bag-mask ventilation can be achieved with 2 rescuers, and 2 rescuers may be required when the victim has significant airway obstruction or poor lung compliance (see Figure 12). One rescuer uses both hands to open the airway and maintain a tight mask-to-face seal while the other rescuer compresses the ventilation bag.[186] Both rescuers should observe the chest to ensure that it rises visibly with each breath.

Gastric Inflation

Gastric inflation can limit effective ventilation.[170] In unresponsive or obtunded patients gastric inflation can be minimized by delivering rescue breaths at low peak inspiratory pressures. Inspiratory pressure can be minimized by delivering the breaths slowly. Pace the ventilation rate and ensure adequate time for exhalation. If the victim is unresponsive, a second trained provider

FIGURE 11. Bag-mask ventilation for infant and child victim. **A,** Bag-mask ventilation for infant. The rescuer is using the E-C clamp technique (the last 3 fingers of one hand lift the jaw and the first 2 fingers hold the mask against the infant's face). **B,** Bag-mask ventilation for child.

A

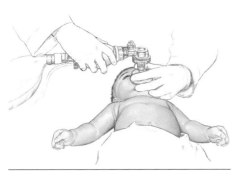

B

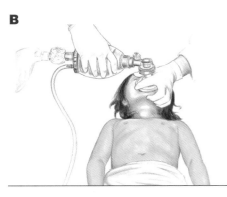

FIGURE 12. Bag-mask ventilation for child victim, 2-rescuer technique.

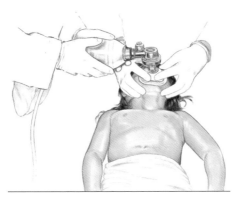

can apply cricoid pressure to reduce gastric inflation.[177] Cricoid pressure may prevent regurgitation (and possible aspiration) of gastric contents in the unconscious victim.[187,188] Do not use excessive pressure on the cricoid cartilage because it may produce tracheal compression and obstruction or distortion of the upper airway anatomy, and do not apply cricoid pressure if the victim is conscious.[189]

If gastric inflation does develop, decompress the stomach with an orogastric or a nasogastric tube. If tracheal and gastric intubation are both planned, ideally you should defer gastric intubation until tracheal intubation has been accomplished. This will reduce the risk of vomiting and laryngospasm.

Ventilation Through a Tracheostomy or Stoma

Anyone responsible for the care of a child with a tracheostomy (including parents, school nurses, and home healthcare providers) should be able to assess and maintain airway patency and provide rescue breathing and bag-mask ventilation through the artificial airway. As with any form of rescue breathing, the key sign of effective ventilation is adequate chest expansion bilaterally. If the tracheostomy becomes obstructed and ventilation cannot be provided through it, remove and replace the tracheostomy tube. If a clean tube is unavailable, provide ventilation at the tracheostomy stoma until a tracheostomy or tracheal tube can be inserted

into the stoma. If the child's upper airway is patent, it may be possible to provide bag-mask ventilation through the nose and mouth using a conventional bag and mask while occluding the superficial tracheal stoma site.

Oxygen

Healthcare providers should administer oxygen to all seriously ill or injured patients with respiratory insufficiency, shock, or trauma as soon as it is available. In these patients inadequate pulmonary gas exchange or inadequate cardiac output limit tissue oxygen delivery.

During cardiac arrest a number of factors contribute to severe progressive tissue hypoxia and the need for supplemental oxygen administration. At best, mouth-to-mouth ventilation provides 16% to 17% oxygen with a maximal alveolar oxygen tension of 80 mm Hg.[157] Even optimal external chest compressions provide only a fraction of normal cardiac output, so blood flow and oxygen delivery to the brain and body are markedly diminished. In addition, CPR is associated with right-to-left pulmonary shunting due to ventilation-perfusion mismatch. Preexisting pulmonary conditions may further compromise oxygenation. The combination of low blood flow and low oxygenation contributes to metabolic acidosis and organ failure. For these reasons oxygen should be administered to children with cardiopulmonary arrest or compromise even if measured arterial oxygen tension is high. Whenever possible, administered oxygen should be humidified to prevent drying and thickening of pulmonary secretions; dried secretions may contribute to obstruction of natural or artificial airways.

Occasionally an infant may require *reduced* inspired oxygen concentration or manipulation of oxygenation and ventilation to control pulmonary blood flow (eg, the neonate with a single ventricle).[190] A review of these unique situations is beyond the scope of this document.

Oxygen may be administered during bag-mask ventilation. In addition, if the victim is breathing spontaneously, oxygen may be delivered by nasal cannula, simple face masks, and non-rebreathing masks.[191-195] The concentration of oxygen delivered is determined by the oxygen flow rate, the type of mask used, and the patient's minute ventilation. As long as the flow of oxygen exceeds the maximum inspiratory flow rate, the prescribed concentration of oxygen will be delivered. If the oxygen flow rate is less than the maximum inspiratory flow rate, room air is entrained, reducing the oxygen concentration delivered to the patient.

Circulation

Assessment: Pulse Check

Cardiac arrest results in the absence of signs of circulation, including a pulse. The pulse check has been the gold standard usually relied on by professional rescuers to evaluate circulation. In adults and children the carotid artery is palpated[196]; in infants the brachial artery is palpated.[197] In the hospital the femoral artery is also palpated.

The 1992 guidelines[134] recommended the pulse check to identify pulseless patients in cardiac arrest who required chest compression. If the rescuer did not detect a pulse in 5 to 10 seconds in an unresponsive, nonbreathing victim, cardiac arrest was presumed to be present and chest compressions were initiated. However, the 1992 guidelines deemphasized the pulse check for infant-child CPR for 2 reasons: (1) several small studies suggested that parents had difficulty finding and counting the pulse even in healthy infants with a strong pulse,[197-199] and (2) the reported complication rate from chest compressions in infants and children is low, so the risk of providing unnecessary chest compressions is low.[200-207]

Since 1992 several published studies have questioned the validity of the pulse check, particularly when used by laypersons, as a test to identify adult cardiac arrest.[196,198,208-219] The validity of the pulse check has been

---

FYI: Assessment for Signs of Circulation by Lay Rescuers

Lay rescuers should assess the victim for signs of circulation as follows:

1. Provide initial rescue breaths to the unresponsive, nonbreathing victim.

2. Look for signs of circulation:

   ▪ With your ear next to the victim's mouth, look, listen, and feel for normal breathing or coughing.

   ▪ Quickly scan the victim for any signs of movement.

3. If the victim is not breathing normally, coughing, or moving, immediately begin chest compressions.

---

evaluated with adult manikin simulation,[213] in unconscious adult patients undergoing cardiopulmonary bypass,[217] unconscious mechanically ventilated adult patients,[214] and conscious adult "test persons."[209,216] These studies concluded that as a diagnostic test for cardiac arrest, the pulse check has serious limitations in accuracy, sensitivity, and specificity.

When lay rescuers check the pulse, they often spend a long time deciding whether a pulse is present; they may fail 1 of every 10 times to recognize the absence of a pulse or cardiac arrest (poor sensitivity). When assessing unresponsive victims who *do* have a pulse, lay rescuers miss the pulse 4 times in 10 (poor specificity). Details of the published studies include the following conclusions[212]:

1. Rescuers take far too much time to check the pulse. Most rescue groups, including laypersons, medical students, paramedics, and physicians, take much longer than the recommended period of 5 to 10 seconds to

check for the carotid pulse in adult victims. In one study half the rescuers required more than 24 seconds to decide whether a pulse was present. Only 15% of the participants correctly confirmed the presence of a pulse within 10 seconds, the maximum time allotted for pulse check.

2. When used as a diagnostic test, the pulse check is extremely inaccurate. In the most comprehensive study documented,[217] the accuracy of the pulse check was described as follows[212]:

   a. Specificity (ability to correctly identify victims who have no pulse and *are* in cardiac arrest) is only 90%. When subjects were pulseless, rescuers thought a pulse was present approximately 10% of the time. When rescuers mistakenly think a pulse *is* present when it is not, they fail to provide chest compressions for 10 of every 100 victims of cardiac arrest. Without a resuscitation attempt, the consequence of such errors is death for 10 of every 100 victims of cardiac arrest.

   b. Sensitivity (ability to correctly recognize victims who *have* a pulse and are *not* in cardiac arrest) is only 55%. When subjects had a pulse, rescuers assessed it as being absent approximately 45% of the time. When rescuers erroneously think a pulse is absent, they provide chest compressions for approximately 4 of 10 victims who do not need them.

   c. Overall accuracy of the pulse check was 65%, with an error rate of 35%.

Data is limited regarding the specificity and sensitivity of the pulse check in pediatric victims of cardiac arrest.[220] Three studies have documented the inability of lay rescuers to find and count a pulse in healthy infants.[197-199] Healthcare providers may also have difficulty reliably separating venous from arterial pulsation during CPR.[221]

Assessment: Check for Signs of Circulation

Healthcare providers should assess the victim for signs of circulation by performing a pulse check while simultaneously evaluating the victim for breathing, coughing, or movement after delivering rescue breaths. Healthcare providers should look for breathing because they are trained to distinguish between agonal breathing and other forms of ventilation not associated with cardiac arrest. This assessment should take no more than 10 seconds. If you do not confidently detect a pulse or other signs of circulation or if the heart rate is less than 60 bpm in an infant or child with signs of poor perfusion, provide chest compressions. It is important to note that unresponsive, nonbreathing infants and children are very likely to have a slow heart rate or no heart rate at all. *Do not delay the initiation of chest compressions to locate a pulse.*

Healthcare providers should learn to palpate the brachial pulse in infants and the carotid pulse in children more than 1 year old. The short, chubby neck of children less than 1 year old makes rapid location of the carotid artery difficult. It is also easy to compress the airway while attempting to palpate a carotid pulse in the infant's neck. The healthcare provider should attempt to palpate the brachial artery when performing the pulse check in infants.[197] The brachial pulse is on the

Critical Concepts:
Assessment of Signs of Circulation by Healthcare Providers

Pulse: more than 60 bpm, confidently felt within 10 seconds (brachial pulse for infant and carotid pulse for child)

Breathing (not agonal)

Coughing

Movement

FIGURE 13. Palpation of central pulse in infant. **A,** Palpation of brachial pulse. **B,** Alternative site: femoral artery.

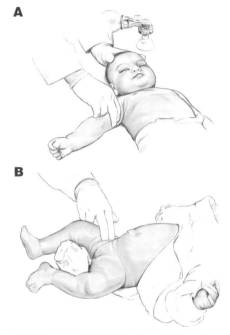

A

B

inside of the upper arm, between the infant's elbow and shoulder. Press the index and middle fingers gently on the inside of the upper arm for no more than 10 seconds when attempting to feel the pulse (Figure 13).

Healthcare providers should learn to locate and palpate the child's carotid artery. It is the most accessible central artery in children and adults. The carotid artery lies on the side of the neck between the trachea and the strap (sternocleido-mastoid) muscles. To feel the artery, locate the victim's Adam's apple with 2 or 3 fingers of one hand while maintaining head tilt with the other hand. Then slide the fingers into the groove on the side closer to you, between the trachea and the sternocleidomastoid muscles, and gently palpate the area over the artery (Figure 14A, B) for no more than 10 seconds (see Critical Concepts box).

If signs of circulation are present but spontaneous breathing is absent, provide rescue breathing at a rate of 20 breaths per minute (once every 3 seconds) until spontaneous breathing resumes. After

provision of approximately 20 breaths (approximately 1 minute), the lone rescuer should activate EMS. If adequate breathing resumes and there is no suspicion of neck trauma, turn the child onto his or her side in the recovery position.

If signs of circulation are absent or the heart rate is less than 60 bpm with signs of poor perfusion, begin chest compressions. This will include a series of compressions coordinated with ventilations. If there are no signs of circulation, the victim is 1 to 8 years of age or older, and an AED is available out of hospital, use the AED. Children 1 to 8 years are about 9 to 25 kg and about 28 to 50 inches (72 to 128 cm) in length.[222] For children less than 8 years of age, use child pads if available. If the child is 8 years or older, use adult pads. (See box on page 167 and Chapter 7). When a monitor/defibrillator is available, assess the ECG rhythm. Hospital defibrillators should deliver appropriate and adjustable child energy doses.

FIGURE 14. Palpation of carotid pulse in child. **A,** Locate the child's Adam's apple with 2 or 3 fingers of one hand while maintaining head tilt with the other hand. **B,** Slide 2 or 3 fingers into the groove on the side of the neck closer to the rescuer, between the trachea and the sternocleidomastoid muscles, and gently palpate the artery.

A

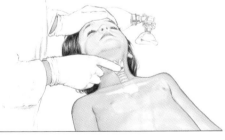

B

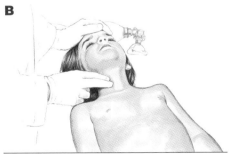

Chest Compressions

Chest compressions are serial, rhythmic compressions of the chest that cause blood to flow to the vital organs (heart, lungs, and brain) in an attempt to keep them viable until ALS can be provided. Chest compressions provide circulation as a result of changes in intrathoracic pressure or direct compression of the heart.[223-227] Chest compressions for infants and children should be provided with ventilations.[228,229]

Compress the lower half of the sternum to a relative depth of approximately one third to one half the anterior-posterior diameter of the chest at a rate of at least 100 compressions per minute for the infant and approximately 100 compressions per minute for the child victim. Be sure to avoid compression of the xiphoid. This relative depth of compression (one third to one half the depth of the chest) differs slightly from that recommended for the newly born. The neonatal resuscitation guidelines call for compression to approximately one third the depth of the chest. The wider range of recommended compression depth and potentially deeper compressions in infants and children is not evidence-based but consensus-based. Chest compressions must be adequate to produce a palpable pulse during resuscitation. Lay rescuers will not attempt to feel a pulse, so they should be taught a compression technique that will most likely result in delivery of effective compressions.

Healthcare providers should evaluate the effectiveness of compressions during CPR. Chest compressions should produce palpable pulses in a central artery (eg, the carotid, brachial, or femoral artery). Although pulses palpated during chest compression may actually represent venous pulsations rather than arterial pulses,[221] pulse assessment by the healthcare provider during CPR remains the most practical quick assessment of the efficacy of chest compressions. Continuous exhaled (end-tidal) carbon dioxide detectors can assist the healthcare provider in evaluating the effectiveness of chest compressions. If chest compres-

FYI: No Pulse Check for Lay Rescuers

The experts and delegates at the 1999 Evidence Evaluation Conference and the Guidelines 2000 Conference reviewed the data and concluded that the pulse check could not be recommended as a tool for lay rescuers to identify victims of cardiac arrest. If rescuers use the pulse check to identify victims of cardiac arrest, they will miss true cardiac arrest at least 10 of 100 times. In addition, rescuers will provide unnecessary chest compressions for many victims who are not in cardiac arrest and do not require such an intervention. This error is less serious but still undesirable. Clearly more worrisome is the potential failure to intervene for a substantial number of victims of cardiac arrest who require immediate intervention to survive.

Therefore, the lay rescuer should not rely on the pulse check to determine the need for chest compressions. Lay rescuers should not perform the pulse check and will not be taught the pulse check in CPR courses. Instead, laypersons will be taught to look for *signs of circulation* (normal breathing, coughing, or movement) in response to rescue breaths. This recommendation applies to victims of any age. Healthcare providers should continue to use the pulse check as one of several signs of circulation. Other signs of circulation include breathing, coughing, or movement in response to rescue breaths. It is anticipated that this guideline change will result in more rapid and accurate identification of cardiac arrest. More important, it should reduce the number of missed opportunities to provide CPR (and early defibrillation using an AED for victims more than 8 years of age) for victims of cardiac arrest.

sions produce inadequate cardiac output and pulmonary blood flow, exhaled carbon dioxide will remain extremely low throughout resuscitation. If an arterial catheter is in place during resuscitation (eg, during chest compressions provided to a patient in the ICU with an arterial monitor in place), chest compressions can be guided by the displayed arterial waveform.

To facilitate optimal chest compressions, the child should be supine on a hard, flat surface. CPR should be performed where the victim is found. If cardiac arrest occurs in a hospital bed, place firm support (a resuscitation board) beneath the patient's back. Optimal support is provided by a resuscitation board that extends from the shoulders to the waist and across the full width of the bed. The use of a wide board is particularly important when providing chest compressions to larger children. If the board is too small, it will be pushed deep into the mattress during compressions, dispersing the force of each compression. Spine boards, preferably with head wells, can be used in ambulances and mobile life support units.[230,231] They provide a firm surface for CPR in the emergency vehicle or on a wheeled stretcher and may also be useful for extricating and immobilizing victims.

Infants with no signs of head or neck trauma may be successfully carried during resuscitation on the rescuer's forearm. The palm of one hand can support the infant's back while the fingers of the other hand compress the sternum. This maneuver effectively lowers the infant's head, allowing the head to tilt back slightly into a neutral position that maintains airway patency. If the infant is carried during CPR, the hard surface is created by the rescuer's forearm, which supports the length of the infant's torso, while the infant's head and neck are supported by the rescuer's hand. Take care to keep the infant's head no higher than the rest of the body. Use the other hand to perform chest compressions. You can lift the infant to provide ventilation (see Figure 15).

FIGURE 15. Chest compression for infant victim supported on rescuer's forearm.

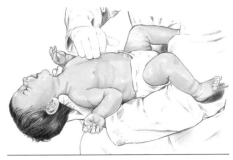

Indications for Chest Compressions

Lay rescuers should provide chest compressions if the infant or child shows no signs of circulation (normal breathing, coughing, or movement) after delivery of rescue breaths. Healthcare providers should provide chest compressions if the infant or child shows no signs of circulation (breathing, coughing, movement, or pulse) or if the heart rate or pulse is less than 60 bpm with signs of poor perfusion after delivery of rescue breaths.

Profound bradycardia in the presence of poor perfusion is an indication for chest compressions because an inadequate heart rate with poor perfusion indicates that cardiac arrest is imminent. Cardiac output in infancy and childhood is largely dependent on heart rate. Although no scientific data has identified an absolute heart rate at which chest compressions should be initiated, the recommendation to provide cardiac compression for a heart rate of less than 60 bpm with signs of poor perfusion is based on ease of teaching and retention of skills.

Chest Compressions in the Infant (Less Than 1 Year of Age)

Two-finger technique (preferred technique for laypersons and lone rescuers):

1. Place the 2 fingers of one hand over the lower half of the sternum[232-235] approximately 1 finger's width below the intermammary line, ensuring that you are not on or near the xiphoid

process.[14] The intermammary line is an imaginary line located between the nipples, over the breastbone (Figure 16).

2. An alternative method of locating the proper compression position is to run 1 finger along the lower costal margin to locate the bony end of the sternum and place 1 finger over the end of the sternum; this will mark the xiphoid process. Then place 2 fingers of your other hand above the xiphoid (moving up the sternum toward the head). The 2 fingers will now be in the appropriate position for chest compressions, avoiding the xiphoid.[14] You may place your other hand under the infant's chest to create a compression surface and slightly elevate the chest so that the neck is neither flexed nor hyperextended and the airway will be maintained in a neutral position.

3. Press down on the sternum, depressing it approximately one third to one

FYI: Differences in Compression-Ventilation Ratio for Newly Born and Infant Resuscitation

Note that the 5:1 ratio of compressions to ventilations recommended for infants differs from the recommended ratio of 3:1 for the newly born or premature infant in the neonatal intensive care unit (ICU). The 3:1 ratio used for the delivery room is based on ease of teaching and skills retention for specifically trained providers in the delivery room, where there is increased emphasis on effective and frequent ventilation for the newly born infant. This compression-ventilation ratio also differs from the 15:2 compression-ventilation ratio recommended for lay or healthcare provider rescuers of adult victims until the airway is secured.

FIGURE 16. Two-finger chest compression technique in infant. Note that the hand that is not performing chest compressions is holding the infant's head in a position that will facilitate the delivery of rescue breaths.

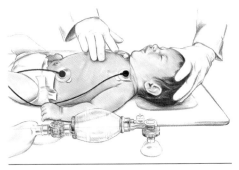

half the depth of the infant's chest. This will correspond to a depth of about ½ to 1 inch (1¼ to 2½ cm), but these measurements are not precise. After each compression completely release the pressure on the sternum and allow the sternum to return to its normal position without lifting your fingers off the chest wall.

4. Deliver compressions in a smooth fashion, with equal time in the compression and relaxation phases. A somewhat shorter time in the compression phase offers theoretical advantages for blood flow in a very young infant animal model of CPR[236] and is discussed in the neonatal guidelines. As a practical matter, with compression rates equal to or greater than 100 per minute (nearly 2 compressions per second), it is unrealistic to think that rescuers will be able to judge or manipulate compression and relaxation phases. In addition, details about such manipulation would increase the complexity of CPR instruction. Rescuers should simply provide compressions in approximately equal compression and relaxation phases for infants and children.

5. Compress the infant's sternum at *a rate of at least 100 times per minute* (this corresponds to a rate slightly less than 2 compressions per second during the groups of 5 compressions).

The compression *rate* refers to the *speed* of compressions, not the actual *number* of compressions delivered per minute. Note that this compression rate will actually result in provision of less than 100 compressions each minute because you will pause to provide 1 ventilation after every fifth compression. The actual *number* of compressions delivered per minute will vary from rescuer to rescuer and will be influenced by the compression rate and speed with which you can position the head, open the airway, and deliver ventilation (see FYI box on this page).[140,237]

6. After 5 compressions open the airway with a head tilt–chin lift (or if trauma is present, use the jaw thrust) and give 1 effective breath. Be sure that the chest rises with the breath. Coordinate compressions and ventilations to avoid simultaneous delivery and ensure adequate ventilation and chest expansion, especially when the airway is unprotected.[238] You may use your other hand (the one not compressing the chest) to maintain the infant's head in a neutral position during the 5 chest compressions. This may help you provide ventilation without the need to reposition the head after each set of 5 compressions. To maintain a neutral head position, place your other hand behind the infant's chest (this will elevate the chest, ensuring that the head is in a neutral position relative to the chest). Alternatively, if there is no sign of head or neck trauma, you can place your other hand on the infant's forehead to maintain head tilt (Figure 16). If there are signs of head or neck trauma, you can place your other hand on the infant's forehead to maintain stability (do not tilt the head).

Continue compressions and breaths in a ratio of 5:1 (for 1 or 2 rescuers).

Two thumb–encircling hands technique (the preferred 2-rescuer technique for healthcare providers when physically feasible):

1. Place both thumbs side by side over the lower half of the infant's sternum, ensuring that the thumbs do not compress on or near the xiphoid process.[14,232-235] The thumbs may overlap in very small infants. Encircle the infant's chest and support the infant's back with the fingers of both hands. Both thumbs should be placed

on the lower half of the infant's sternum, approximately 1 finger's width below the intermammary line. The intermammary line is an imaginary line located between the nipples, over the breastbone (Figure 17).

2. With your hands encircling the chest, use both thumbs to depress the sternum approximately one third to one half the depth of the infant's chest. This will correspond to a depth of approximately ½ to 1 inch (1¼ to 2½ cm), but these measurements are not precise. After each compression completely release the pressure on the sternum and allow the sternum to return to its normal position without lifting your thumbs off the chest wall.

3. Deliver compressions in a smooth fashion, with approximately equal time in the compression and relaxation phases. See "Chest Compressions in the Infant," Step 4, page 156.

4. Compress the sternum at *a rate equal to or greater than 100 times per minute* (this corresponds to a rate slightly less than 2 compressions per second during the groups of 5 compressions). The compression *rate* refers to the *speed* of compressions, not the actual number of compressions delivered per minute. Cardiac output in infancy and childhood is largely dependent on heart rate (see the FYI box on this page).[140,237]

5. After 5 compressions, pause briefly for the second rescuer to open the air-

FIGURE 17. Two thumb–encircling hands chest compression technique for infant (2 rescuers).

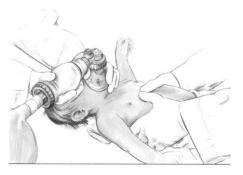

way with a head tilt–chin lift (or if trauma is suspected, with a jaw thrust) and give 1 effective breath (the chest should rise with the breath). Compressions and ventilations should be coordinated to avoid simultaneous delivery and ensure adequate ventilation and chest expansion, especially when the airway is unprotected.[238]

Continue compressions and breaths in a ratio of 5:1 (for 1 or 2 rescuers).

Chest Compressions in the Child (Approximately 1 to 8 Years of Age)

1. Place the heel of one hand over the lower half of the sternum, ensuring that you do not compress on or near the xiphoid process. Lift your fingers to avoid pressing on the child's ribs (Figure 18).

2. Depress the sternum approximately one third to one half the depth of the child's chest. This corresponds to a compression depth of approximately 1 to 1½ inches (2½ to 4 cm), but these measurements are not precise. After the compression, release the pressure on the sternum, allowing it to return to its normal position, but do not remove your hand from the surface of the chest.

3. Compress the sternum at *a rate of approximately 100 times per minute* (this corresponds to a rate slightly less than 2 compressions per second during the groups of 5 compressions). The compression *rate* refers to the *speed* of compressions, not the actual number of compressions delivered per minute (see previous FYI box).[140,237]

4. After 5 compressions, open the airway and give 1 effective rescue breath. Be sure the chest rises with the breath.

5. Return your hand immediately to the correct position on the sternum and give 5 chest compressions.

6. Continue compressions and breaths in a ratio of 5:1 (for 1 or 2 rescuers).

FIGURE 18. One-hand chest compression technique in child. Note that the hand that is not performing chest compressions is holding the child's head in a position that will facilitate the delivery of rescue breaths.

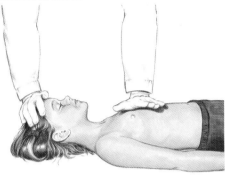

A number of reasonable techniques are available to teach proper hand position for chest compression. The technique used should locate the lower half of the sternum, avoiding force on or near the xiphoid process and asymmetric force on the ribs. Emphasis should be placed on optimizing mechanics to depress the chest rhythmically approximately one third to one half the depth of the chest at a rate of approximately 100 times per minute and coordinating with rescue breaths to ensure delivery of adequate ventilation in between compressions without delay.

In large children and children *8 years of age or older,* the adult 2-handed method of chest compression should be used to achieve an adequate depth of compression, as follows (for further information, see Chapter 6, "Adult CPR"):

1. Place the heel of one hand on the lower half of the sternum. Place the heel of your other hand on top of the back of the first hand.

2. Interlock the fingers of both hands and lift the fingers to avoid pressure on the child's ribs.

3. Position yourself vertically above the victim's chest and, with your arm straight, press down on the sternum to depress it approximately 1½ to 2 inches (4 to 5 cm). Release the pressure com-

pletely after each compression, allowing the sternum to return to its normal position, but do not remove your hands from the surface of the chest.

4. Compress the sternum at *a rate of approximately 100 times per minute* (this corresponds to a rate of slightly less than 2 compressions per second during the groups of 15 compressions). The compression *rate* refers to the *speed* of compressions, not the actual number of compressions delivered per minute (see FYI box on preceding page).[140,237]

5. *If the trachea is not intubated:* after 15 compressions, open the airway with the head tilt–chin lift (if trauma to the head and neck is suspected, use the jaw-thrust maneuver to open the airway) and give 2 effective breaths. Be sure the chest rises with each breath.

   If the trachea is intubated: compressions and ventilations may be asynchronous. Be sure the chest rises with each breath.

6. Continue compressions and breaths in a ratio of 15:2 for 1 or 2 rescuers until the airway is secured (intubated), then change to a ratio of 5 compressions to 1 ventilation (see "Compression-Ventilation Ratio," on the next page).

Coordination of Compressions and Rescue Breathing

External chest compressions for infants and children should always be accompanied by rescue breathing. When 2 rescuers are providing CPR for an infant or child with an unsecured airway, the rescuer providing the compressions should pause after every fifth compression to allow the second rescuer to provide 1 effective ventilation. This pause is necessary until the airway is secured (intubated). Once the airway is secured (the trachea is intubated), the pause is no longer necessary. However, coordination of compressions and ventilation may facilitate adequate ventilation even after tracheal intubation and is emphasized in the newly born. Compressions may be initiated immediately after chest inflation and may augment active exhalation during CPR.

Although the technique of simultaneous compression and ventilation may augment coronary perfusion pressure in some settings,[239-242] it may produce barotrauma and decrease ventilation and is not recommended. Priority is given to ensuring adequate ventilation and avoidance of potentially harmful excessive barotrauma in children.[241]

Reassess the victim after 20 cycles of compressions and ventilations (slightly more than 1 minute) and every few minutes thereafter for any sign of resumption of spontaneous breathing or signs of circulation. The number 20 is easy to remember, so it is used to provide a guideline interval for reassessment rather than an indication of the absolute number of cycles delivered in exactly 1 minute. In the delivery room setting, more frequent assessments of heart rate — approximately every 30 seconds — are recommended for the newly born.

In infants it may be difficult for the lone rescuer to coordinate rapid compressions and ventilations in a 5:1 ratio with a rate of at least 100 compressions per minute.[237,243,244] To minimize interruptions in chest compressions, if no trauma is present the rescuer can maintain airway patency during compressions by using the hand that is not performing compressions to maintain a head tilt (Figures 16 and 18).

Effective chest expansion should be visible with each breath you provide. If the chest does not rise, use the hand performing chest compressions to perform a chin lift (or jaw thrust) to open the airway when rescue breaths are delivered. Then return the hand to the sternum-compression position to resume compressions after the breath is delivered. If trauma is present, the hand that is not performing

compressions should maintain head stability during chest compressions.

In children head tilt alone is often inadequate to maintain airway patency. Usually both of the rescuer's hands are required to perform the head tilt–chin lift maneuver (or jaw thrust) with each ventilation. The time needed to position the hands for each breath, locate landmarks, and reposition the hand to perform compressions may reduce the total number of compressions provided in 1 minute. Therefore, when moving the hand performing the compressions back to the sternum, visualize and return your hand to the approximate location used in the previous sequence of compressions.

Compression-Ventilation Ratio

Ideal compression-ventilation ratios for infants and children have not been established. From an educational standpoint, a single universal compression-ventilation ratio for victims of all ages and all rescuers providing BLS and ALS interventions would be desirable. Studies of monitored rescuers have demonstrated that the 15:2 compression-ventilation ratio delivers more compressions per minute, and the 5:1 compression-ventilation ratio delivers more ventilations per minute.[140,237]

There is consensus among resuscitation councils that pediatric guidelines should recommend a compression-ventilation ratio of 3:1 for newly born infants and 5:1 for infants and children up to 8 years of age. A 15:2 compression-ventilation ratio is now recommended for older children (8 years and older) and adults for 1- or 2-rescuer CPR until the airway is secure (intubated). The rationale for maintaining age-specific differences in compression-ventilation ratios during resuscitation includes the following:

- Respiratory problems are the most common cause of pediatric arrest, and most victims of pediatric cardiopulmonary arrest are hypoxic and hypercarbic. Therefore, effective ventilation should be emphasized.

- Physiological respiratory rates in infants and children are faster than in adults.

- Current providers are trained in and accustomed to these ratios. Any change from the current guidelines in a fundamental aspect of resuscitation steps should be supported by a high level of scientific evidence.

The actual number of delivered interventions (compressions and ventilations) per minute will vary from rescuer to rescuer and will depend on the compression rate, the amount of time the rescuer spends opening the airway and providing ventilation, and rescuer fatigue.[237,245,246] At present there is insufficient evidence to justify changing the current recommendations for compression-ventilation ratios in infants and children to a universal ratio.

Emerging evidence in *adult* victims of cardiac arrest suggests that the provision of longer sequences of uninterrupted chest compressions (a compression-ventilation ratio greater than 5:1) may be easier to teach and retain.[137] In addition, animal data suggests that longer sequences of uninterrupted chest compressions may improve coronary perfusion.[247,248] Finally, longer sequences of compressions may allow more efficient second-rescuer interventions in the out-of-hospital EMS setting.[243] These observations have led to a recommendation for a 15:2 compression-ventilation ratio for 1- and 2-rescuer CPR in older children (8 years and older) and adults. However, for resuscitation of infants and children, emphasis remains on delivery of ventilations, so a 5:1 compression-ventilation ratio continues to be recommended for resuscitation of infants and children less than 8 years of age. In the in-patient setting it is appropriate for a unit or institution to select the pediatric ratio of 5:1 for resuscitation of all pediatric patients (for 1- or 2-rescuer CPR, whether or not the airway is secured), even those more than 8 years of age, to simplify in-hospital protocols and training.

Partial CPR: Is Something Better Than Nothing?

Clinical studies have established that outcomes are dismal when the pediatric victim of cardiac arrest remains in arrest until the arrival of EMS personnel. In comparison, excellent outcomes are typical when the child is successfully resuscitated before the arrival of EMS personnel.[6,12,13,35,42,53,249-251] In such cases some of these patients were apparently resuscitated with "partial CPR," consisting of chest compressions or rescue breathing only.

In some published surveys healthcare providers have expressed reluctance to perform mouth-to-mouth ventilation for unknown victims of cardiopulmonary arrest.[252-254] This reluctance has also been expressed by some potential lay rescuers who were surveyed,[35,255] although reluctance has not been expressed about resuscitation of infants and children.

The effectiveness of partial or "compression-only" or "no-ventilation" CPR has been studied in animal models of *acute VF* sudden cardiac arrest and in some clinical trials of *adult* out-of-hospital cardiac arrest. Some evidence in adult animal models and limited adult clinical trials suggests that positive-pressure ventilation may not be essential during the initial 6 to 12 minutes of an *acute adult VF* cardiac arrest.[27,256-262] Spontaneous gasping and passive chest recoil may provide some ventilation during that time without the need for active rescue breathing.[258,261] In addition, cardiac output during chest compression is only approximately 25% of normal, so the ventilation necessary to maintain optimal ventilation-perfusion relationships may be minimal.[263,264] *However, it does not appear that these observations can be applied to resuscitation of infants and children.*

Well-controlled animal studies have established that simulated bystander CPR with chest compressions plus rescue breathing is superior to chest compressions alone or rescue breathing alone for asphyxial cardiac arrest and severe asphyxial hypoxic-ischemic shock (pulseless cardiac arrest). However, chest compression–only CPR and rescue breathing–only CPR have been shown to be effective early in animal models of pulseless arrest, and the use of either of these forms of "partial CPR" was found to be superior to no bystander CPR.

Preliminary evidence suggests that both chest compressions and active rescue breathing are necessary for optimal resuscitation of the asphyxial arrests most commonly encountered in children.[228,229] For pediatric cardiac arrest, the lay rescuer should provide immediate chest compressions and rescue breathing. If the lay rescuer is unwilling or unable to provide rescue breathing or chest compressions, it is better to provide either chest compressions or rescue breathing than no bystander CPR.

— End of BLS Sequence —

Circulatory Adjuncts and Mechanical Devices for Chest Compression

The use of mechanical devices to provide chest compressions during CPR is not recommended for children. These devices have been designed and tested for use in adults, but their safety and efficacy in children have not been studied. Active compression-decompression CPR (ACD-CPR) has been shown to increase cardiac output compared with standard CPR in adult animal models.[265,266] ACD-CPR maintains coronary perfusion during compression and decompression in humans[267,268] and provides ventilation if the airway is patent.[267,269] In clinical trials ACD-CPR has produced variable results, including improved short-term outcome (eg, return of spontaneous circulation and survival for 24 hours).[270-273] But these improved outcomes are not consistent,[274] and no long-term survival benefits of ACD-CPR have been reported in most trials. On the basis of these variable clinical results, ACD-CPR is considered an optional technique for *adult* CPR. *This technique cannot be recommended for use in children because it has not been studied in this age group.*

Interposed abdominal compression CPR (IAC-CPR) has been shown to increase blood flow in laboratory and computer models[275-277] of adult CPR. IAC-CPR has been shown to improve hemodynamics of CPR and return of spontaneous circulation for *adult* patients in some clinical in-hospital settings[278,279] with no evidence of excessive harm. The technique is slightly more complex than standard CPR, however, and it does require an additional rescuer. IAC-CPR has been recommended as an alternative technique for trained adult healthcare providers in-hospital. This technique cannot be recommended for use in children because it has not been studied in this age group.

Relief of Foreign-Body Airway Obstruction

BLS providers should be able to recognize and relieve severe or complete FBAO. Three maneuvers to remove foreign bodies are suggested: back blows, chest thrusts, and abdominal thrusts. There are some differences between resuscitation councils as to the sequence of actions used to relieve FBAO; the published data does not support the effectiveness of one sequence over another. There is consensus that lack of protection of the upper abdominal organs by the rib cage renders infants and young children at risk for iatrogenic trauma from abdominal thrusts.[280] Therefore, the use of abdominal thrusts is not recommended for relief of FBAO in infants.

Epidemiology and Recognition of FBAO (Choking)

Most reported cases of FBAO in adults are caused by impacted food and occur while the victim is eating. Most reported episodes of choking in infants and children occur during eating or play, when parents or child-care providers are present. The choking event is therefore commonly witnessed, and the rescuer usually intervenes when the victim is conscious/responsive.

Signs of severe or complete FBAO in infants and children include the *sudden* onset of respiratory distress associated with weak or silent coughing, inability to speak, stridor (a high-pitched, noisy sound or wheezing), and increasing respiratory difficulty. These signs and symptoms of airway obstruction may also be caused by infections such as epiglottitis and croup, which produce in-airway edema. Signs of FBAO (rather than infectious airway obstruction) typically develop very abruptly, with no other signs of illness or infection (such as fever, signs of congestion, hoarseness, drooling, lethargy, or limpness). If the child has an *infectious* cause of airway obstruction, the Heimlich maneuver, back blows, and chest thrusts will *not* relieve the airway obstruction. The child must be taken immediately to an emergency facility.

Priorities for Teaching Relief of Severe or Complete FBAO

When FBAO produces signs of severe or *complete* airway obstruction, act quickly to relieve the obstruction. If partial obstruction is present and the child is coughing forcefully, do not interfere with the child's spontaneous coughing and breathing efforts. Try to relieve the obstruction only if the cough is or becomes ineffective (loss of sound), respiratory difficulty increases and is accompanied by stridor, or the victim becomes unresponsive. Activate the EMS system as quickly as possible if the child is having difficulty breathing. If more than 1 rescuer is present, the second rescuer activates the EMS system while the first rescuer attends to the child.

If a *responsive infant* shows signs of complete FBAO, deliver a combination of back blows and chest thrusts until the object is expelled or the victim becomes unresponsive. Although the data in this age group is limited, Heimlich thrusts are not recommended because they may damage the relatively large and unprotected liver. Reports of gastric rupture

---

Critical Concepts: Signs of Severe or Complete Airway Obstruction

In a conscious choking child the following are signs of severe or complete airway obstruction that require immediate action:

- **"Universal choking sign"**: the child clutches his or her neck with the thumb and index finger (Figure 19)

- Inability to speak

- Weak, ineffective coughs

- High-pitched sounds or no sounds while inhaling

- Increased difficulty breathing (breathing with distress)

- Cyanosis

Note: You do *not* need to act if the victim can cough forcefully and speak. Do not interfere at this point because a strong cough is the most effective way to remove a foreign body. Stay with the victim and monitor his or her condition. If the partial obstruction persists, activate the EMS or emergency response system.

---

and abdominal injury in adults have contributed to this concern.[281,282]

If a *responsive child* (1 to 8 years of age) shows signs of severe or complete FBAO, provide a series of Heimlich subdiaphragmatic abdominal thrusts.[283,284] These thrusts increase intrathoracic pressure, creating artificial "coughs" that force air and the foreign body out of the airway.

Epidemiological data[10,285] does not distinguish between FBAO fatalities in which the victims are responsive when first encountered and those in which the victims are unresponsive when initially encountered. The likelihood that a cardiac arrest or unresponsiveness will be

---

caused by an unsuspected FBAO is thought to be low.[10,286] However, the impact of averting a cardiac arrest in a *responsive victim* with severe or complete airway obstruction would be significant.

Healthcare providers should continue to perform abdominal thrusts for responsive *adults and children* with complete FBAO and alternating back blows and chest thrusts for responsive *infants* with complete FBAO. Healthcare providers should also be taught relief of FBAO in *unresponsive* infants, children, and adults. These sequences of actions for healthcare providers are unchanged from the 1992 guidelines.

Relief of FBAO in the Responsive Infant: Back Blows and Chest Thrusts

The following sequence is used to clear an FBAO from the airway of an infant. Back blows (Figure 20A) are delivered while the infant is supported in the prone position, straddling the rescuer's forearm, with the head lower than the trunk. After 5 back blows, if the object has not been expelled, give up to 5 chest thrusts (Figure 20B). These chest thrusts consist of chest compressions over the lower half of the sternum, 1 finger's width below the intermammary line. This landmark is

FIGURE 19. Universal choking sign.

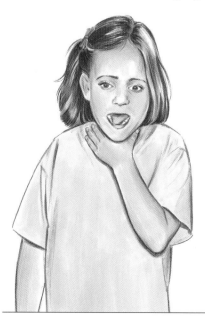

the same location used to provide chest compressions during CPR. Chest thrusts are delivered while the infant is supine, held on the rescuer's forearm, with the infant's head lower than the body.

Perform the following steps to relieve airway obstruction (the rescuer is usually seated or kneeling with the infant on the rescuer's lap):

1. Hold the infant prone with the head slightly lower than the chest, resting on your forearm. Support the infant's head by firmly supporting the jaw. Take care to avoid compressing the soft tissues of the infant's throat. Rest your forearm on your thigh to support the infant.

2. Deliver up to 5 back blows forcefully in the middle of the back between the infant's shoulder blades, using the heel of the hand. Each blow should be delivered with sufficient force to attempt to dislodge the foreign body.

3. After delivering up to 5 back blows, place your free hand on the infant's back, supporting the occiput of the infant's head with the palm of your hand. The infant will be adequately cradled between your 2 forearms, with the palm of one hand supporting the face and jaw while the palm of the other hand supports the occiput.

4. Turn the infant as a unit while carefully supporting the head and neck. Hold the infant in the supine position with your forearm resting on your thigh. Keep the infant's head lower than the trunk.

5. Provide up to 5 quick downward chest thrusts in the same location as chest compressions — lower third of the sternum, approximately 1 finger's width below the intermammary line. Chest thrusts are delivered at a rate of approximately 1 per second, each with the intention of creating enough of an "artificial cough" to dislodge the foreign body.

6. Repeat the sequence of up to 5 back blows and up to 5 chest thrusts until the object is removed or the victim becomes unresponsive.

Relief of FBAO in the Responsive Child: Abdominal Thrusts (Heimlich Maneuver)

The rescuer should perform the following steps to relieve complete airway obstruction in the child who is standing or sitting:

1. Stand or kneel behind the victim, arms directly under the victim's axillae, encircling the victim's chest.

2. Place the flat, thumb side of one fist against the victim's abdomen in the midline slightly above the navel and well below the tip of the xiphoid process.

3. Grasp the fist with the other hand and exert a series of up to 5 quick inward and upward thrusts (Figure 21). Do not touch the xiphoid process or the lower margins of the rib cage because force applied to these structures may damage internal organs.[280,294,295]

FIGURE 20. Relief of severe or complete FBAO in infant. **A,** Back blows. **B,** Chest thrusts.

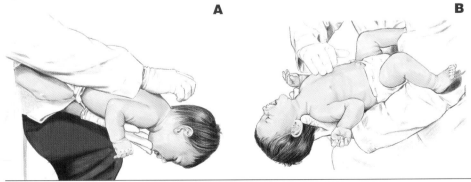

4. Each thrust should be a separate, distinct movement, delivered with the intent to relieve the obstruction. Continue the series of up to 5 thrusts until the foreign body is expelled or the patient becomes unresponsive.

Relief of FBAO in the Unresponsive Infant or Child

Blind finger sweeps should *not* be performed in infants and children because the foreign body may be pushed back into the airway, causing further obstruction or injury to the supraglottic area.[296,297] When abdominal thrusts or chest thrusts are provided to the unresponsive/unconscious, nonbreathing victim, open the victim's mouth by grasping both the tongue and lower jaw between the thumb and finger and lifting (tongue-jaw lift).[148] This action draws the tongue away from the back of the throat and may itself partially relieve the obstruction. If you see a foreign body, carefully remove it.

If the infant victim becomes unresponsive, perform the following sequence:

1. Open the victim's airway using a tongue-jaw lift and look for an object in the pharynx (see Figure 22). If an object is visible, remove it. Do not perform a blind finger sweep.

2. Open the airway with a head tilt–chin lift and attempt to provide rescue breaths. If the breaths are not effective, reposition the head and reattempt ventilation.

3. If the breaths are still not effective, perform the sequence of up to 5 back blows and up to 5 chest thrusts.

4. Repeat steps 1 through 3 until the object is dislodged and the airway is patent or for approximately 1 minute. If the airway obstruction is not relieved after approximately 1 minute, activate the EMS system.

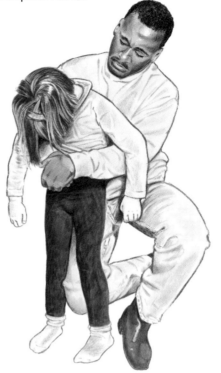

FIGURE 21. Abdominal thrusts performed for responsive child with severe or complete FBAO.

5. If breaths are effective, check for signs of circulation and continue CPR as needed, or place the infant in the recovery position if the infant shows adequate breathing and signs of circulation.

If the child victim becomes unresponsive, place the victim in the supine position and perform the following sequence:

1. Open the victim's airway using a tongue-jaw lift and look for an object in the pharynx. If an object is visible, remove it. Do not perform a blind finger sweep.

2. Open the airway with a head tilt–chin lift and attempt to provide rescue breaths. If breaths are not effective, reposition the head and reattempt ventilation.

3. If the breaths are still not effective, kneel beside the victim or straddle the victim's hips and prepare to perform the Heimlich maneuver (abdominal thrusts) as follows:

a. Place the heel of one hand on the child's abdomen in the midline slightly above the navel and well below the rib cage and xiphoid process. Place the other hand on top of the first.

b. Press both hands onto the abdomen with a quick inward and upward thrust (Figure 23). Direct each thrust upward in the midline and not to either side of the abdomen. If necessary, perform a series of up to 5 thrusts. Each thrust should be a separate and distinct movement of sufficient force to attempt to dislodge the airway obstruction.

4. Repeat steps 1 through 3 until the object is retrieved or rescuer breaths are effective. If the airway obstruction is not cleared after 1 minute, activate the EMS system.

5. Once effective breaths are delivered, assess for signs of circulation and provide additional CPR as needed or place the child in the recovery position if the child demonstrates adequate breathing and signs of circulation.

BLS in Special Situations

BLS for the Trauma Victim

The principles of resuscitation of the seriously injured child are the same as those for any pediatric patient with poten-

FIGURE 22. Tongue-jaw lift for unresponsive child with severe or complete FBAO.

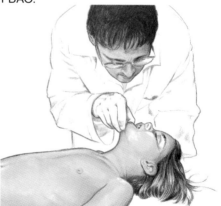

tial cardiorespiratory deterioration. Some aspects of pediatric trauma care require emphasis, however, because improper resuscitation is a major cause of preventable pediatric trauma death.[298-300] *Common errors in pediatric trauma resuscitation include failure to open and maintain the airway with cervical spine protection, inadequate or overzealous fluid resuscitation, and failure to recognize and treat internal bleeding.* Ideally a qualified surgeon should be involved early in the course of resuscitation. In regions with developed EMS systems, children with multisystem trauma should be rapidly transported to trauma centers with pediatric expertise.

The relative value of aeromedical transport compared with ground transport of children with multiple trauma is unclear and should be evaluated by individual EMS systems.[301-303] The preferred mode of transport will likely depend on EMS system characteristics.

BLS support requires meticulous attention to airway, breathing, and circulation from the moment of injury. The airway may become obstructed by soft tissues, blood, or dental fragments. These causes of airway obstruction should be anticipated and treated if they occur. Airway

---

FIGURE 23. Abdominal thrusts performed for supine, unresponsive child.

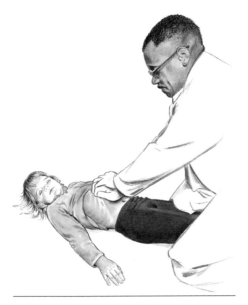

---

control includes spinal immobilization, which is continued during transport and stabilization in an ALS facility. This is best accomplished by a combined jaw-thrust and spinal stabilization maneuver, using only the amount of manual control necessary to prevent cranial-cervical motion (see Figure 24). The head tilt–chin lift is contraindicated because it may worsen existing cervical spinal injury. Rescuers should ensure that the neck is maintained in a neutral position because the prominent occiput of the child predisposes the neck to slight flexion when the child is placed on a flat surface.[231,304,305]

It may be difficult to immobilize the cervical spine of an infant or young child in a neutral position. Spinal immobilization of young children on a backboard that contains a recess for the head is recommended. If such a board is unavailable, the effect of a head recess can be simulated by placing a layer of towels or sheets ½ to 1 inch high on the board so that it elevates the torso (from shoulders to buttocks) and maintains the neck in neutral alignment.[230,231,306,307] The neck and airway should be in neutral position when the head rests on the backboard. Semirigid cervical collars are available in a wide range of sizes to help immobi-

lize children of various sizes. The child's head and neck should be further immobilized with linen rolls and tape, with secondary immobilization of the child on a spine board.

If 2 rescuers are present, the first rescuer opens the airway with a jaw-thrust maneuver while the second rescuer ensures that the cervical spine is absolutely stabilized in a neutral position. Avoid traction on or movement of the neck because it might convert a partial spinal cord injury to a complete one. Once the airway is controlled, immobilize the cervical spine as described above. Throughout immobilization and during transport, support oxygenation and ventilation.[308]

BLS for the Submersion Victim

Submersion is a leading cause of death in children worldwide. *The duration and severity of hypoxia sustained during submersion is the single most important determinant of outcome. CPR, particularly rescue breathing, should be attempted as soon as the unresponsive submersion victim is pulled from the water.* If possible, rescue breathing should be provided even while the victim is still in the water if the rescuer's safety is ensured.

Many infants and children submerged for brief periods of time will respond to stimulation or rescue breathing alone.[12] If the child does not have signs of circulation (breathing, coughing, or movement) after initial rescue breaths are provided, begin chest compressions.

FIGURE 24. Spine immobilization with airway opening in child with potential head and neck trauma.

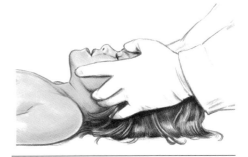

In 1994 the Institute of Medicine reviewed the recommendations of the AHA regarding resuscitation of near-drowning victims and supported the emphasis on initial establishment of effective ventilation.[282] There is no evidence that water acts as an obstructive foreign body, and time should not be wasted in attempting to remove water from the victim's lungs using abdominal thrusts or other FBAO maneuvers. Such maneuvers will delay CPR and the critically important support of airway and ventilation.[282] They may also produce complications.

Additional special resuscitation situations are discussed in Chapter 11, "Special Resuscitation Situations."

Family Presence During Resuscitation

According to surveys in the United States and the United Kingdom,[309-314] most family members would like to be present during the attempted resuscitation of a loved one. Parents and those who care for chronically ill children are often knowledgeable about and comfortable with medical equipment and emergency procedures. Family members with no medical background report that being at the side of a loved one and saying good-bye during the final moments of life is extremely comforting.[309,315,316] Parents or family members often fail to ask if they can be present, but healthcare providers should offer the opportunity whenever possible.[312,315,317,318]

Family members present during resuscitation report that their presence helped them adjust to the death of their loved one,[309,311] and most indicate they would choose to be present again.[309] Standardized psychological examinations suggest that family members present during resuscitation show less anxiety and depression and more constructive grief behavior than family members not present during resuscitation.[313]

When family members are present during resuscitative efforts, resuscitation team members should be sensitive to their presence. If possible, a member of the healthcare team should remain with the family to answer questions, clarify information, and offer comfort.[319]

In the prehospital setting family members are typically present during resuscitation of a loved one. Prehospital care providers are often too busy to give undivided attention to the needs of family members.

But brief explanations and the opportunity to remain with the loved one can be comforting. Some EMS systems provide follow-up visits to family members after unsuccessful resuscitation.

Termination of Resuscitative Efforts

Despite the best efforts of healthcare providers, most children who experience a cardiac arrest do not survive and never demonstrate return of spontaneous circulation. Return of spontaneous circulation is unlikely if the child fails to respond to effective BLS and ALS and 2 or more doses of epinephrine.[1,35,52] Special resuscitation circumstances, local resources, and underlying conditions and prognoses create a complex decision matrix for the resuscitation team. In general, in the absence of recurring or refractory VF or VT, history of a toxic drug exposure, or a primary hypothermic injury, the resuscitation team should discontinue resuscitative efforts after 30 minutes, especially if there is no return of spontaneous circulation. For further discussion, see Chapter 12, "CPR and Defibrillation: The Human Dimension."

Maximizing the Effectiveness of PBLS Training

CPR is the critical link in the Chain of Survival, particularly for infants and children. For many years the AHA and members of the International Liaison Committee on Resuscitation (ILCOR) have promoted the goal of appropriate bystander (lay rescuer) response to every witnessed cardiopulmonary emergency, such as a choking child, a child in respiratory distress, or an infant or a child in cardiac arrest. Although immediate bystander CPR can result in resuscitation even before the arrival of emergency personnel,[12,13] bystander CPR is not provided for a majority of victims of cardiac arrest.[1,35] Witnesses may fail to initiate resuscitation for several reasons; the most obvious is that they have not learned CPR.

CPR courses have evolved over the last decade into instructor-based, classroom-based programs. Yet this approach is not effective in teaching the critical psychomotor skills of CPR. Several studies have documented the failure of lay rescuers to perform CPR after participating in these traditional courses.[286,320] In 1998 these findings led the AHA to convene the National ECC Educational Conference to discuss how to improve CPR skills performance and retention. The experts came to 2 major conclusions:

- Current CPR programs for lay rescuers contain too much cognitive material and do not provide enough hands-on practice time.

- CPR programs for lay rescuers should focus on acquisition of specific psychomotor skills and retention of those skills over time.

Core Objectives

The core objectives for the PBLS course and modules are simple. After participation in a BLS course the rescuer who assists an unresponsive victim will be able to

1. Recognize a situation in which resuscitation is appropriate

2. Activate the EMS system when appropriate

3. Get and use an AED for adult victims and child victims more than 8 years old

4. Provide effective ventilations (chest rise after bag-mask, mouth-to-mouth, mouth-to-mask, and mouth-to–barrier device breathing). All healthcare pro-

viders should be capable of providing bag-mask ventilation for infants and children.

5. Provide effective chest compressions that generate a palpable pulse

6. Perform all skills in a manner that is safe for the victim, rescuer, and bystanders

The participant should remember how to perform these skills for 2 years after training.

If participants are to achieve core objectives, CPR programs must be simplified. They must focus on skills acquisition rather than cognitive knowledge. Training programs that attempt to teach large amounts of material fail to achieve core educational objectives (eg, the psychomotor skills of CPR), with poor participant skills retention and performance.[57] By comparison, focused training programs emphasizing skills acquisition result in superior levels of skills performance.[58,286-288]

This compelling data mandates consideration of the potential negative effects of science changes on teaching CPR. Such consideration influenced debates about guidelines changes. Interventions that could produce even modest improvements in survival were more readily endorsed if they were easy to teach and would simplify CPR instruction. Conversely, interventions that would have a negative impact on CPR training (eg, complex instruction and skills that would require extensive practice) had to be supported by higher levels of evidence of effectiveness to justify their introduction.

Course instructors should focus on ensuring participant mastery of core objectives. Skills practice time must be maximized and lecture time minimized. Resuscitation councils should evaluate skills acquisition by participants and use the information to continuously improve resuscitation programs.

Audio and Visual CPR Performance Aids for BLS Interventions

CPR is a complex psychomotor task that is difficult to teach, learn, remember, and perform. Not surprisingly, observed CPR performance is often poor (inadequate compression depth, inadequate compression rate, etc). The use of audio and visual CPR performance aids during training can improve acquisition of CPR psychomotor skills. The use of audio prompts (eg, an audiotape with the appropriate cadence of "compress-compress-compress-breathe") improves CPR performance in both clinical and laboratory settings.[244,247,287,321,322] Use of these devices should be considered in areas where CPR is performed infrequently.

Summary

The epidemiology and outcome of pediatric cardiopulmonary arrest and the priorities, techniques, and sequence of pediatric resuscitation assessments and interventions differ from those for adults. Current guidelines have been updated after extensive multinational evidence-based review and discussion over several years. Areas of controversy in current guidelines and recommendations made by consensus are detailed. A large degree of uniformity exists in the current guidelines advocated by the AHA, Heart and Stroke Foundation of Canada, European Resuscitation Council, Australian Resuscitation Council, and Resuscitation Council of Southern Africa. Differences are currently based on local and regional preferences, training networks, and customs rather than scientific controversy.

Summary of Key Concepts

- ✔ The outcome of pulseless cardiac arrest in infants and children is poor. Therefore, healthcare providers should prevent arrest when possible by reducing risk of sudden infant death, trauma, and submersion.

- ✔ Cardiopulmonary arrest in infants and children is most often the result of progressive respiratory failure or shock. Respiratory arrest often precedes cardiac arrest. If the infant or child develops respiratory arrest and the rescuer intervenes and provides rescue breathing, it may be possible to prevent cardiac arrest.

- ✔ Ideally CPR is initiated simultaneously with activation of the emergency response system. When a lone rescuer finds an unresponsive infant or child, the rescuer should perform approximately 1 minute of CPR and then phone 911 or the emergency response system (phone fast).

- ✔ If the lone rescuer encounters an infant or child who collapses suddenly and the rescuer has reason to believe that sudden cardiac arrest has occurred, the rescuer should phone 911 (or the emergency response system) and then return to the victim to perform CPR.

- ✔ Open the airway using the head tilt–chin lift maneuver (or jaw thrust without head tilt for patients suspected of having spinal injuries).

- ✔ Mouth-to-mouth-and-nose, mouth-to-nose, and mouth-to-mouth breathing are acceptable rescue breathing techniques to provide ventilation for the infant.

- ✔ Lay rescuers with a duty to respond and healthcare providers should use standard precautions and barrier devices when available to deliver rescue breaths to the unresponsive, nonbreathing victim.

- ✔ Healthcare providers should be proficient in bag-mask ventilation.

- ✔ Tracheal intubation should be attempted only by those proficient in the technique, using secondary confirmation techniques to detect tube misplacement and displacement.

- ✔ Healthcare providers should perform a pulse check while checking for other signs of circulation (breathing, coughing, or movement).

✔ The ratio of 5 compressions to 1 ventilation is recommended for both 1- and 2-rescuer CPR for the infant (outside the delivery room) or child victim.

✔ The compression rate for 1- and 2-rescuer CPR is at least 100 compressions per minute for infant victims and approximately 100 compressions per minute for child victims.

✔ The BLS sequence of action for infants and children is

1. Assess responsiveness.

2. If the victim is unresponsive, open the airway (using head tilt–chin lift or jaw thrust), and assess breathing (look, listen, and feel).

3. If the victim is not breathing, provide rescue breathing.

4. Check for signs of circulation (pulse check for healthcare providers only, breathing, coughing, or movement).

5. If there are no signs of circulation, provide chest compressions (at a rate of at least 100 compressions per minute for infants and approximately 100 compressions per minute for children with a compression-ventilation ratio of 5:1). If the child is 1 to 8 years of age or older in the prehospital setting, use an AED as soon as it is available. Use child pads for children 1 to 8 (if available) and adult pads for victims 8 years of age and older. In the hospital setting, attach a monitor/defibrillator/pacer as soon as one is available.

6. After approximately 1 minute of rescue support, phone 911 or other emergency response number (if not already done).

✔ For victims in respiratory arrest, rescuers should initially provide 2 slow rescue breaths followed by 1 breath every 3 seconds (20 breaths per minute).

✔ Forceful or excessive ventilation during CPR may cause gastric inflation, regurgitation, and aspiration.

✔ Cricoid pressure is helpful in preventing gastric inflation in the unresponsive victim.

Critical Concepts:
2003 Recommendation for Use of AEDs in Children 1 to 8 Years of Age

AED technology has changed rapidly since the 2000 Guidelines were published. Several manufacturers now market AEDs that accommodate both adult electrode pads and pediatric cable-pad systems that attenuate the delivered energy to a dose more appropriate for children under the age of 8 years. Clinical experience with the devices has yet to be published. Data from two recent large studies of the effectiveness of the AED rhythm analysis algorithms in pediatric patients have been published since the ECC Guidelines 2000 were drafted.[323,324]

Intense interest in the topic of AED use for pediatric arrest victims prompted the AHA, with the International Liaison Committee on Resuscitation (ILCOR), to conduct an evaluation of the technical advances and the AED rhythm analysis data. The following conclusions are part of an advisory statement that has been prepared to revise the ECC Guidelines 2000 recommendation for use of AEDs in children under the age of 8 years.[325]

■ AEDs may be used for children 1 to 8 years of age with no signs of circulation. Ideally the device should deliver a child dose. The arrhythmia detection algorithm used in the device should demonstrate high specificity for pediatric shockable rhythms (ie, will not recommend shock delivery for nonshockable rhythms): *Class IIb*.

■ Currently there is insufficient evidence to support a recommendation for or against the use of AEDs in infants <1 year of age.

■ For a single rescuer responding to a child without signs of circulation, 1 minute of CPR continues to be recommended before any other action, such as activating EMS or attaching an AED.

■ Defibrillation is recommended for documented VF/pulseless VT: *Class I*.

The use of AEDs and adult pads in children approximately 8 years of age and older (and approximately ≥25 kg in weight or 128 cm in height) carries a Class IIb recommendation. This recommendation is based on some evidence of accuracy of AED diagnostic algorithms in older children and adolescents[323,326,327] and on the fact that a shock of 150 to 200 J to an 8-year-old child with a median weight of 25 kg would result in a 6 to 8 J/kg shock. This dose is higher than the 2 to 4 J/kg defibrillation dose recommended in the PALS Guidelines but is less than 10 J/kg. The consensus of the experts is that there is little potential for myocardial damage with an initial dose that is less than 10 J/kg.

Note that the Subcommittee on Pediatric Resuscitation recommends that healthcare providers who routinely care for children at risk for arrhythmias and cardiac arrest (eg, in-hospital settings) should continue to use defibrillators capable of appropriate energy adjustment.

For more information on the 2003 revision of the ECC Guidelines 2000 recommendations for use of AEDs in children 1 to 8 years of age, visit the AHA ECC website (**www.americanheart.org/cpr**).

Review Questions

1. You are in the clinic, and a mother walks in carrying her limp infant in her arms. She says, "I think he stopped breathing on the way here." What should be your first step in the BLS sequence of action?

   a. check for breathing

   b. check for signs of circulation

   c. check for responsiveness

   d. open the airway

2. You have volunteered to care for several infants during a charity event at a local school. You and another volunteer are placing the infants in cribs for naps. The other volunteer knows that you are a healthcare provider and asks you to name the best position in which to place infants for sleep. What is your response?

   a. place all infants prone (on their stomachs) so if they vomit they will not aspirate

   b. place all healthy infants supine (on their backs) to sleep to reduce the risk of sudden infant death syndrome

   c. place all infants in a semi-upright position to reduce the risk of vomiting and sleep apnea

   d. place all infants face-down on soft, fluffy surfaces to cushion the infant's head and neck

3. Paramedics have transported a young infant with a history of apnea to the Emergency Department. When they arrive in the Emergency Department you note that the infant is breathing slowly, is not responsive to stimulation, and has poor color. You transfer the infant to a gurney in the pediatric resuscitation room, open the infant's airway, and note that the infant is breathing slowly and shallowly at a rate of approximately 6 breaths per minute. What should your next action be?

   a. immediately provide rescue breaths with a bag-mask device and oxygen

   b. immediately check for a pulse and other signs of circulation to determine if chest compressions are needed

   c. administer oxygen but do not provide ventilations or compressions

   d. attempt to relieve foreign-body airway obstruction

4. You are alone and have provided effective positive-pressure breaths using a bag and mask for an unresponsive 3-year-old child with agonal respirations and poor perfusion. You then check the carotid pulse and detect a pulse that is approximately 55 bpm. What should your next action be?

   a. continue rescue breathing only at a rate of approximately 20 breaths per minute

   b. administer 100% oxygen and place the child in the recovery position

   c. phone 911 or other emergency response number

   d. begin chest compressions at a rate of approximately 100 compressions per minute

5. What is the correct BLS sequence for lone rescuers for out-of-hospital resuscitation of infants and children who are found to be unresponsive?

   a. phone the emergency response number immediately, then return to the victim, and check for signs of circulation; if there are no signs of circulation, open the airway and check for breathing; if there is no breathing, give rescue breaths

   b. open the airway and check for breathing; if there is no effective breathing, give 2 rescue breaths, check for signs of circulation, and if there are no signs of circulation, begin chest compressions and phone 911 after approximately 1 minute

   c. phone 911 or the emergency response number, open the airway, and check for breathing; if there is no breathing, give 2 rescue breaths, check for signs of circulation; if there are no signs of circulation, begin chest compressions

   d. open the airway and give rescue breaths, then check for signs of circulation; if there are no signs of circulation, leave the victim to phone 911, then return to the victim to begin chest compressions

6. You find an infant who is unresponsive. You have sent a colleague to phone the emergency response number. You perform a head tilt–chin lift and look, listen, and feel for breathing. If the infant is not breathing, what should you do next?

   a. give 2 rapid breaths to make the chest rise

   b. give 2 slow breaths to make the chest rise

   c. give 1 slow breath and try not to make the chest rise

   d. give 1 rapid breath just until the chest barely rises

   e. begin chest compressions

7. You are attempting to assess signs of circulation in a 6-year-old child. After you provide 2 rescue breaths, the child is unresponsive and not breathing, coughing, or moving. Where should you feel for the pulse of an unresponsive child victim?

   a. the radial pulse

   b. the carotid pulse

   c. the femoral pulse

   d. the brachial pulse

8. You are at a lake and have just helped pull a 4-year-old from the water. The child is limp and blue and does not respond to stimulation of any kind. What should you do immediately?

   a. send someone to phone 911 while you open the airway and prepare to provide rescue breathing

   b. try to eliminate water from the airway using a Heimlich abdominal thrust

   c. begin chest compressions

   d. attach an AED as soon as it is available before providing rescue breaths

9. At the scene you are caring for a 7-year-old child who fell 20 feet from a rooftop. She is unresponsive, and you direct bystanders to phone 911. Your next step in the BLS sequence of action should be

   a. jaw thrust without head tilt

   b. check for signs of circulation

   c. head tilt–chin lift

   d. begin chest compressions

10. You are performing rescue breathing for an infant with respiratory arrest. You ensure that you are delivering a proper rescue breath by

    a. observing a change in the victim's color

    b. checking the victim regularly for signs of circulation

    c. seeing the victim's chest rise during rescue breathing

    d. checking the airway frequently

How did you do?

1, c; **2,** b; **3,** a; **4,** d; **5,** b; **6,** b; **7,** b; **8,** a; **9,** a; **10,** c.

References

1. Young KD, Seidel JS. Pediatric cardiopulmonary resuscitation: a collective review. *Ann Emerg Med.* 1999;33:195-205.

2. Hoyert DL, Kochanek KD, Murphy SL. Deaths: final data for 1997. *Natl Vital Stat Rep.* 1999;47:1-104.

3. Eisenberg M, Bergner L, Hallstrom A. Epidemiology of cardiac arrest and resuscitation in children. *Ann Emerg Med.* 1983;12:672-674.

4. Gausche M, Seidel JS, Henderson DP, Ness B, Ward PM, Wayland BW, Almeida B. Pediatric deaths and emergency medical services (EMS) in urban and rural areas. *Pediatr Emerg Care.* 1989;5:158-162.

5. Torphy DE, Minter MG, Thompson BM. Cardiorespiratory arrest and resuscitation of children. *Am J Dis Child.* 1984;138:1099-1102.

6. Friesen RM, Duncan P, Tweed WA, Bristow G. Appraisal of pediatric cardiopulmonary resuscitation. *Can Med Assoc J.* 1982;126:1055-1058.

7. Walsh CK, Krongrad E. Terminal cardiac electrical activity in pediatric patients. *Am J Cardiol.* 1983;51:557-561.

8. Zaritsky A. Cardiopulmonary resuscitation in children. *Clin Chest Med.* 1987;8:561-571.

9. *1999 Injury Facts.* Itasca, Ill: National Safety Council; 1999.

10. Fingerhut LA, Cox CS, Warner M. International comparative analysis of injury mortality: findings from the ICE (International Collaborative Effort) on Injury Statistics, Vital and Health Statistics of the Centers for Disease Control and Prevention. *Adv Data.* 1998 Oct 7:1-20.

11. Peters K, Kochanek K, Murphy S. Deaths: final data for 1996. *Natl Vital Stat Rep.* 1998;47:1-100.

12. Kyriacou DN, Arcinue EL, Peek C, Kraus JF. Effect of immediate resuscitation on children with submersion injury. *Pediatrics.* 1994;94:137-142.

13. Hickey RW, Cohen DM, Strausbaugh S, Dietrich AM. Pediatric patients requiring CPR in the prehospital setting. *Ann Emerg Med.* 1995;25:495-501.

14. Clements F, McGowan J. Finger position for chest compressions in cardiac arrest in infants. *Resuscitation.* 2000;44:43-46.

15. Whitelaw CC, Slywka B, Goldsmith LJ. Comparison of a 2-finger versus 2-thumb method for chest compressions by healthcare providers in an infant mechanical model. *Resuscitation.* 2000;43:213-216.

16. Eckenhoff JE. Some anatomic considerations of the infant larynx influencing endotracheal anesthesia. *Anesthesiology.* 1951;12:401-410.

17. Coté CJ, Ryan J, Todres ID, Goudsouzian NG, eds. *A Practice of Anesthesia for Infants and Children.* 2nd ed. Philadelphia, Pa: WB Saunders; 1993.

18. Nadkarni V. Ventricular fibrillation in the asphyxiated piglet model. In: Quan L, Franklin WH, eds. *Ventricular Fibrillation: A Pediatric Problem.* Armonk, NY: Futura Publishers; 2000:43-54.

19. Bayes de Luna A, Coumel P, Leclercq JF. Ambulatory sudden cardiac death: mechanisms of production of fatal arrhythmia on the basis of data from 157 cases. *Am Heart J.* 1989;117: 151-159.

20. Cummins RO, Chamberlain DA, Abramson NS, Allen M, Baskett P, Becker L, Bossaert L, Delooz H, Dick W, Eisenberg M, et al. Recommended guidelines for uniform reporting of data from out-of-hospital cardiac arrest: the Utstein Style. Task Force of the American Heart Association, the European Resuscitation Council, the Heart and Stroke Foundation of Canada, and the Australian Resuscitation Council. *Ann Emerg Med.* 1991;20:861-874.

21. Cummins RO. From concept to standard-of-care? Review of the clinical experience with automated external defibrillators. *Ann Emerg Med.* 1989;18:1269-1275.

22. Larsen MP, Eisenberg MS, Cummins RO, Hallstrom AP. Predicting survival from out-of-hospital cardiac arrest: a graphic model. *Ann Emerg Med.* 1993;22:1652-1658.

23. White RD, Vukov LF, Bugliosi TF. Early defibrillation by police: initial experience with measurement of critical time intervals and patient outcome. *Ann Emerg Med.* 1994;23: 1009-1013.

24. Ladwig KH, Schoefinius A, Danner R, Gurtler R, Herman R, Koeppel A, Hauber P. Effects of early defibrillation by ambulance personnel on short- and long-term outcome of cardiac arrest survival: the Munich experiment. *Chest.* 1997; 112:1584-1591.

25. Stiell IG, Wells GA, Field BJ, Spaite DW, De Maio VJ, Ward R, Munkley DP, Lyver MB, Luinstra LG, Campeau T, Maloney J, Dagnone E. Improved out-of-hospital cardiac arrest survival through the inexpensive optimization of an existing defibrillation program: OPALS study phase II. Ontario Prehospital Advanced Life Support. *JAMA.* 1999;281:1175-1181.

26. White RD, Hankins DG, Bugliosi TF. Seven years' experience with early defibrillation by police and paramedics in an emergency medical services system. *Resuscitation.* 1998;39: 145-151.

27. Van Hoeyweghen RJ, Bossaert LL, Mullie A, Calle P, Martens P, Buylaert WA, Delooz H, Belgian Cerebral Resuscitation Study Group. Quality and efficiency of bystander CPR. *Resuscitation.* 1993;26:47-52.

28. Bossaert L, Van Hoeyweghen R, the Cerebral Resuscitation Study Group. Bystander cardiopulmonary resuscitation (CPR) in out-of-hospital cardiac arrest. *Resuscitation.* 1989; 17(suppl):S55-S69.

29. Nadkarni V, Hazinski MF, Zideman D, Kattwinkel J, Quan L, Bingham R, Zaritsky A, Bland J, Kramer E, Tiballs J. Pediatric resuscitation: an advisory statement from the Pediatric Working Group of the International Liaison Committee on Resuscitation. *Circulation.* 1997;95:2185-2195.

30. Slonim AD, Patel KM, Ruttimann UE, Pollack MM. Cardiopulmonary resuscitation in pediatric intensive care units. *Crit Care Med.* 1997;25:1951-1955.

31. Richman PB, Nashed AH. The etiology of cardiac arrest in children and young adults: special considerations for ED management. *Am J Emerg Med.* 1999;17:264-270.

32. Kuisma M, Suominen P, Korpela R. Paediatric out-of-hospital cardiac arrests: epidemiology and outcome. *Resuscitation.* 1995;30:141-150.

33. Kuisma M, Maatta T, Repo J. Cardiac arrests witnessed by EMS personnel in a multitiered system: epidemiology and outcome. *Am J Emerg Med.* 1998;16:12-16.

34. Finer NN, Horbar JD, Carpenter JH. Cardiopulmonary resuscitation in the very low birth weight infant: the Vermont Oxford Network experience. *Pediatrics.* 1999;104: 428-434.

35. Sirbaugh PE, Pepe PE, Shook JE, Kimball KT, Goldman MJ, Ward MA, Mann DM. A prospective, population-based study of the demographics, epidemiology, management, and outcome of out-of-hospital pediatric cardiopulmonary arrest. *Ann Emerg Med.* 1999; 33:174-184.

36. Zaritsky A. Outcome following cardiopulmonary resuscitation in the pediatric intensive care unit. *Crit Care Med.* 1997;25:1937-1938.

37. Saugstad OD. Practical aspects of resuscitating asphyxiated newborn infants. *Eur J Pediatr.* 1998;157(suppl 1):S11-S15.

38. Palme-Kilander C. Methods of resuscitation in low-Apgar-score newborn infants: a national survey. *Acta Paediatr.* 1992;81:739-744.

39. World Health Organization. *The World Health Report: Report of the Director-General.* 1995. Geneva, Switzerland: World Health Organization; 1995.

40. Kattwinkel J, Niermeyer S, Nadkarni V, Tibballs J, Phillips B, Zideman D, Van Reempts P, Osmond M. An advisory statement from the Pediatric Working Group of the International Liaison Committee on Resuscitation. *Pediatrics.* 1999;103:e56.

41. Appleton GO, Cummins RO, Larson MP, Graves JR. CPR and the single rescuer: at what age should you "call first" rather than "call fast"? *Ann Emerg Med.* 1995;25:492-494.

42. Mogayzel C, Quan L, Graves JR, Tiedeman D, Fahrenbruch C, Herndon P. Out-of-hospital ventricular fibrillation in children and adolescents: causes and outcomes. *Ann Emerg Med.* 1995;25:484-491.

43. Dieckmann RA, Vardis R. High-dose epinephrine in pediatric out-of-hospital cardiopulmonary arrest. *Pediatrics.* 1995;95:901-913.

44. Losek JD, Hennes H, Glaeser PW, Smith DS, Hendley G. Prehospital countershock treatment of pediatric asystole. *Am J Emerg Med.* 1989; 7:571-575.

45. Safranek DJ, Eisenberg MS, Larsen MP. The epidemiology of cardiac arrest in young adults. *Ann Emerg Med.* 1992;21:1102-1106.

46. Schindler MB, Bohn D, Cox PN, McCrindle BW, Jarvis A, Edmonds J, Barker G. Outcome of out-of-hospital cardiac or respiratory arrest in children. *N Engl J Med.* 1996;335: 1473-1479.

47. Ronco R, King W, Donley DK, Tilden SJ. Outcome and cost at a children's hospital following resuscitation for out-of-hospital cardiopulmonary arrest. *Arch Pediatr Adolesc Med.* 1995;149:210-214.

48. Hazinski MF, Chahine AA, Holcomb GW III, Morris JA Jr. Outcome of cardiovascular collapse in pediatric blunt trauma. *Ann Emerg Med.* 1994;23:1229-1235.

49. Innes PA, Summers CA, Boyd IM, Molyneux EM. Audit of paediatric cardiopulmonary resuscitation. *Arch Dis Child.* 1993;68:487-491.

50. Losek JD, Hennes H, Glaeser P, Hendley G, Nelson DB. Prehospital care of the pulseless, nonbreathing pediatric patient. *Am J Emerg Med.* 1987;5:370-374.

51. Zaritsky A, Nadkarni V, Getson P, Kuehl K. CPR in children. *Ann Emerg Med.* 1987;16: 1107-1111.

52. O'Rourke PP. Outcome of children who are apneic and pulseless in the emergency room. *Crit Care Med.* 1986;14:466-468.

53. Quan L, Gore EJ, Wentz K, Allen J, Novack AH. Ten-year study of pediatric drownings and near-drownings in King County, Washington: lessons in injury prevention. *Pediatrics.* 1989; 83:1035-1040.

54. Childhood injuries in the United States. Division of Injury Control, Center for Environmental Health and Injury Control, Centers for Disease Control. *Am J Dis Child.* 1990;144:627-646.

55. Adgey AA, Johnston PW, McMechan S. Sudden cardiac death and substance abuse. *Resuscitation.* 1995;29:219-221.

56. Ackerman MJ. The long QT syndrome. *Pediatr Rev.* 1998;19:232-238.

57. Brennan RT, Braslow A. Skill mastery in cardiopulmonary resuscitation training classes. *Am J Emerg Med.* 1995;13:505-508.

58. Handley JA, Handley AJ. Four-step CPR: improving skill retention. *Resuscitation.* 1998;36:3-8.

59. Newacheck PW, Strickland B, Shonkoff JP, Perrin JM, McPherson M, McManus M, Lauver C, Fox H, Arango P. An epidemiologic profile of children with special health care needs. *Pediatrics.* 1998;102:117-123.

60. McPherson M, Arango P, Fox H, Lauver C, McManus M, Newacheck PW, Perrin JM, Shonkoff JP, Strickland B. A new definition of children with special health care needs. *Pediatrics.* 1998;102:137-140.

61. Committee on Pediatric Emergency Medicine, American Academy of Pediatrics. Emergency preparedness for children with special health care needs. *Pediatrics.* 1999;104:e53.

62. Spaite DW, Conroy C, Tibbitts M, Karriker KJ, Seng M, Battaglia N, Criss EA, Valenzuela TD, Meislin HW. Use of emergency medical services by children with special health care needs. *Prehosp Emerg Care.* 2000;4:19-23.

63. Schultz-Grant LD, Young-Cureton V, Kataoka-Yahiro M. Advance directives and do not resuscitate orders: nurses' knowledge and the level of practice in school settings. *J Sch Nurs.* 1998;14:4-10,12-13.

64. Seidel JS. Emergency medical services and the pediatric patient: are the needs being met? II: training and equipping emergency medical services providers for pediatric emergencies. *Pediatrics.* 1986;78:808-812.

65. Seidel JS. EMS-C in urban and rural areas: the California experience. In: *Emergency Medical Services for Children: Report of the 97th Ross Conference on Pediatric Research.* Columbus, Ohio: Ross Laboratories; 1989:808-812.

66. Applebaum D. Advanced prehospital care for pediatric emergencies. *Ann Emerg Med.* 1985; 14:656-659.

67. Zaritsky A, French JP, Schafermeyer R, Morton D. A statewide evaluation of pediatric prehospital and hospital emergency services. *Arch Pediatr Adolesc Med.* 1994;148:76-81.

68. Graham CJ, Stuemky J, Lera TA. Emergency medical services preparedness for pediatric emergencies. *Pediatr Emerg Care.* 1993;9: 329-331.

69. Cook RT Jr. The Institute of Medicine report on emergency medical services for children: thoughts for emergency medical technicians, paramedics, and emergency physicians. *Pediatrics.* 1995;96:199-206.

70. Makhmudova NM, Urinbaev MZ, Pak MA, Abukov MI, Faizieva NP. Organization of emergency medical services for the children in Tashkent [in Russian]. *Sov Zdravookhr.* 1990:55-59.

71. Foltin GL. Critical issues in urban emergency medical services for children. *Pediatrics.* 1995; 96:174-179.

72. Brooks JG. Sudden infant death syndrome. *Pediatr Ann.* 1995;24:345-383.

73. Altemeier WA III. A pediatrician's view: crib death and managed care. *Pediatr Ann.* 1995;24: 345-346.

74. Dwyer T, Ponsonby AL. SIDS epidemiology and incidence. *Pediatr Ann.* 1995;24:350-352, 354-356.

75. Willinger M. SIDS prevention. *Pediatr Ann.* 1995;24:358-364.

76. Valdes-Dapena M. The postmortem examination. *Pediatr Ann.* 1995;24:365-372.

77. McClain ME, Shaefer SJ. Supporting families after sudden infant death. *Pediatr Ann.* 1995; 24:373-378.

78. Filiano JJ, Kinney HC. Sudden infant death syndrome and brainstem research. *Pediatr Ann.* 1995;24:379-383.

79. American Academy of Pediatrics Task Force on Infant Positioning and SIDS. Positioning and sudden infant death syndrome (SIDS): update. *Pediatrics.* 1996;98:1216-1218.

80. American Academy of Pediatrics AAP Task Force on Infant Positioning and SIDS. Positioning and SIDS. *Pediatrics.* 1992;89: 1120-1126.

81. Willinger M, Hoffman HJ, Hartford RB. Infant sleep position and risk for sudden infant death syndrome: report of meeting held January 13 and 14, 1994, National Institutes of Health, Bethesda, MD. *Pediatrics.* 1994;93:814-819.

82. Mitchell EA, Scragg R. Observations on ethnic differences in SIDS mortality in New Zealand. *Early Hum Dev.* 1994;38:151-157.

83. Blair PS, Fleming PJ, Bensley D, Smith I, Bacon C, Taylor E, Berry J, Golding J, Tripp J, Confidential Enquiry into Stillbirths and Deaths Regional Coordinators and Researchers. Smoking and the sudden infant death syndrome: results from 1993-5 case-control study for confidential inquiry into stillbirths and deaths in infancy. *BMJ.* 1996;313:195-198.

84. Danesco E, Miller T, Spicer R. Incidence and costs of 1987-1994 childhood injuries: demographic breakdowns. *Pediatrics.* 2000;105:e27.

85. Guyer B, Ellers B. Childhood injuries in the United States: mortality, morbidity, and cost. *Am J Dis Child.* 1990;144:649-652.

86. Cushman R, James W, Waclawik H. Physicians promoting bicycle helmets for children: a randomized trial. *Am J Public Health.* 1991; 81:1044-1046.

87. Centers for Disease Control. Fatal injuries to children: United States, 1986. *JAMA.* 1990; 264:952-953.

88. The National Committee for Injury Prevention and Control. Injury prevention: meeting the challenge. *Am J Prev Med.* 1989;5:1-303.

89. Giguere JF, St-Vil D, Turmel A, Di Lorenzo M, Pothel C, Manseau S, Mercier C. Airbags and children: a spectrum of C-spine injuries. *J Pediatr Surg.* 1998;33:811-816.

90. Bourke GJ. Airbags and fatal injuries to children. *Lancet.* 1996;347:560.

91. Hazinski MF, Eddy VA, Morris JA Jr. Children's traffic safety program: influence of early elementary school safety education on family seat belt use. *J Trauma.* 1995;39:1063-1068.

92. Patel DR, Greydanus DE, Rowlett JD. Romance with the automobile in the 20th century: implications for adolescents in a new millennium. *Adolesc Med.* 2000;11:127-139.

93. Harre N, Field J. Safe driving education programs at school: lessons from New Zealand. *Aust N Z J Public Health.* 1998;22:447-450.

94. Brown RC, Gains MJ, Greydanus DE, Schonberg SK. Driver education: position paper of the Society for Adolescent Medicine. *J Adolesc Health.* 1997;21:416-418.

95. Robertson LS. Crash involvement of teenaged drivers when driver education is eliminated from high school. *Am J Public Health.* 1980;70:599-603.

96. Margolis LH, Kotch J, Lacey JH. Children in alcohol-related motor vehicle crashes. *Pediatrics.* 1986;77:870-872.

97. O'Malley PM, Johnston LD. Drinking and driving among US high school seniors, 1984-1997. *Am J Public Health.* 1999;89:678-684.

98. Lee JA, Jones-Webb RJ, Short BJ, Wagenaar AC. Drinking location and risk of alcohol-impaired driving among high school seniors. *Addict Behav.* 1997;22:387-393.

99. Quinlan KP, Brewer RD, Sleet DA, Dellinger AM. Characteristics of child passenger deaths and injuries involving drinking drivers. *JAMA.* 2000;283:2249-2252.

100. Margolis LH, Foss RD, Tolbert WG. Alcohol and motor vehicle-related deaths of children as passengers, pedestrians, and bicyclists. *JAMA.* 2000;283:2245-2248.

101. DiGuiseppi CG, Rivara FP, Koepsell TD, Polissar L. Bicycle helmet use by children: evaluation of a community-wide helmet campaign. *JAMA.* 1989;262:2256-2261.

102. Thompson RS, Rivara FP, Thompson DC. A case-control study of the effectiveness of bicycle safety helmets. *N Engl J Med.* 1989; 320:1361-1367.

103. DiGuiseppi CG, Rivara FP, Koepsell TD. Attitudes toward bicycle helmet ownership and use by school-age children. *Am J Dis Child.* 1990;144:83-86.

104. Byard RW, Lipsett J. Drowning deaths in toddlers and preambulatory children in South Australia. *Am J Forensic Med Pathol.* 1999; 20:328-332.

105. Sachdeva RC. Near drowning. *Crit Care Clin.* 1999;15:281-296.

106. Fergusson DM, Horwood LJ. Risks of drowning in fenced and unfenced domestic swimming pools. *N Z Med J.* 1984;97: 777-779.

107. Forjuoh SN, Coben JH, Dearwater SR, Weiss HB. Identifying homes with inadequate smoke detector protection from residential fires in Pennsylvania. *J Burn Care Rehabil.* 1997;18:86-91.

108. Marshall SW, Runyan CW, Bangdiwala SI, Linzer MA, Sacks JJ, Butts JD. Fatal residential fires: who dies and who survives? *JAMA.* 1998;279:1633-1637.

109. Division of Injury, Epidemiology, and Control, Center for Environmental Health and Injury Control, Centers for Disease Control. Cost of injury–United States: a report to Congress. *MMWR.* 1989;38:743-746.

110. Hall J, Quincy M, Karter M. National Safety Council tabulations of National Center for Health Statistics mortality data. 1999.

111. *An Evaluation of Residential Smoke Detector Performance Under Actual Field Conditions.* Washington, DC: Federal Emergency Management Agency; 1980.

112. Fingerhut LA, Ingram DD, Feldman JJ. Firearm homicide among black teenage males in metropolitan counties: comparison of death rates in two periods, 1983 through 1985 and 1987 through 1989. *JAMA.* 1992;267: 3054-3058.

113. Fingerhut LA. Firearm mortality among children, youth, and young adults 1-34 years of age, trends and current status: United States, 1985-90. *Adv Data.* 1993:1-20.

114. Beaman V, Annest JL, Mercy JA, Kresnow M, Pollock DA. Lethality of firearm-related injuries in the United States population. *Ann Emerg Med.* 2000;35:258-266.

115. Weil DS, Hemenway D. Loaded guns in the home: analysis of a national random survey of gun owners. *JAMA.* 1992;267:3033-3037.

116. Callahan CM, Rivara FP. Urban high school youth and handguns: a school-based survey. *JAMA.* 1992;267:3038-3042.

117. Cohen LR, Potter LB. Injuries and violence: risk factors and opportunities for prevention during adolescence. *Adolesc Med.* 1999;10: 125-135.

118. Simon TR, Crosby AE, Dahlberg LL. Students who carry weapons to high school: comparison with other weapon-carriers. *J Adolesc Health.* 1999;24:340-348.

119. Brent DA, Perper JA, Allman CJ, Moritz GM, Wartella ME, Zelenak JP. The presence and accessibility of firearms in the homes of adolescent suicides: a case-control study. *JAMA.* 1991;266:2989-2995.

120. Svenson JE, Spurlock C, Nypaver M. Pediatric firearm-related fatalities: not just an urban problem. *Arch Pediatr Adolesc Med.* 1996;150:583-587.

121. Wintemute GJ, Parham CA, Beaumont JJ, Wright M, Drake C. Mortality among recent purchasers of handguns. *N Engl J Med.* 1999;341:1583-1589.

122. Kellermann AL, Rivara FP, Somes G, Reay DT, Francisco J, Banton JG, Prodzinski J, Fligner C, Hackman BB. Suicide in the home in relation to gun ownership. *N Engl J Med.* 1992;327:467-472.

123. Kellermann AL, Rivara FP, Rushforth NB, Banton JG, Reay DT, Francisco JT, Locci AB, Prodzinski J, Hackman BB, Somes G. Gun ownership as a risk factor for homicide in the home. *N Engl J Med.* 1993;329: 1084-1091.

124. Christoffel KK. Toward reducing pediatric injuries from firearms: charting a legislative and regulatory course. *Pediatrics.* 1991;88: 294-305.

125. American Academy of Pediatrics Committee on Injury and Poison Prevention. Firearm injuries affecting the pediatric population. *Pediatrics.* 1992;89:788-970.

126. Christoffel KK. Pediatric firearm injuries: time to target a growing population. *Pediatr Ann.* 1992;21:430-436.

127. Rivara FP, Grossman DC, Cummings P. Injury prevention: second of two parts. *N Engl J Med.* 1997;337:613-618.

128. Reilly JS. Prevention of aspiration in infants and young children: federal regulations. *Ann Otol Rhinol Laryngol.* 1990;99:273-276.

129. Harris CS, Baker SP, Smith GA, Harris RM. Childhood asphyxiation by food: a national analysis and overview. *JAMA.* 1984;251: 2231-2235.

130. Rimell FL, Thome A Jr, Stool S, Reilly JS, Rider G, Stool D, Wilson CL. Characteristics of objects that cause choking in children. *JAMA.* 1995;274:1763-1766.

131. Kuisma M, Alaspaa A. Out-of-hospital cardiac arrests of non-cardiac origin: epidemiology and outcome. *Eur Heart J.* 1997;18: 1122-1128.

132. Mejicano GC, Maki DG. Infections acquired during cardiopulmonary resuscitation: estimating the risk and defining strategies for prevention. *Ann Intern Med.* 1998;129: 813-828.

133. Dracup K, Moser DK, Doering LV, Guzy PM. Comparison of cardiopulmonary resuscitation training methods for parents of infants at high risk for cardiopulmonary arrest. *Ann Emerg Med.* 1998;32:170-177.

134. Emergency Cardiac Care Committee and Subcommittees, American Heart Association. Guidelines for cardiopulmonary resuscitation and emergency cardiac care, VI: pediatric advanced life support. *JAMA.* 1992;268: 2262-2275.

135. American Heart Association, International Liaison Committee on Resuscitation (ILCOR). Guidelines 2000 for cardiopulmonary resuscitation and emergency cardiovascular care: International consensus on science. *Circulation.* 2000;102(suppl I): I-1–I-384.

136. Eisenburger P, Safar P. Life supporting first aid training of the public: review and recommendations. *Resuscitation.* 1999;41:3-18.

137. Assar D, Chamberlain D, Colquhoun M, Donnelly P, Handley AJ, Leaves S, Kern KB, Mayor S. A rationale for staged teaching of basic life support. *Resuscitation.* 1998;39: 137-143.

138. Amith G. Revising educational requirements: challenging four hours for both basic life support and automated external defibrillators. *New Horiz.* 1997;5:167-172.

139. Palmisano JM, Akingbola OA, Moler FW, Custer JR. Simulated pediatric cardiopulmonary resuscitation: initial events and response times of a hospital arrest team. *Respir Care.* 1994;39:725-729.

140 Whyte SD, Wyllie JP. Paediatric basic life support: a practical assessment. *Resuscitation.* 1999;41:153-157.

141. Whyte SD, Sinha AK, Wyllie JP. Neonatal resuscitation: a practical assessment. *Resuscitation.* 1999;40:21-25.

142. Ward P, Johnson LA, Mulligan NW, Ward MC, Jones DL. Improving cardiopulmonary resuscitation skills retention: effect of two checklists designed to prompt correct performance. *Resuscitation.* 1997;34:221-225.

143. Hazinski MF. Is pediatric resuscitation unique? Relative merits of early CPR and ventilation versus early defibrillation for young victims of prehospital cardiac arrest. *Ann Emerg Med.* 1995;25:540-543.

144. Ruben HM, Elam JO, Ruben AM, Greene DG. Investigation of upper airway problems in resuscitation, I: studies of pharyngeal x-rays and performance by laymen. *Anesthesiology.* 1961;22:271-279.

145. Safar P, Escarrage LA. Compliance in apneic anesthetized adults. *Anesthesiology.* 1959;20: 283-289.

146. Elam JO, Greene DG, Schneider MA, Ruben HM, Gordon AS, Hustead RF, Benson DW, Clements JA, Ruben A. Head-tilt method of oral resuscitation. *JAMA.* 1960;172:812-815.

147. Guildner CW. Resuscitation: opening the airway: a comparative study of techniques for opening an airway obstructed by the tongue. *JACEP.* 1976;5:588-590.

148. Roth B, Magnusson J, Johansson I, Holmberg S, Westrin P. Jaw lift: a simple and effective method to open the airway in children. *Resuscitation.* 1998;39:171-174.

149. Baskett P, Nolan J, Parr M. Tidal volumes which are perceived to be adequate for resuscitation. *Resuscitation.* 1996;31:231-234.

150. Ruppert M, Reith MW, Widmann JH, Lackner CK, Kerkmann R, Schweiberer L, Peter K. Checking for breathing: evaluation of the diagnostic capability of emergency medical services personnel, physicians, medical students, and medical laypersons. *Ann Emerg Med.* 1999;34:720-729.

151. Noc M, Weil MH, Sun S, Tang W, Bisera J. Spontaneous gasping during cardiopulmonary resuscitation without mechanical ventilation. *Am J Respir Crit Care Med.* 1994;150: 861-864.

152. Poets CF, Meny RG, Chobanian MR, Bonofiglo RE. Gasping and other cardiorespiratory patterns during sudden infant deaths. *Pediatr Res.* 1999;45:350-354.

153. Handley AJ, Becker LB, Allen M, van Drenth A, Kramer EB, Montgomery WH. Single rescuer adult basic life support: an advisory statement from the Basic Life Support Working Group of the International Liaison Committee on Resuscitation (ILCOR). *Resuscitation.* 1997;34:101-108.

154. Fulstow R, Smith GB. The new recovery position: a cautionary tale. *Resuscitation.* 1993;26:89-91.

155. Doxey J. Comparing Resuscitation Council (UK) recovery position with recovery position of 1992 European Resuscitation Council guidelines: a user's perspective. *Resuscitation.* 1998;1997:39:161-169.

156. Turner S, Turner I, Chapman D, Howard P, Champion P, Hatfield J, James A, Marshall S, Barber S. A comparative study of the 1992 and 1997 recovery positions for use in the UK. *Resuscitation.* 1998;39:153-160.

157. Wenzel V, Idris AH, Banner MJ, Fuerst RS, Tucker KJ. The composition of gas given by mouth-to-mouth ventilation during CPR. *Chest.* 1994;106:1806-1810.

158. Htin KJ, Birenbaum DS, Idris AH, Banner MJ, Gravenstein N. Rescuer breathing pattern significantly affects O_2 and CO_2 received by patient during mouth-to-mouth ventilation. *Crit Care Med.* 1998;26:A56.

159. Zideman DA. Paediatric and neonatal life support. *Br J Anaesth.* 1997;79:178-187.

160. Tonkin SL, Davis SL, Gunn TR. Nasal route for infant resuscitation by mothers. *Lancet.* 1995;345:1353-1354.

161. Dembofsky CA, Gibson E, Nadkarni V, Rubin S, Greenspan JS. Assessment of infant cardiopulmonary resuscitation rescue breathing technique: relationship of infant and caregiver facial measurements. *Pediatrics.* 1999;103:E17.

162. Segedin E, Torrie J, Anderson B. Nasal airway versus oral route for infant resuscitation. *Lancet.* 1995;346:382.

163. Wilson-Davis SL, Tonkin SL, Gunn TR. Air entry in infant resuscitation: oral or nasal routes? *J Appl Physiol.* 1997;82:152-155.

164. Miller MJ, Martin RJ, Carlo WA, Fouke JM, Strohl KP, Fanaroff AA. Oral breathing in newborn infants. *J Pediatr.* 1985;107:465-469.

165. Moss ML. The veloepiglottic sphincter and obligate nose breathing in the neonate. *J Pediatr.* 1965;67:330-331.

166. Nowak AJ, Casamassimo PS. Oral opening and other selected facial dimensions of children 6 weeks to 36 months of age. *J Oral Maxillofac Surg.* 1994;52:845-847.

167. Stocks J, Godfrey S. Nasal resistance during infancy. *Respir Physiol.* 1978;34:233-246.

168. Rodenstein DO, Perlmutter N, Stanescu DC. Infants are not obligatory nasal breathers. *Am Rev Respir Dis.* 1985;131:343-347.

169. Terndrup TE, Kanter RK, Cherry RA. A comparison of infant ventilation methods performed by prehospital personnel. *Ann Emerg Med.* 1989;18:607-611.

170. Berg MD, Idris AH, Berg RA. Severe ventilatory compromise due to gastric distention during pediatric cardiopulmonary resuscitation. *Resuscitation.* 1998;36:71-73.

171. Melker RJ. Asynchronous and other alternative methods of ventilation during CPR. *Ann Emerg Med.* 1984;13:758-761.

172. Melker RJ, Banner MJ. Ventilation during CPR: two-rescuer standards reappraised. *Ann Emerg Med.* 1985;14:397-402.

173. Goldman SL, McCann EM, Lloyd BW, Yup G. Inspiratory time and pulmonary function in mechanically ventilated babies with chronic lung disease. *Pediatr Pulmonol.* 1991;11: 198-201.

174. Weiler N, Heinrichs W, Dick W. Assessment of pulmonary mechanics and gastric inflation pressure during mask ventilation. *Prehospital Disaster Med.* 1995;10:101-105.

175. Wenzel V, Idris AH, Banner MJ, Kubilis PS, Band R, Williams JL Jr, Lindner KH. Respiratory system compliance decreases after cardiopulmonary resuscitation and stomach inflation: impact of large and small tidal volumes on calculated peak airway pressure. *Resuscitation.* 1998;38:113-118.

176. Petito SP, Russell WJ. The prevention of gastric inflation: a neglected benefit of cricoid pressure. *Anaesth Intensive Care.* 1988;16: 139-143.

177. Moynihan RJ, Brock-Utne JG, Archer JH, Feld LH, Kreitzman TR. The effect of cricoid pressure on preventing gastric insufflation in infants and children. *Anesthesiology.* 1993;78: 652-656.

178. *Medical Treatment Effectiveness Research 1990.* Rockville, Md: US Agency for Health Care Policy and Research; 1990.

179. Terndrup TE, Warner DA. Infant ventilation and oxygenation by basic life support providers: comparison of methods. *Prehospital Disaster Med.* 1992;7:35-40.

180. Hess D, Ness C, Oppel A, Rhoads K. Evaluation of mouth-to-mask ventilation devices. *Respir Care.* 1989;34:191-195.

181. Mondolfi AA, Grenier BM, Thompson JE, Bachur RG. Comparison of self-inflating bags with anesthesia bags for bag-mask ventilation in the pediatric emergency department. *Pediatr Emerg Care.* 1997;13:312-316.

182. Field D, Milner AD, Hopkin IE. Efficiency of manual resuscitators at birth. *Arch Dis Child.* 1986;61:300-302.

183. Milner AD. Resuscitation at birth. *Eur J Pediatr.* 1998;157:524-527.

184. Hirschman AM, Kravath RE. Venting vs ventilating: a danger of manual resuscitation bags. *Chest.* 1982;82:369-370.

185. Finer NN, Barrington KJ, Al-Fadley F, Peters KL. Limitations of self-inflating resuscitators. *Pediatrics.* 1986;77:417-420.

186. Jesudian MC, Harrison RR, Keenan RL, Maull KI. Bag-valve-mask ventilation: two rescuers are better than one: preliminary report. *Crit Care Med.* 1985;13:122-123.

187. Salem MR, Wong AY, Mani M, Sellick BA. Efficacy of cricoid pressure in preventing gastric inflation during bag-mask ventilation in pediatric patients. *Anesthesiology.* 1974;40: 96-98.

188. Sellick BA. Cricoid pressure to control regurgitation of stomach contents during induction of anesthesia. *Lancet.* 1961;404-406.

189. Hartsilver EL, Vanner RG. Airway obstruction with cricoid pressure. *Anaesthesia.* 2000;55:208-211.

190. Shime N, Hashimoto S, Hiramatsu N, Oka T, Kageyama K, Tanaka Y. Hypoxic gas therapy using nitrogen in the preoperative management of neonates with hypoplastic left heart syndrome. *Pediatr Crit Care Med.* 2000; 1:38-41.

191. Palme C, Nystrom B, Tunell R. An evaluation of the efficiency of face masks in the resuscitation of newborn infants. *Lancet.* 1985;1: 207-210.

192. Finer NN, Bates R, Tomat P. Low flow oxygen delivery via nasal cannula to neonates. *Pediatr Pulmonol.* 1996;21:48-51.

193. Vain NE, Prudent LM, Stevens DP, Weeter MM, Maisels MJ. Regulation of oxygen concentration delivered to infants via nasal cannulas. *Am J Dis Child.* 1989;143:1458-1460.

194. Locke RG, Wolfson MR, Shaffer TH, Rubenstein SD, Greenspan JS. Inadvertent administration of positive end-distending pressure during nasal cannula flow. *Pediatrics.* 1993;91:135-138.

195. Mettey R, Masson G, Hoppeler A. Use of nasal cannula to induce positive expiratory pressure in neonatology [in French]. *Arch Fr Pediatr.* 1984;41:117-121.

196. Mather C, O'Kelly S. The palpation of pulses. *Anaesthesia.* 1996;51:189-191.

197. Cavallaro DL, Melker RJ. Comparison of two techniques for detecting cardiac activity in infants. *Crit Care Med.* 1983;11:189-190.

198. Whitelaw CC, Goldsmith LJ. Comparison of two techniques for determining the presence of a pulse in an infant. *Acad Emerg Med.* 1997;4:153-154.

199. Lee CJ, Bullock LJ. Determining the pulse for infant CPR: time for a change? *Mil Med.* 1991;156:190-193.

200. Bush CM, Jones JS, Cohle SD, Johnson H. Pediatric injuries from cardiopulmonary resuscitation. *Ann Emerg Med.* 1996;28:40-44.

201. Spevak MR, Kleinman PK, Belanger PL, Primack C, Richmond JM. Cardiopulmonary resuscitation and rib fractures in infants: a postmortem radiologic-pathologic study. *JAMA.* 1994;272:617-618.

202. Kaplan JA, Fossum RM. Patterns of facial resuscitation injury in infancy. *Am J Forensic Med Pathol.* 1994;15:187-191.

203. Feldman KW, Brewer DK. Child abuse, cardiopulmonary resuscitation, and rib fractures. *Pediatrics.* 1984;73:339-342.

204. Nagel EL, Fine EG, Krischer JP, Davis JH. Complications of CPR. *Crit Care Med.* 1981;9:424.

205. Powner DJ, Holcombe PA, Mello LA. Cardiopulmonary resuscitation-related injuries. *Crit Care Med.* 1984;12:54-55.

206. Parke TR. Unexplained pneumoperitoneum in association with basic cardiopulmonary resuscitation efforts. *Resuscitation.* 1993; 26:177-181.

207. Kramer K, Goldstein B. Retinal hemorrhages following cardiopulmonary resuscitation. *Clin Pediatr.* 1993;32:366-368.

208. Brearley S, Shearman CP, Simms MH. Peripheral pulse palpation: an unreliable physical sign. *Ann R Coll Surg Engl.* 1992;74:169-171.

209. Bahr J, Klingler H, Panzer W, Rode H, Kettler D. Skills of lay people in checking the carotid pulse. *Resuscitation.* 1997;35:23-26.

210. Ochoa FJ, Ramalle-Gomara E, Carpintero JM, Garcia A, Saralegui I. Competence of health professionals to check the carotid pulse. *Resuscitation.* 1998;37:173-175.

211. Flesche CW, Zucker TP, Lorenz C, Neruda B, Tarnow J. The carotid pulse check as a diagnostic tool to assess pulselessness during adult basic life support. *Euroanaesthesia.* 1995;95.

212. Cummins RO, Hazinski MF. Cardiopulmonary resuscitation techniques and instruction: when does evidence justify revision? *Ann Emerg Med.* 1999;34:780-784.

213. Flesche CW, Neruda B, Breuer S, Tarnow J. Basic cardiopulmonary resuscitation skills: a comparison of ambulance staff and medical students in Germany. *Resuscitation.* 1994; 28:S25.

214. Flesche CW, Neruda B, Noetges T, Tarnow J. Do cardiopulmonary skills among medical students meet current standards and patients' needs? *Resuscitation.* 1994;28:S25.

215. Monsieurs KG, De Cauwer HG, Bossaert LL. Feeling for the carotid pulse: is five seconds enough? *Resuscitation.* 1996;31:S3.

216. Flesche CW, Breuer S, Mandel LP, Breivik H, Tarnow J. The ability of health professionals to check the carotid pulse. *Circulation.* 1994;90:I-288.

217. Eberle B, Dick WF, Schneider T, Wisser G, Doetsch S, Tzanova I. Checking the carotid pulse check: diagnostic accuracy of first responders in patients with and without a pulse. *Resuscitation.* 1996;33:107-116.

218. Lundin M, Wiksten JP, Perakyla T, Lindfors O, Savolainen H, Skytta J, Lepantalo M. Distal pulse palpation: is it reliable? *World J Surg.* 1999;23:252-255.

219. Liberman M, Lavoie A, Mulder D, Sampalis J. Cardiopulmonary resuscitation: errors made by pre-hospital emergency medical personnel. *Resuscitation.* 1999;42:47-55.

220. Theophilopoulos DT, Burchfield DJ. Accuracy of different methods for heart rate determination during simulated neonatal resuscitations. *J Perinatol.* 1998;18:65-67.

221. Connick M, Berg RA. Femoral venous pulsations during open-chest cardiac massage. *Ann Emerg Med.* 1994;24:1176-1179.

222. Lubitz DS, Seidel JS, Chameides L, Luten RC, et al. A rapid method for estimating weight and resuscitation drug dosages from length in the pediatric age group. *Ann Emerg Med.* 1988;17:576-581.

223. Maier GW, Tyson GS Jr, Olsen CO, Kernstein KH, Davis JW, Conn EH, Sabiston DC Jr, Rankin JS. The physiology of external cardiac massage: high-impulse cardiopulmonary resuscitation. *Circulation.* 1984;70:86-101.

224. Kouwenhoven WB, Jude JR, Knickerbocker GG. Closed-chest cardiac massage. *JAMA.* 1960;173:1064-1067.

225. Kern KB, Hilwig R, Ewy GA. Retrograde coronary blood flow during cardiopulmonary resuscitation in swine: intracoronary Doppler evaluation. *Am Heart J.* 1994;128:490-499.

226. Tucker KJ, Khan J, Idris A, Savitt MA. The biphasic mechanism of blood flow during cardiopulmonary resuscitation: a physiologic comparison of active compression-decompression and high-impulse manual external cardiac massage. *Ann Emerg Med.* 1994;24:895-906.

227. Forney J, Ornato JP. Blood flow with ventilation alone in a child with cardiac arrest. *Ann Emerg Med.* 1980;9:624-626.

228. Berg RA, Hilwig RW, Kern KB, Babar I, Ewy GA. Simulated mouth-to-mouth ventilation and chest compressions (bystander cardiopulmonary resuscitation) improves outcome in a swine model of prehospital pediatric asphyxial cardiac arrest. *Crit Care Med.* 1999;27:1893-1899.

229. Johnson JC. Quality assurance in EMS. In: Roush WR, Aranosian RD, Blair TMH, Handal KA, Kellow RC, Steward RD, eds. *Principles of EMS Systems: A Comprehensive Text for Physicians.* Dallas, Tex: American College of Emergency Physicians; 1989.

230. Nypaver M, Treloar D. Neutral cervical spine positioning in children. *Ann Emerg Med.* 1994;23:208-211.

231. Herzenberg JE, Hensinger RN, Dedrick DK, Phillips WA. Emergency transport and positioning of young children who have an injury of the cervical spine: the standard backboard may be hazardous. *J Bone Joint Surg Am.* 1989;71:15-22.

232. Finholt DA, Kettrick RG, Wagner HR, Swedlow DB. The heart is under the lower third of the sternum: implications for external cardiac massage. *Am J Dis Child.* 1986; 140:646-649.

233. Phillips GW, Zideman DA. Relation of infant heart to sternum: its significance in cardiopulmonary resuscitation. *Lancet.* 1986;1:1024-1025.

234. Orlowski JP. Optimum position for external cardiac compression in infants and young children. *Ann Emerg Med.* 1986;15:667-673.

235. Shah NM, Gaur HK. Position of heart in relation to sternum and nipple line at various ages. *Indian Pediatr.* 1992;29:49-53.

236. Dean JM, Koehler RC, Schleien CL, Berkowitz I, Michael JR, Atchison D, Rogers MC, Traystman RJ. Age-related effects of compression rate and duration in cardiopulmonary resuscitation. *J Appl Physiol.* 1990;68:554-560.

237. Kinney SB, Tibballs J. An analysis of the efficacy of bag-valve-mask ventilation and chest compression during different compression-ventilation ratios in manikin-simulated paediatric resuscitation. *Resuscitation.* 2000;43: 115-120.

238. Burchfield D, Erenberg A, Mullett MD, Keenan WJ, Denson SE, Kattwinkel J, Bloom R. Why change the compression and ventilation rates during CPR in neonates? Neonatal Resuscitation Steering Committee, American Heart Association and American Academy of Pediatrics. *Pediatrics.* 1994;93: 1026-1027.

239. Chandra N, Rudikoff M, Weisfeldt ML. Simultaneous chest compression and ventilation at high airway pressure during cardiopulmonary resuscitation. *Lancet.* 1980;1:175-178.

240. Babbs CF, Tacker WA, Paris RL, Murphy RJ, Davis RW. CPR with simultaneous compression and ventilation at high airway pressure in 4 animal models. *Crit Care Med.* 1982;10: 501-504.

241. Hou SH, Lue HC, Chu SH. Comparison of conventional and simultaneous compression-ventilation cardiopulmonary resuscitation in piglets. *Jpn Circ J.* 1994;58:426-432.

242. Barranco F, Lesmes A, Irles JA, Blasco J, Leal J, Rodriguez J, Leon C. Cardiopulmonary resuscitation with simultaneous chest and abdominal compression: comparative study in humans. *Resuscitation.* 1990;20:67-77.

243. Wik L, Steen PA. The ventilation/compression ratio influences the effectiveness of two rescuer advanced cardiac life support on a manikin. *Resuscitation.* 1996;31:113-119.

244. Milander MM, Hiscok PS, Sanders AB, Kern KB, Berg RA, Ewy GA. Chest compression and ventilation rates during cardiopulmonary resuscitation: the effects of audible tone guidance. *Acad Emerg Med.* 1995;2:708-713.

245. Nadkarni V, Tice L, Randall D, Corddry D. Metabolic effects on rescuer of varying compression-ventilation ratios during infant, pediatric, and adult CPR. *Crit Care Med.* 1999; 27:A43.

246. Nadkarni V, Goodie B, Tice L, Cox T, Rose MJ. Evaluation of a universal compression/ventilation ratio for one-rescuer CPR in infant, pediatric, and adult manikins. *Crit Care Med.* 1997;25:A61.

247. Kern KB, Sanders AB, Raife J, Milander MM, Otto CW, Ewy GA. A study of chest compression rates during cardiopulmonary resuscitation in humans: the importance of rate-directed chest compressions. *Arch Intern Med.* 1992;152:145-149.

248. Kern KB, Hilwig RW, Berg RA, Ewy GA. Efficacy of chest compression-only BLS CPR in the presence of an occluded airway. *Resuscitation.* 1998;39:179-188.

249. Biggart MJ, Bohn DJ. Effect of hypothermia and cardiac arrest on outcome of near-drowning accidents in children. *J Pediatr.* 1990;117: 179-183.

250. Fiser DH, Wrape V. Outcome of cardiopulmonary resuscitation in children. *Pediatr Emerg Care.* 1987;3:235-238.

251. Kemp AM, Sibert JR. Outcome in children who nearly drown: a British Isles study. *BMJ.* 1991;302:931-933.

252. Ornato JP, Hallagan LF, McMahan SB, Peeples EH, Rostafinski AG. Attitudes of BCLS instructors about mouth-to-mouth resuscitation during the AIDS epidemic. *Ann Emerg Med.* 1990;19:151-156.

253. Brenner BE, Van DC, Cheng D, Lazar EJ. Determinants of reluctance to perform CPR among residents and applicants: the impact of experience on helping behavior. *Resuscitation.* 1997;35:203-211.

254. Hew P, Brenner B, Kaufman J. Reluctance of paramedics and emergency medical technicians to perform mouth-to-mouth resuscitation. *J Emerg Med.* 1997;15:279-284.

255. Locke CJ, Berg RA, Sanders AB, Davis MF, Milander MM, Kern KB, Ewy GA. Bystander cardiopulmonary resuscitation: concerns about mouth-to-mouth contact. *Arch Intern Med.* 1995;155:938-943.

256. Berg RA, Kern KB, Sanders AB, Otto CW, Hilwig RW, Ewy GA. Bystander cardiopulmonary resuscitation: is ventilation necessary? *Circulation.* 1993;88:1907-1915.

257. Berg RA, Wilcoxson D, Hilwig RW, Kern KB, Sanders AB, Otto CW, Eklund DK, Ewy GA. The need for ventilatory support during bystander CPR. *Ann Emerg Med.* 1995;26: 342-350.

258. Berg RA, Kern KB, Hilwig RW, Berg MD, Sanders AB, Otto CW, Ewy GA. Assisted ventilation does not improve outcome in a porcine model of single-rescuer bystander cardiopulmonary resuscitation. *Circulation.* 1997;95:1635-1641.

259. Berg RA, Kern KB, Hilwig RW, Ewy GA. Assisted ventilation during "bystander" CPR in a swine acute myocardial infarction model does not improve outcome. *Circulation.* 1997;96:4364-4371.

260. Chandra NC, Gruben KG, Tsitlik JE, Brower R, Guerci AD, Halperin HH, Weisfeldt ML, Permutt S. Observations of ventilation during resuscitation in a canine model. *Circulation.* 1994;90:3070-3075.

261. Tang W, Weil MH, Sun S, Kette D, Kette F, Gazmuri RJ, O'Connell F, Bisera J. Cardiopulmonary resuscitation by precordial compression but without mechanical ventilation. *Am J Respir Crit Care Med.* 1994;150: 1709-1713.

262. Noc M, Weil MH, Tang W, Turner T, Fukui M. Mechanical ventilation may not be essential for initial cardiopulmonary resuscitation. *Chest.* 1995;108:821-827.

263. Weil MH, Rackow EC, Trevino R, Grundler W, Falk JL, Griffel MI. Difference in acid-base state between venous and arterial blood during cardiopulmonary resuscitation. *N Engl J Med.* 1986;315:153-156.

264. Sanders AB, Otto CW, Kern KB, Rogers JN, Perrault P, Ewy GA. Acid-base balance in a canine model of cardiac arrest. *Ann Emerg Med.* 1988;17:667-671.

265. Lindner KH, Pfenninger EG, Lurie KG, Schurmann W, Lindner IM, Ahnefeld FW. Effects of active compression-decompression resuscitation on myocardial and cerebral blood flow in pigs. *Circulation.* 1993;88: 1254-1263.

266. Chang MW, Coffeen P, Lurie KG, Shultz J, Bache RJ, White CW. Active compression-decompression CPR improves vital organ perfusion in a dog model of ventricular fibrillation. *Chest.* 1994;106:1250-1259.

267. Shultz JJ, Coffeen P, Sweeney M, Detloff B, Kehler C, Pineda E, Yakshe P, Adler SW, Chang M, Lurie KG. Evaluation of standard and active compression-decompression CPR in an acute human model of ventricular fibrillation. *Circulation.* 1994;89:684-693.

268. Baubin M, Haid C, Hamm P, Gilly H. Measuring forces and frequency during active compression decompression cardiopulmonary resuscitation: a device for training, research and real CPR. *Resuscitation.* 1999;43:17-24.

269. Cohen TJ, Tucker KJ, Lurie KG, Redberg RF, Dutton JP, Dwyer KA, Schwab TM, Chin MC, Gelb AM, Scheinman MM, et al, Cardiopulmonary Resuscitation Working Group. Active compression-decompression: a new method of cardiopulmonary resuscitation. *JAMA.* 1992;267:2916-2923.

270. Plaisance P, Adnet F, Vicaut E, Hennequin B, Magne P, Prudhomme C, Lambert Y, Cantineau JP, Leopold C, Ferracci C, Gizzi M, Payen D. Benefit of active compression-decompression cardiopulmonary resuscitation as a prehospital advanced cardiac life support: a randomized multicenter study. *Circulation.* 1997;95:955-961.

271. Mauer D, Schneider T, Dick W, Withelm A, Elich D, Mauer M. Active compression-decompression resuscitation: a prospective, randomized study in a two-tiered EMS system with physicians in the field. *Resuscitation.* 1996;33:125-134.

272. Mauer DK, Nolan J, Plaisance P, Sitter H, Benoit H, Stiell IG, Sofianos E, Keiding N, Lurie KG. Effect of active compression-decompression resuscitation (ACD-CPR) on survival: a combined analysis using individual patient data. *Resuscitation.* 1999;41:249-256.

273. Stiell IG, Hebert PC, Wells GA, Laupacis A, Vandemheen K, Dreyer JF, Eisenhauer MA, Gibson J, Higginson LA, Kirby AS, Mahon JL, Maloney JP, Weitzman BN. The Ontario trial of active compression-decompression cardiopulmonary resuscitation for in-hospital and prehospital cardiac arrest. *JAMA*. 1996; 275:1417-1423.

274. Skogvoll E, Wik L. Active compression-decompression cardiopulmonary resuscitation: a population-based, prospective randomised clinical trial in out-of-hospital cardiac arrest. *Resuscitation*. 1999;42:163-172.

275. Babbs CF. CPR techniques that combine chest and abdominal compression and decompression: hemodynamic insights from a spreadsheet model. *Circulation*. 1999;100: 2146-2152.

276. Lurie KG. Recent advances in mechanical methods of cardiopulmonary resuscitation. *Acta Anaesthesiol Scand Suppl*. 1997;111: 49-52.

277. Tang W, Weil MH, Schock RB, Sato Y, Lucas J, Sun S, Bisera J. Phased chest and abdominal compression-decompression: a new option for cardiopulmonary resuscitation. *Circulation*. 1997;95:1335-1340.

278. Lindner KH, Wenzel V. New mechanical methods for cardiopulmonary resuscitation (CPR): literature study and analysis of effectiveness [in German]. *Anaesthesist*. 1997;46: 220-230.

279. Sack JB, Kesselbrenner MB. Hemodynamics, survival benefits, and complications of interposed abdominal compression during cardiopulmonary resuscitation. *Acad Emerg Med*. 1994;1:490-497.

280. Majumdar A, Sedman PC. Gastric rupture secondary to successful Heimlich manoeuvre. *Postgrad Med J*. 1998;74:609-610.

281. Fink JA, Klein RL. Complications of the Heimlich maneuver. *J Pediatr Surg*. 1989;24: 486-487.

282. Rosen P, Stoto M, Harley J. The use of the Heimlich maneuver in near drowning: Institute of Medicine report. *J Emerg Med*. 1995;13:397-405.

283. Heimlich HJ. A life-saving maneuver to prevent food-choking. *JAMA*. 1975;234:398-401.

284. Day RL, Crelin ES, DuBois AB. Choking: the Heimlich abdominal thrust vs back blows: an approach to measurement of inertial and aerodynamic forces. *Pediatrics*. 1982;70: 13-119.

285. National Center for Health Statistics and National Safety Council. *Data on Odds of Death Due to Choking*. 1998.

286. Braslow A, Brennan RT, Newman MM, Bircher NG, Batcheller AM, Kaye W. CPR training without an instructor: development and evaluation of a video self-instruc-tional system for effective performance of cardiopulmonary resuscitation. *Resuscitation*. 1997;34:207-220.

287. Todd KH, Braslow A, Brennan RT, Lowery DW, Cox RJ, Lipscomb LE, Kellermann AL. Randomized, controlled trial of video self-instruction versus traditional CPR training. *Ann Emerg Med*. 1998;31:364-369.

288. Todd KH, Heron SL, Thompson M, Dennis R, O'Connor J, Kellermann AL. Simple CPR: a randomized, controlled trial of video self-instructional cardiopulmonary resuscitation training in an African American church congregation. *Ann Emerg Med*. 1999;34:730-737.

289. Langhelle A, Sunde K, Wik L, Steen PA. Airway pressure with chest compressions versus Heimlich manoeuvre in recently dead adults with complete airway obstruction. *Resuscitation*. 2000;44:105-108.

290. Sternbach G, Kiskaddon RT. Henry Heimlich: a life-saving maneuver for food choking. *J Emerg Med*. 1985;3:143-148.

291. Redding JS. The choking controversy: critique of evidence on the Heimlich maneuver. *Crit Care Med*. 1979;7:475-479.

292. Gordon AS, Belton MK, Ridolpho PF. Emergency management of foreign body obstruction. In: Safar P, Elam JO, eds. *Advances in Cardiopulmonary Resuscitation*. New York, NY: Springer-Verlag, Inc; 1977: 39-50.

293. Guildner CW, Williams D, Subitch T. Airway obstructed by foreign material: the Heimlich maneuver. *JACEP*. 1976;5:675-677.

294. Bintz M, Cogbill TH. Gastric rupture after the Heimlich maneuver. *J Trauma*. 1996;40: 59-160.

295. Cowan M, Bardole J, Dlesk A. Perforated stomach following the Heimlich maneuver. *Am J Emerg Med*. 1987;5:121-122.

296. Kabbani M, Goodwin SR. Traumatic epiglottis following blind finger sweep to remove a pharyngeal foreign body. *Clin Pediatr*. 1995; 34:495-497.

297. Hartrey R, Bingham RM. Pharyngeal trauma as a result of blind finger sweeps in the choking child. *J Accid Emerg Med*. 1995; 12:52-54.

298. Dykes EH, Spence LJ, Young JG, Bohn DJ, Filler RM, Wesson DE. Preventable pediatric trauma deaths in a metropolitan region. *J Pediatr Surg*. 1989;24:107-110.

299. Esposito TJ, Sanddal ND, Dean JM, Hansen JD, Reynolds SA, Battan K. Analysis of preventable pediatric trauma deaths and inappropriate trauma care in Montana. *J Trauma*. 1999;47:243-251.

300. Suominen P, Rasanen J, Kivioja A. Efficacy of cardiopulmonary resuscitation in pulseless paediatric trauma patients. *Resuscitation*. 1998;36:9-13.

301. Koury SI, Moorer L, Stone CK, Stapczynski JS, Thomas SH. Air vs ground transport and outcome in trauma patients requiring urgent operative interventions. *Prehosp Emerg Care*. 1998;2:289-292.

302. Brathwaite CE, Rosko M, McDowell R, Gallagher J, Proenca J, Spott MA. A critical analysis of on-scene helicopter transport on survival in a statewide trauma system. *J Trauma*. 1998;45:140-144.

303. Moront ML, Gotschall CS, Eichelberger MR. Helicopter transport of injured children: system effectiveness and triage criteria. *J Pediatr Surg*. 1996;31:1183-1186.

304. Markenson D, Foltin G, Tunik M, Cooper A, Giordano L, Fitton A, Lanotte T. The Kendrick extrication device used for pediatric spinal immobilization. *Prehosp Emerg Care*. 1999; 3:66-69.

305. Curran C, Dietrich AM, Bowman MJ, Ginn-Pease ME, King DR, Kosnik E. Pediatric cervical-spine immobilization: achieving neutral position? *J Trauma*. 1995;39:729-732.

306. Huerta C, Griffith R, Joyce SM. Cervical spine stabilization in pediatric patients: evaluation of current techniques. *Ann Emerg Med*. 1987;16:1121-1126.

307. Treloar DJ, Nypaver M. Angulation of the pediatric cervical spine with and without cervical collar. *Pediatr Emerg Care*. 1997; 13:5-8.

308. Soud T, Pieper P, Hazinski MF. Pediatric trauma. In: Hazinski MF. *Nursing Care of the Critically Ill Child*. St Louis, Mo: Mosby – Year Book; 1992:842-843.

309. Doyle CJ, Post H, Burney RE, Maino J, Keefe M, Rhee KJ. Family participation during resuscitation: an option. *Ann Emerg Med*. 1987;16:673-675.

310. Hanson C, Strawser D. Family presence during cardiopulmonary resuscitation: Foote Hospital emergency department's nine-year perspective. *J Emerg Nurs*. 1992;18:104-106.

311. Barratt F, Wallis DN. Relatives in the resuscitation room: their point of view. *J Accid Emerg Med*. 1998;15:109-111.

312. Meyers TA, Eichhorn DJ, Guzzetta CE. Do families want to be present during CPR? A retrospective survey. *J Emerg Nurs*. 1998;24: 400-405.

313. Robinson SM, Mackenzie-Ross S, Campbell Hewson GL, Egleston CV, Prevost AT. Psychological effect of witnessed resuscitation on bereaved relatives. *Lancet*. 1998; 352:614-617.

314. Boie ET, Moore GP, Brummett C, Nelson DR. Do parents want to be present during invasive procedures performed on their children in the emergency department? A survey of 400 parents. *Ann Emerg Med*. 1999;34: 70-74.

315. Boyd R. Witnessed resuscitation by relatives. *Resuscitation.* 2000;43:171-176.

316. Hampe SO. Needs of the grieving spouse in a hospital setting. *Nurs Res.* 1975;24:113-120.

317. Offord RJ. Should relatives of patients with cardiac arrest be invited to be present during cardiopulmonary resuscitation? *Intensive Crit Care Nurs.* 1998;14:288-293.

318. Shaner K, Eckle N. Implementing a program to support the option of family presence during resuscitation. *Assoc Care Child Health (ACCH) Advocate.* 1997;3:3-7.

319. Eichhorn DJ, Meyers TA, Mitchell TG, Guzzetta CE. Opening the doors: family presence during resuscitation. *J Cardiovasc Nurs.* 1996;10:59-70.

320. Moser DK, Coleman S. Recommendations for improving cardiopulmonary resuscitation skills retention. *Heart Lung.* 1992;21:372-380.

321. Doherty A, Damon S, Hein K, Cummins RO. Evaluation of CPR prompt and home learning system for teaching CPR to lay rescuers. *Circulation.* 1998;98(suppl I):I-410.

322. Starr LM. Electronic voice boosts CPR responses. *Occup Health Saf.* 1997;66:30-37.

323. Cecchin F, Jorgenson DB, Berul CI, Perry JC, Zimmerman AA, Duncan BW, Lupinetti FM, Snyder D, Lyster TD, Rosenthal GL, Cross B, Atkins DL. Is arrhythmia detection by automatic external defibrillator accurate for children? Sensitivity and specificity of an automatic external defibrillator algorithm in 696 pediatric arrhythmias. *Circulation.* 2001;103:2483-2488.

324. Atkinson E, Mikysa B, Conway JA, Parker M, Christian K, Deshpande J, Knilans TK, Smith J, Walker C, Stickney RE, Hampton DR, Hazinski MF. Specificity and sensitivity of automated external defibrillator rhythm analysis in infants and children. *Ann Emerg Med.* In press.

325. Samson RA, Berg RA, Bingham R, Biarent D, Coovadia A, Hazinski MF, Hickey RW, Nadkarni V, Nichol G, Tibballs J, Reis AG, Tse S, Zideman D, Potts J, Uzark K, Atkins D. Use of automated external defibrillators for children: an update: an advisory statement from the Pediatric Advanced Life Support Task Force, International Liaison Committee on Resuscitation. *Circulation.* 2003;107:3250-3255.

326. Hazinski MF, Walker C, Smith J, Deshpande J. Specificity of automatic external defibrillator rhythm analysis in pediatric tachyarrhythmias [abstract]. *Circulation.* 1997;96(suppl I):I-561.

327. Atkins DL, Hartley LL, York DK. Accurate recognition and effective treatment of ventricular fibrillation by automated external defibrillators in adolescents. *Pediatrics.* 1998;101(pt 1):393-397.

Appendix: Safety Checklist

This Safety Checklist was designed to help you make your home or work environment as safe as possible for infants and children. It can be used to inspect your home, the childcare center where your children stay after school, or any other place where children spend time. Take time to go around your house and see just how safe your home is for a child and learn how you can make it safer.

If you already follow the suggested safety precaution, check the box in the first column. If you need to purchase a certain item to make your home safer, the box on the far right will be shaded, indicating the need to purchase a "Safety Item." Check the shaded box when you have purchased the appropriate safety items.

	I follow this safety precaution (✔ = yes)	Purchase of safety item is required for all shaded boxes (✔ = item purchased)
Car Safety		
1. Ensure that every person in the car "buckles up" correctly.		
2. Have children less than 12 years old ride in the BACK seat with appropriate child restraints or lap-shoulder restraints.		
3. Use a rear-facing infant safety seat until infants weigh at least 20 lb and are 1 year old. ■ Secure all car seats in the BACK seat of the car. ■ Secure the seat following the manufacturer's instructions. ■ Test for tightness by pushing the seat forward, backward, and side to side. Tighten the belt to ensure that the seat does not move more than ½ inch (1 cm). ■ For proper adjustment, the seat belt buckle and latch plate (if needed) must be located well below the frame or toward the center of the seat.		**Safety item — infant safety seat**
4. Wait until a child weighs 20 lb (9 kg) and is at least 1 year old and can sit with good head control before using a convertible seat or toddler seat in the forward-facing position. Place these seats in the BACK seat of the car.		**Safety item — child safety seat**
5. Use a belt-positioning booster seat for children weighing 40 to 80 lb (18 to 36 kg). Secure the seat with a 3-point seat belt (lap and shoulder belt) in the BACK seat of the car. ■ If a shield is provided, fasten it close to the child's body. ■ Properly install the tether harness if required.		**Safety item — belt-positioning booster seat**

	I follow this safety precaution (✔ = yes)	Purchase of safety item is required for all shaded boxes (✔ = item purchased)
Car Safety *(continued)*		
6. Children cannot be properly restrained with a lap-shoulder belt until they are at least 4 feet 9 inches (58 inches or 148 cm) tall, weigh 80 lb (36 kg), and can sit in the automobile seat with their knees bent over the edge. Always use a combination lap-shoulder belt to restrain children sitting in an automobile seat. ■ The shoulder belt should fit across the shoulder and breastbone. If it crosses the face and neck, use a belt-positioning booster seat to ensure that the belt is properly placed. Do not hook the shoulder belt under the child's arm. ■ All children 12 years old or younger should ride in the BACK seat.		
General Indoor Safety		
7. Place a sticker with emergency telephone numbers near or on the telephone. Include numbers for the EMS system, police, fire department, local hospital or physician, the poison control center in your area, and your telephone number.		**Safety item — phone sticker with emergency response numbers**
8. Install smoke detectors on the ceiling in the hallway outside sleeping or napping areas and on each floor at the head of stairs. Test the alarm monthly and replace batteries twice a year (for example, in the fall and spring when the time changes to and from daylight saving time).		**Safety item — smoke detector**
9. Ensure that there are 2 unobstructed emergency exits from the home, childcare center, classroom, or other facility where children are likely to be present.		
10. Develop and practice a fire escape plan.		
11. Ensure that a working fire extinguisher is on the premises.		**Safety item — fire extinguisher**
12. All space heaters are approved; in safe condition; out of a child's reach; placed at least 3 feet from curtains, papers, and furniture; and have protective covers.		
13. All wood-burning stoves are inspected yearly and vented properly. Place stoves out of a child's reach.		

	I follow this safety precaution (✔ = yes)	Purchase of safety item is required for all shaded boxes (✔ = item purchased)
General Indoor Safety *(continued)*		
14. Ensure that electric cords are not frayed or overloaded. Place out of a child's reach.		
15. Install "shock stops" (plastic outlet plugs) or outlet covers on all electric outlets.		Safety item — **plastic outlet plugs**
16. To prevent falls, always keep one hand on the infant while he or she is on a high surface such as a changing table.		
17. Position healthy full-term infants on their back or side to sleep. *Do not place infants on their stomach to sleep.*		
18. The crib is safe. ■ The crib mattress fits snugly with no more than 2 fingers' breadth between the mattress and crib railing. ■ The distance between crib slats is less than 2⅜ inches (so the infant's head won't get caught).		
19. Check the strength of stairs, railings, porches, and balconies.		
20. Light hallways and stairways to prevent falls.		
21. Use toddler gates at the top and bottom of stairs. (Do not use accordion-type gates with wide spaces at the top. They can entrap a child's head and cause strangulation.)		Safety item — **toddler gates (NOT accordion-type)**
22. Do not let your child use an infant walker.		
23. To prevent falls, place locks (available at hardware stores) on all windows. Put gates on the lower part of open windows.		Safety item — **window locks, gates**
24. Store medicines and vitamins out of a child's reach and in child-resistant containers.		Safety item — **child-resistant containers**
25. Store cleaning products out of a child's reach and sight. ■ Store and label all household poisons in their original containers in high locked cabinets (not under sinks). ■ Do not store chemicals or poisons in soda bottles. ■ Store cleaning products separately from food.		

	I follow this safety precaution (✔ = yes)	Purchase of safety item is required for all shaded boxes (✔ = item purchased)
General Indoor Safety *(continued)*		
26. Install safety latches or locks on cabinets that contain potentially **dangerous items and are within a child's reach.**		☐ **Safety item — safety latches or locks on cabinets**
27. Keep purses containing vitamins, medications, cigarettes, matches, jewelry, and calculators (which have easy-to-swallow button batteries) out of a child's reach.		
28. Install a lock or hook-and-eye latch on the door leading to the basement or garage to prevent children from entering those areas. Place a lock at the top of the door frame.		☐ **Safety item — latch on basement, garage doors**
29. Keep potentially harmful plants out of a child's reach. (Many plants are poisonous. Consult your poison control center.)		
30. Be sure that toy chests have lightweight lids, no lids, or safe-closing hinges.		
Kitchen Safety		
31. To minimize the risk of burns: ■ Keep hot liquids, foods, and cooking utensils out of a child's reach. ■ Place hot liquids and food away from the edge of the table. ■ Cook on the back burners when possible and turn pot handles toward the center of the stove. ■ Avoid using tablecloths and place mats that can be yanked off, spilling hot liquids or food. ■ Keep high chairs and stools away from the stove. ■ Do not keep snacks near the stove. ■ Teach young children the meaning of the word *hot*.		
32. Keep all foods and small items (including balloons) that can choke a child out of reach. Test toys for size with a toilet-paper roll (if it fits inside the roll, it can choke a small child).		
33. Keep knives and other sharp objects out of a child's reach.		
Bathroom Safety		
34. Bathe children in no more than 1 or 2 inches of water. Stay with infants and young children throughout the bath.		

	I follow this safety precaution (✓ = yes)	Purchase of safety item is required for all shaded boxes (✓ = item purchased)
Bathroom Safety *(continued)*		
35. Use skidproof mats or stickers in the bathtub.		▢ Safety item — bath mats or stickers
36. Adjust the maximum temperature of the water heater to 120° to 130°F (48.9° to 54.4°C) or medium heat (test with a thermometer).		
37. Keep electrical appliances (radios, hair dryers, space heaters, etc) out of the bathroom or unplugged, away from water, and out of a child's reach.		
Firearms		
38. If firearms are stored in the home, they must be locked and inaccessible to children. Store guns individually locked and unloaded, and store ammunition separately.		▢ Safety item — trigger lock, lock-boxes for firearms
Outdoor Safety		
39. Playground equipment is assembled and anchored correctly according to manufacturer's instructions over a level, cushioned surface such as sand or wood chips.		
40. Your child knows the rules of safe bicycling. ▪ Wear a protective helmet. ▪ Use the correct size bicycle. ▪ Ride on the right side of the road (*with* traffic). ▪ Use hand signals and wear bright or reflective clothing.		▢ Safety item — bicycle helmet
41. Do not allow children to play with fireworks.		
42. Your child is properly protected while roller skating or skateboarding. ▪ Child wears helmet and protective padding on knees and elbows. ▪ Child skates only in rinks or parks that are free of traffic.		▢ Safety item — helmet and protective padding
43. Your child is properly protected while riding on sleds or snow disks. ▪ Child sleds only in daylight and only in a safe, supervised area away from motor vehicles.		
44. Your child is properly protected while participating in contact sports. ▪ Proper adult instruction and supervision are provided. ▪ Teammates are of similar weight and size. ▪ Appropriate safety equipment is used.		▢ Safety item — safety equipment for contact sports

	I follow this safety precaution (✔ = yes)	Purchase of safety item is required for all shaded boxes (✔ = item purchased)
Outdoor Safety *(continued)*		
45. To reduce the risk of animal bites: ■ Teach your child how to handle and care for a pet. ■ Teach your child never to try to separate fighting animals, even when a familiar pet is involved. ■ Teach your child to avoid unfamiliar animals.		
46. If you have a home swimming pool, be sure the pool is totally enclosed with fencing at least 5 feet high and that all gates are self-closing and self-latching. There should be no direct access (without a locked gate) from the home into the pool area. In addition ■ Children must *always* be supervised by an adult when swimming. Never allow a child to swim alone. ■ Change young children from swimsuits into street clothes and remove all toys from the pool area at the end of swim time. ■ All adults and older children should learn CPR. ■ Pools on nearby properties should be protected from use by unsupervised children.		**Safety item — 5-foot fence around swimming pool with self-closing, self-latching gate**

Note: Much of the safety information presented in this course is based on the SAFEHOME program developed by the Massachusetts Department of Public Health as part of its Statewide Comprehensive Injury Prevention Program and the Children's Traffic Safety Program at Vanderbilt University in Nashville, Tenn. The SAFEHOME program was funded by the Federal Division of Maternal and Child Health. The Children's Traffic Safety Program was funded by the Department of Transportation and the Tennessee Governor's Highway Safety Program.

You are at the health club, and you hear a commotion in the weight room. You quickly respond and find a 52-year-old man who has collapsed while exercising. You note that he is unresponsive and send a worker to phone 911. You open the man's airway and discover that he is not breathing. You have no barrier device. Will you perform mouth-to-mouth breathing on this stranger? If not, what are your options?

Safety During CPR Training and Actual Rescue

Overview

Safety during CPR training and in actual rescue situations has gained increased attention in the years since the outbreak of the HIV epidemic. The general public may have concerns or misinformation about the possibility of disease transmission. The following recommendations should minimize the possible risk of infection to instructors and students during CPR training and actual performance of CPR. Recommendations for manikin decontamination and rescuer safety were originally established in 1978 by the Centers for Disease Control (CDC)[1] and updated twice by the AHA, the American Red Cross, and the CDC.[2,3]

Disease Transmission During CPR Training

The risk of disease transmission during CPR training is extremely low. *The use of manikins during CPR training has never been shown to be responsible for an outbreak of infection, and a literature search through March 2000 revealed no reports of infection associated with CPR training.*[3,4] The 1980s, however, saw a dramatic increase in inquiries about the possible role of CPR training manikins in transmitting infectious diseases such as HIV, hepatitis B virus (HBV), herpes viruses, and various upper and lower respiratory infections such as influenza, infectious mononucleosis, and tuberculosis. *To date, an estimated 70 million people in the United States have had direct*

Learning Objectives

At the end of this chapter you will be able to

1. Discuss the risk of disease transmission during perform-ance of CPR

2. List methods for reducing the chances of disease transmission during performance of CPR

3. Discuss the risk of disease transmission during manikin practice

4. List methods for reducing the chances of disease transmis-sion during manikin practice

5. Discuss the benefits of using face shields versus face masks during CPR

6. List the procedures for isolation of body substances during positive-pressure ventilations

---

contact with manikins in CPR training courses with no reported infectious complications.[4]

Under certain circumstances infectious agents can live on manikin surfaces, pre-senting the possibility of disease trans-mission. Therefore, manikin surfaces should be cleaned and disinfected in a consistent manner after each use and after each class.[5]

Two important practices are needed to minimize risk of transmission of infec-tious agents during CPR training. First, rescuers should avoid any contact with saliva or body fluids that may be present on manikins. A rescuer's hands and oral mucosa can become contaminated if he or she touches a manikin that has not been properly cleaned between uses. This type of contamination can occur in any of several ways: if a student touches a manikin around the mouth before the manikin is properly cleaned, if students practice mouth-to-mouth ventilation on a manikin that has not been properly cleaned, or if rescuers place their fingers inside the mouth of the manikin during practice sessions (eg, to demonstrate a finger sweep). Most contamination can be prevented with adequate cleansing of the manikin between each use in a prac-tice session.

During mouth-to-mouth ventilation prac-tice, however, students often forget that the inside of the manikin's mouth is con-taminated by saliva unless it is cleaned or replaced after every use. If students touch the inside of the manikin's mouth, they should wash their hands thoroughly before continuing practice. Otherwise, bacteria can be transmitted from the hands of those students to other students or to their own oral, nasal, or ocular mucosa.

Second, the internal parts of the manikin, such as valve mechanisms and artificial lungs, invariably become contaminated during practice and must be thoroughly cleaned between each use. If these parts are not dismantled and cleaned or replaced after class, they may become sources of contamination for subsequent classes. There is no evidence, however, that manikin valve mechanisms produce aerosols even when air is forcibly expelled during chest compression.

Because of the wide variety of manikins that are commercially available, it is impossible to detail here the cleaning required for each model and type of manikin. Instructors and training agencies should carefully follow the manufacturers' recommendations for use and maintenance of manikins.[5-7]

The resistance levels of micro-organisms such as HIV, HBV, and *herpesvirus* have not been fully characterized. Several intermediate-level disinfectants, however, can be used to kill these micro-organisms on manikins. Solutions containing iodine are *not* recommended for cleansing because the solutions may stain or otherwise damage plastic materials. Solutions containing formaldehyde or glutaraldehyde also are not recommended because they leave an undesirable residue and odors.[8]

To date there is no evidence that HIV can be transmitted by casual personal contact, indirect contact with inanimate surfaces, or via an airborne route.[4] It is also clear that HBV and HIV are more susceptible to disinfectant chemicals than previously thought.[9] HIV, the primary retroviral agent that causes AIDS, is comparatively fragile and is inactivated in less than 10 minutes at room temperature by a number of disinfectants, including agents recommended for manikin cleaning.[10-13]

If current recommendations published by the AHA and manikin manufacturers for manikin cleaning and decontamination are followed carefully, risk of transmission of HIV and HBV, as well as risk of bacterial and fungal infections, should be minimized. The guidelines are discussed in detail in the *Instructor's Manual for Basic Life Support*.

The risk of transmission of any infectious disease during manikin practice appears to be low. Although millions of people worldwide have used training manikins in the past 30 years, no documented cases of transmission of bacterial, fungal, or viral disease by a CPR training manikin were included in a recent review article[4] or a literature search through March 2000. In the absence of evidence of infectious disease transmission, the lifesaving potential of CPR should be vigorously emphasized and broad-scale CPR training continued.

Disease Transmission During Actual Performance of CPR

Healthcare workers and public safety personnel must often perform ventilations on persons they do not know. By comparison, a layperson is far less likely to perform CPR than a healthcare provider during any given day or week. If the layperson does perform CPR, it will most likely be in the home, where 70% to 80% of respiratory and cardiac arrests occur[2] and the victim is known to the rescuer.

The actual risk of disease transmission during mouth-to-mouth ventilation is quite small. Only 15 reports of CPR-related infection were published between 1960 and 1998,[4] and no reports have been published in scientific journals from 1998 through March 2000.[4,14] At last report (1998)[4] the cases of disease transmission during CPR included *Helicobacter pylori*,[15] *Mycobacterium tuberculosis*,[16] meningococcus,[17] herpes simplex,[18-20] *Shigella*,[21] *Streptococcus*,[22] *Salmonella*,[23] and *Neisseria gonorrhoeae*.[4] No reports on transmission of HIV, hepatitis B virus (HBV), hepatitis C virus, or cytomegalovirus were found.[4] Nevertheless, despite the remote chances of its occurring, fears about disease transmission are common in this era of universal precautions.

Laypersons, physicians, nurses, and even BLS instructors may be reluctant to perform mouth-to-mouth ventilation.[24-30] The most commonly stated reason for not performing mouth-to-mouth ventilation is fear of contracting AIDS. In one survey only 5% of 975 respondents reported a willingness to perform chest compression with mouth-to-mouth ventilation on a stranger, whereas 68% would "definitely" perform chest compression alone if it was offered as an effective alternative CPR technique.[19] The attitude of rescuers who have chosen to perform mouth-to-mouth ventilation is much different regarding fear of infectious disease. Of bystanders who performed CPR in one study, 92% stated that they had no fear of infectious disease.[31] Of 425 interviewed rescuers from the same group, 99.5% indicated that if called on they would perform CPR again.[31] Researchers have found that there is little reluctance by lay rescuers to perform CPR on family members, even in the presence of vomitus or alcohol on the breath.[32]

The rescuer who responds to an emergency for an unknown victim should be guided by his or her moral and ethical values and knowledge of risks that may exist in various rescue situations. The rescuer should assume that any emergency situation involving exposure to certain body fluids has the potential for disease transmission for both the rescuer and victim. If the rescuer is unwilling or unable to perform mouth-to-mouth breathing, chest compressions alone should be attempted because they may increase the chances for survival. This is particularly true if the victim is exhibiting gasping breaths or if the time to defibrillation is likely to be short.[33-37]

The greatest concern over the risk of disease transmission should be directed to persons who perform CPR frequently, particularly healthcare providers, both in and out of hospital. Providers of out-of-hospital emergency health care include paramedics, emergency medical technicians, law enforcement personnel, firefighters, lifeguards, and others whose jobs require them to provide first-response medical care, including CPR. If appropriate precautions are taken to prevent exposure to blood or other body fluids, the risk of disease transmission from infected persons to providers of out-of-hospital emergency health care should be no higher than that for those providing emergency care in hospital.

The probability that any rescuer, lay or professional, will become infected with HBV or HIV as a result of performing CPR is minimal.[38] Transmission of HBV and HIV between healthcare workers and patients as a result of blood exchange or penetration of the skin by blood-contaminated instruments has been documented[39]; however, transmission of HBV and HIV infection during mouth-to-mouth resuscitation has not been documented.[4,40] There is experimental evidence that some face masks are impermeable to the HIV-1 virus.[41]

Direct mouth-to-mouth breathing will likely result in the exchange of saliva between victim and rescuer. HBV-positive saliva, however, has not been shown to be infectious, even to oral mucous membranes, through contamination of shared musical instruments or through HBV carriers.[38] In addition, saliva has not been implicated in the transmission of HIV after bites, percutaneous inoculation, or contamination of cuts and open wounds with saliva from HIV-infected patients.[42,43] The theoretical risk of infection is greater for salivary or aerosol transmission of herpes simplex, *Neisseria meningitidis,* and airborne diseases such as tuberculosis and other respiratory infections. Rare instances of transmission of herpes during CPR have been reported.[20]

The emergence of multidrug-resistant tuberculosis[44,45] and the risk of transmission of tuberculosis to emergency workers[46] are cause for concern. Rescuers with impaired immune systems may be particularly at risk. In most instances transmission of tuberculosis requires prolonged close exposure such as that which occurs in households, but transmission to emergency workers can occur during resuscitative efforts by either the airborne route[46] or direct contact. The magnitude of risk is unknown but probably low. If

a caregiver performs mouth-to-mouth resuscitation on a person suspected of having tuberculosis, the caregiver should be evaluated for tuberculosis using standard approaches based on the caregiver's baseline skin test results.[47] Caregivers with negative baseline skin test results should be retested 12 weeks later. Preventive therapy should be considered for all persons with positive test results and should be given to all converters.[47,48] The optimal preventive therapeutic agent has not been established for areas where multidrug-resistant tuberculosis is common or following exposure to known multidrug-resistant tuberculosis. Some authorities suggest using 2 or more agents.[49]

Performance of mouth-to-mouth resuscitation or invasive procedures can result in the exchange of blood between victim and rescuer. This is especially true in trauma cases or if either victim or rescuer has breaks in the skin on or around the lips or soft tissues of the oral mucosa. Thus, a theoretical risk of HBV and HIV transmission during mouth-to-mouth resuscitation exists, but disease transmission has not been documented.[4,50]

Barrier Devices: Face Masks and Face Shields

To absolutely minimize the risk of disease transmission between victim and rescuer, rescuers with a duty to provide CPR should follow the precautions and guidelines established by the Centers for Disease Control and Prevention[38] and the Occupational Safety and Health Administration. These precautions include the use of barriers such as latex gloves and manual ventilation equipment such as a bag-mask system with valves capable of diverting the victim's expired air away from the rescuer. Rescuers who have an infection that may be transmitted by blood or saliva should not perform mouth-to-mouth resuscitation if circumstances allow other immediate and effective methods of ventilation.

The perceived risk of disease transmission during CPR has reduced the willingness of some laypersons to initiate mouth-to-mouth ventilation for unknown victims of cardiac arrest. Public education is vital to alleviate this fear. In addition, if such a concern is identified, rescuers should be encouraged to learn mouth-to–barrier device (face mask or face shield) ventilation.

A lone rescuer who is unwilling or unable to initiate mouth-to-mouth ventilation should at least access the EMS system, open the airway, and perform chest compressions until the arrival of a rescuer who is willing to provide ventilation or until ventilation can be initiated by skilled rescuers (arriving BLS ambulance providers or paramedics) with the necessary barrier devices.

Several studies confirm that there is a risk of transmission of pathogens (disease-causing organisms) during exposure to blood, saliva, and other body fluids. [8,18-21,23,51,52] OSHA supports this observation. Several devices have been developed to minimize the risk of rescuers being exposed to pathogens. BLS course participants should be taught to use a barrier device (face shield or face mask) when a mouth-to-mask device is unavailable and mouth-to-mouth ventilation would place the rescuer at risk. The face mask may be a more effective barrier to oral bacteria than the face shield. In fact, all face masks with a 1-way valve prevent the transmission of bacteria to the rescuer side of the mask. Conversely, the rescuer side of face shields became contaminated in 6 of 8 tests.[53]

Because the efficacy of face shields has not been proved, during CPR training those with a duty to respond should learn how to use masks with 1-way valves and other manual ventilation devices.[15,16] Masks without a 1-way valve and inline filters (including those with S-shaped devices) offer little if any protection and should not be considered for routine use.[15,16] Intubation with tracheal tubes and other airway adjuncts obviates the need for mouth-to-mouth resuscitation and enables ventilation that equals or is more effective than that provided by the use of masks alone.[54-59] Early intubation is encouraged when equipment and trained professionals are available. Resuscitation equipment that is contaminated by blood or other body fluids should be discarded or thoroughly cleaned and disinfected after each use.[60]

Summary

The risk of disease transmission during training and performance of CPR in an actual rescue is minimal. During training and resuscitations, however, healthcare providers have a responsibility to follow the first principle of medical care: "do no harm." The simple practice of infection control during CPR training and the isolation of body substances during performance of CPR will help prevent transmission of disease and facilitate the well-being of both victim and rescuer in the case of sudden cardiac death.

Summary of Key Concepts

Take time to review the key concepts covered in this chapter:

- The chance of disease transmission is very low during training and in actual rescues.

- Manikins should be cleaned and disinfected after each use according to the manufacturer's specifications and AHA recommendations.

- Students should never place their fingers in the mouth of a manikin during practice sessions unless the mouth is cleaned or replaced between uses.

- If rescuers are unwilling to perform mouth-to-mouth rescue breathing on a cardiac arrest victim, compressions alone may help save the victim's life.

- When possible, a barrier device should be used to perform rescue breathing.

- In a study of rescuers who performed mouth-to-mouth rescue breathing in actual cardiac arrests, 99.5% indicated that they would do it again if needed.

- Mouth-to-mask breathing is more effective than bag-mask breathing in delivering adequate tidal volumes.

Review Questions

1. A 43-year-old man has collapsed on a bus. You perform mouth-to-mouth breathing and cardiac compressions. Afterward a relative of the man tells you that the victim is HIV positive. Which of the following best describes your chance of contracting AIDS from this contact?

   a. very high

   b. high

   c. moderate

   d. very low

2. You are a dispatcher. You receive a call from the scene of a cardiac arrest. You try to give phone-assisted instructions in CPR, but the caller refuses to perform mouth-to-mouth breathing for fear of contracting an infectious disease. What is the next best action that you can take at this time?

   a. convince the caller to overcome his or her fear

   b. direct the caller to open the airway and then perform chest compressions only

   c. tell the caller to search for a neighbor who is willing to perform mouth-to-mouth breathing

   d. advise the caller that he or she has a legal responsibility to act

3. You and a friend are practicing CPR on a manikin. You note that your friend performs a finger sweep deep into the manikin's airway immediately after you have practiced mouth-to-mouth ventilation on the same manikin. What advice should you give her?

   a. tell her to wash her hands before continuing practice

   b. don't worry; this does not present a risk of disease transmission

   c. don't worry; this is a routine activity during CPR training

   d. tell her she should soak her hand in bleach for 10 minutes

4. You are an EMT responding to a cardiac arrest call. The best way to prevent any risk of contracting an infection during rescue breathing is to

   a. perform compressions-only CPR

   b. use a barrier device or bag mask

   c. place a cloth between you and the victim

   d. use the mouth-to-nose breathing technique

How did you do?

Answers: **1,** d; **2,** b; **3,** a; **4,** b.

References

1. *Centers for Disease Control. Recommendations for Decontaminating Manikins Used in Cardiopulmonary Resuscitation: Hepatitis Surveillance, Report 42.* Atlanta, Ga: Centers for Disease Control; 1978:34-36.

2. AHA Emergency Cardiac Care Committee and Subcommittees. Guidelines for cardiopulmonary resuscitation and emergency cardiac care. *JAMA.* 1992;268:2171-2295.

3. Risk of infection during CPR training and rescue: supplemental guidelines. The Emergency Cardiac Care Committee of the American Heart Association. *JAMA.* 1989;262:2714-2715.

4. Mejicano GC, Maki DG. Infections acquired during cardiopulmonary resuscitation: estimating the risk and defining strategies for prevention. *Ann Intern Med.* 1998;129:813-828.

5. Stern A, Dickinson E. Don't be a dummy: staying safe with mannequin training. *J Emerg Med Serv.* 1994;19:85-86.

6. Corless IB, Lisker A, Buckheit RW. Decontamination of an HIV-contaminated CPR manikin. *Am J Public Health.* 1992;82:1542-1543.

7. Q & A: disinfecting Resusci Annes. *Healthcare Hazardous Materials Management.* 1992;5:11.

8. Bond WW, Favero MS, Petersen NJ, Ebert JW. Inactivation of hepatitis B virus by intermediate-to-high-level disinfectant chemicals. *J Clin Microbiol.* 1983;18:535-538.

9. Favero MS, Bond WW. Sterilization, disinfection and antisepsis in the hospital. In: Balows A, Hausler WJ Jr, Hermann KL, Eisenberg HD, Shadomy HJ, eds. *Manual of Clinical Microbiology.* 5th ed. Washington, DC: American Society for Microbiology; 1991: 183-200.

10. Resnick L, Veren K, Salahuddin SZ, Tondreau S, Markham PD. Stability and inactivation of HTLV-III/LAV under clinical and laboratory environments. *JAMA.* 1986;255:1887-1891.

11. Martin LS, McDougal JS, Loskoski SL. Disinfection and inactivation of the human T lymphotropic virus type III/ lymphadenopathy-associated virus. *J Infect Dis.* 1985; 152:400-403.

12. McDougal JS, Cort SP, Kennedy MS, Cabridilla CD, Feorino PM, Francis DP, Hicks D, Kalyanaraman VS, Martin LS. Immunoassay for the detection and quantitation of infectious human retrovirus, lymphadenopathy-associated virus (LAV). *J Immunol Methods.* 1985;76:171-183.

13. Spire B, Dormont D, Barre-Sinoussi F, Montagnier L, Chermann JC. Inactivation of lymphadenopathy-associated virus by heat, gamma rays, and ultraviolet light. *Lancet.* 1985;1:188-189.

14. Sun D, Bennett RB, Archibald DW. Risk of acquiring AIDS from salivary exchange through cardiopulmonary resuscitation courses and mouth-to-mouth resuscitation. *Semin Dermatol.* 1995;14:205-211.

15. Simmons M, Deao D, Moon L, Peters K, Cavanaugh S. Bench evaluation: three face-shield CPR barrier devices. *Respir Care.* 1995;40:618-623.

16. Pulmonary resuscitators. *Health Devices.* 1989;18:333-352.

17. Feldman HA. Some recollections of the meningococcal disease: the first Harry F. Dowling lecture. *JAMA.* 1972;220:1107-1112.

18. Finkelhor RS, Lampman JH. Herpes simplex infection following cardiopulmonary resuscitation. *JAMA.* 1980;243:650.

19. Mannis MJ, Wendel RT. Transmission of herpes simplex during cardiopulmonary resuscitation training. *Compr Ther.* 1984;10:15-17.

20. Hendricks AA, Shapiro EP. Primary herpes simplex infection following mouth-to-mouth resuscitation. *JAMA.* 1980;243:257-258.

21. Todd MA, Bell JS. Shigellosis from cardiopulmonary resuscitation. *JAMA.*1980;243:331.

22. Valenzuela TD, Hooten TM, Kaplan EL, Schlievert P. Transmission of 'toxic strep' syndrome from an infected child to a firefighter during CPR. *Ann Emerg Med.* 1991;20:90-92.

23. Ahmad F, Senadhira DC, Charters J, Acquilla S. Transmission of salmonella via mouth-to-mouth resuscitation. *Lancet.* 1990;335:787-788.

24. Ornato JP, Hallagan LF, McMahan SB, Peeples EH, Rostafinski AG. Attitudes of BCLS instructors about mouth-to-mouth resuscitation during the AIDS epidemic. *Ann Emerg Med.* 1990;19:151-156.

25. Brenner BE, Kauffman J. Reluctance of internists and medical nurses to perform mouth-to-mouth resuscitation. *Arch Intern Med.* 1993;153:1763-1769.

26. Locke CJ, Berg RA, Sanders AB, Davis MF, Milander MM, Kern KB, Ewy GA. Bystander cardiopulmonary resuscitation: concerns about mouth-to-mouth. *Arch Intern Med.* 1995;155: 938-943.

27. Brenner B, Stark B, Kauffman J. The reluctance of house staff to perform mouth-to-mouth resuscitation in the inpatient setting: what are the considerations? *Resuscitation.* 1994;28:185-193.

28. Brenner B, Kauffman J, Sachter JJ. Comparison of the reluctance of house staff of metropolitan and suburban hospitals to perform mouth-to-mouth resuscitation. *Resuscitation.* 1996;32:5-12.

29. Michael AD, Forrester JS. Mouth-to-mouth ventilation: the dying art. *Am J Emerg Med.* 1992;10:156-161.

30. Bierens JJ, Berden HJ. Basic-CPR and AIDS: are volunteer life-savers prepared for a storm? *Resuscitation.* 1996;32:185-191.

31. Axelsson A, Herlitz J, Ekstrom L, Holmberg S. Bystander-initiated cardiopulmonary resuscitation out-of-hospital: a first description of the bystanders and their experiences. *Resuscitation.* 1996;33:3-11.

32. McCormack AP, Damon SK, Eisenberg MS. Disagreeable physical characteristics affecting bystander CPR. *Ann Emerg Med.* 1989;18: 283-285.

33. Berg RA, Kern KB, Sanders AB, Otto CW, Hilwig RW, Ewy GA. Bystander cardiopulmonary resuscitation: is ventilation necessary? *Circulation.* 1993;88(4 Pt 1):1907-1915.

34. Chandra NC, Gruben KG, Tsitlik JE, Brower R, Guerci AD, Halperin HH, Weisfeldt ML, Permutt S. Observations of ventilation during resuscitation in a canine model. *Circulation.* 1994;90:3070-3075.

35. Tang W, Weil MH, Sun S, Kette D, Kette F, Gazmuri RJ, O'Connell F, Bisera J. Cardiopulmonary resuscitation by precordial compression but without mechanical ventilation. *Am J Respir Crit Care Med.* 1994;150:1709-1713.

36. Noc M, Weil MH, Tang W, Turner T, Fukui M. Mechanical ventilation may not be essential for initial cardiopulmonary resuscitation. *Chest.* 1995;108:821-827.

37. Becker LB, Berg RA, Pepe PE, Idris AH, Aufderheide TP, Barnes TA, Stratton SJ, Chandra NC. A reappraisal of mouth-to-mouth ventilation during bystander-initiated cardiopulmonary resuscitation: a statement from healthcare professionals from the Ventilation Working Group of the Basic Life Support and Pediatric Life Support Subcommittees, American Heart Association. *Resuscitation.* 1997;35:189-201.

38. Centers for Disease Control and National Institute for Occupational Health and Safety. Guidelines for prevention of transmission of human immunodeficiency virus and hepatitis B virus to health-care and public-safety workers: a response to P. L. 100-607 The Health Omnibus Programs Extension Act of 1988. *MMWR Suppl.* 1989;38:3-37.

39. Marcus R. Surveillance of health care workers exposed to blood from patients infected with the human immunodeficiency virus. *N Engl J Med.* 1988;319:1118-1123.

40. Sande MA. Transmission of AIDS: the case against casual contagion. *N Engl J Med.* 1986; 314:380-382.

41. Lightsey DM, Shah PK, Forrester JS, Micheal TA. A human immunodeficiency virus-resistant airway for cardiopulmonary resuscitation. *Am J Emerg Med.* 1992;10:73-77.

42. Friedland GH, Saltzman BR, Rogers MF, Kahl PA, Lesser ML, Mayers MM, Klein RS. Lack of transmission of HTLV-III/LAV infection to household contacts of patients with AIDS or AIDS-related complex with oral candidiasis. *N Engl J Med.* 1986;314:344-349.

43. Fox PC, Wolff A, Yeh CK, Atkinson JC, Baum BJ. Saliva inhibits HIV-1 infectivity. *J Am Dent Assoc.* 1988;116:635-637.

44. Centers for Disease Control. Outbreak of multidrug-resistant tuberculosis: Texas, California, and Pennsylvania. *MMWR.* 1990;39:369-372.

45. Centers for Disease Control. Epidemiologic notes and reports: nosocomial transmission of multidrug-resistant tuberculosis among HIV-infected persons: Florida and New York, 1988-1991. *MMWR.* 1991;40:585-591.

46. Haley CE, McDonald RC, Rossi L, Jones WD Jr, Haley RW, Luby JP. Tuberculosis epidemic among hospital personnel. *Infect Control Hosp Epidemiol.* 1989;10:204-210.

47. Dooley SW Jr, Castro KG, Hutton MD, Mullan RJ, Polder JA, Snider DE Jr. Guidelines for preventing the transmission of tuberculosis in healthcare settings, with special focus on HIV-related issues. *MMWR.* 1990;39:1-29.

48. Centers for Disease Control. The use of preventive therapy for tuberculosis infection in the United States: recommendations of the Advisory Committee for Elimination of Tuberculosis. *MMWR Recommendations and Reports.* 1990;39:9-12.

49. Steinberg JL, Nardell EA, Kass EH. Antibiotic prophylaxis after exposure to antibiotic-resistant Mycobacterium tuberculosis. *Rev Infect Dis.* 1988;10:1208-1219.

50. Piazza M, Chirianni A, Picciotto L, Guadagnino V, Orlando R, Cataldo PT. Passionate kissing and microlesions of the oral mucosa: possible role in AIDS transmission. *JAMA.* 1989;261:244-245.

51. Heilman KM, Muschenheim C. Primary cutaneous tuberculosis resulting from mouth-to-mouth respiration. *N Engl J Med.* 1965;273:1035-1036.

52. Occupational Safety and Health Administration of Labor. Occupational exposure to bloodborne pathogens-final rule. *Fed Regist.* 1991;56:64004-64182.

53. Cydulka RK, Connor PJ, Myers TF, Pavza G, Parker M. Prevention of oral bacterial flora transmission by using mouth-to-mask ventilation during CPR. *J Emerg Med.* 1991;9:317-321.

54. Rumball CJ, MacDonald D. The PTL, Combitube, laryngeal mask, and oral airway: a randomized prehospital comparative study of ventilatory device effectiveness and cost effectiveness in 470 cases of cardiopulmonary arrest. *Prehosp Emerg Care.* 1997;1:1-10.

55. Staudinger T, Brugger S, Watschinger B, Roggla M, Dielacher C, Lobl T, Fink D, Klauser R, Frass M. Emergency intubation with the Combitube: comparison with the endotracheal airway. *Ann Emerg Med.* 1993;22:1573-1575.

56. Staudinger T, Brugger S, Roggla M, Rintelen C, Atherton GL, Johnson JC, Frass M. [Comparison of the Combitube with the endotracheal tube in cardiopulmonary resuscitation in the prehospital phase]. *Wien Klin Wochenschr.* 1994;106:412-415.

57. Atherton GL, Johnson JC. Ability of paramedics to use the Combitube in prehospital cardiac arrest. *Ann Emerg Med.* 1993;22:1263-1268.

58. Bartlett RL, Martin SD, McMahon JM Jr, Schafermeyer RW, Vukich DJ, Hornung CA. A field comparison of the pharyngeotracheal lumen airway and the endotracheal tube. *J Trauma.* 1992;32:280-284.

59. Frass M, Frenzer R, Rauscha F, Schuster E, Glogar D. Ventilation with the esophageal tracheal combitube in cardiopulmonary resuscitation: promptness and effectiveness. *Chest.* 1988;93:781-784.

60. Recommendation for prevention of HIV transmission in health-care settings. *MMWR Suppl.* 1987;36:1S-18S.

You are an emergency medical technician-basic (EMT-B) responding to a call about a nearby near-drowning. You arrive at the lake and find a young man swimming weakly and struggling to stay afloat in the water 50 yards from shore. You and your partner launch a dinghy into the water and quickly row out to the victim. Before you reach him the swimmer suddenly sinks below the surface. You manage to find him and pull him safely into the boat.

The victim is unresponsive. You open his airway and note that he is taking agonal breaths. You provide 2 slow breaths with a mouth-to-mask device and check for signs of circulation. He has no pulse or other signs of circulation. You start compressions while your partner dries the man's chest and attaches the AED. The AED indicates "no shock advised," but the victim still has no signs of circulation. You continue CPR while your partner rows the boat to shore.

Just as you arrive at the shore, the victim begins to move and cough and you note a carotid pulse. The young man becomes responsive during transport to the hospital. You think "Just in time! He's going to be all right."

Special Resuscitation Situations

Overview

Special situations that can lead to cardio-pulmonary arrest may require changes in the sequence or specific aspects of resuscitation. This chapter reviews several of these special resuscitation situations, including hypothermia, submersion (near-drowning), trauma, electric shock and lightning strike, and pregnancy. As healthcare providers you should note the differences in triage, emphasis, and technique and be prepared to modify your approach to resuscitation accordingly.

Hypothermia

Severe hypothermia (body temperature below 30°C [86°F]) is associated with marked depression of cerebral blood flow and oxygen requirement, reduced cardiac output, and decreased arterial pressure.[1,2] Victims may appear to be clinically dead because of marked depression of brain function.[2-4] Full resuscitation with intact neurologic recovery may be possible, but it is unusual.[5-10]

Hypothermia may make the assessment of the victim's breathing and circulation difficult, but do not withhold lifesaving procedures on the basis of clinical presentation.[2] Transport victims as soon as possible to a center where monitored rewarming is possible.

Severe accidental hypothermia is a serious and preventable health problem. Hypothermia in inner-city areas has a high

Learning Objectives

After reading this chapter you should be able to

1. Discuss the potential effect of hypothermia on a rescuer's ability to palpate a pulse and the implications this information has on pulse check for these victims

2. Describe BLS management of a cardiac arrest victim who is hypothermic

3. Explain safety considerations associated with the rescue of a near-drowning victim

4. Describe BLS management of a near-drowning victim who is in cardiac arrest

5. Describe BLS management of a trauma victim who is in cardiac arrest

6. Explain safety considerations associated with a rescue of a victim of electric shock

7. Describe BLS management of a cardiac arrest associated with electric shock or lightning strike

8. Describe BLS management of a pregnant victim in cardiac arrest

9. Describe special considerations for managing a victim of cardiac arrest

10. Describe special considerations for managing a cardiac arrest associated with asphyxia

association with mental illness, poverty, and drug and alcohol use.[11] In some rural areas more than 90% of hypothermic deaths are associated with elevated blood alcohol levels.[12] Successful treatment of hypothermia requires optimal training of emergency personnel and appropriate resuscitation methods at each institution.

Basic Life Support

When the victim is cold, respiratory rate and pulse will be slow, breathing will be shallow, and peripheral vasoconstriction will make pulses difficult to feel. For these reasons assess breathing and, later, the pulse for a period of 30 to 45 seconds to confirm respiratory arrest, pulseless cardiac arrest, or bradycardia profound enough to require chest compressions. If the victim is not breathing, initiate rescue breathing, ideally with bag-mask and supplemental warmed, humidified oxygen. If the victim is pulseless with no detectable sign of circulation, begin chest compressions immediately. Do not withhold BLS until the victim is rewarmed.[13]

To prevent further core heat loss in the victim, remove wet garments from the victim; insulate or shield him or her from wind, heat, or cold; and if possible ventilate with warm, humidified oxygen.[2,5,14,15]

If the hypothermic victim is *not* in cardiac arrest, it is appropriate to apply external warming devices to truncal areas only (warm packs to neck, armpits, and groin). After stabilization prepare the patient carefully for transport to a hospital. All other field interventions require ACLS capability.

Treatment for severe hypothermia (a temperature less than 30°C [86°F]) in the field remains controversial. Many providers do not have the time or equipment to adequately assess the victim or provide controlled warming, so rapid transport is generally recommended.

Provide prehospital rewarming with humidified oxygen or warm fluids when available to help prevent temperature afterdrop.[2,5,11,12,14] Assessment of core temperature in the field with either tympanic membrane sensors or rectal probes is recommended (for EMS systems so equipped) but should not delay transfer.

To prevent VF, avoid rough movement and excess activity. Transport the patient in the horizontal position to avoid aggravating hypotension.

If the hypothermic victim is in cardiac arrest, the BLS treatment protocol should still target airway, breathing, and circulation, but a modified approach is required. AEDs should be available on virtually all BLS rescue units. If VF is detected, deliver up to 3 shocks to attempt defibrillation.[13] If VF persists after 3 shocks, stop efforts to defibrillate and immediately begin CPR, rewarming, and stabilization for transportation. If the victim's core temperature is less than 30°C (86°F), successful conversion to normal sinus rhythm may not be possible until rewarming is accomplished.[14]

Some clinicians believe that patients who appear dead after prolonged exposure to cold temperatures should not be considered dead until they are near normal core temperature and are still unresponsive to CPR.[2,14] However, when the victim of unwitnessed cardiac arrest is found in a cold environment, it may be difficult to determine if the arrest was due to hypothermia or if hypothermia followed a normothermic arrest. For example, a middle-aged man who suffers a normothermic cardiac arrest while shoveling snow may cool down after the arrest. The victim may also sustain additional organ insult.

Critical Concepts:
BLS Care for Hypothermia

General BLS principles for the management of hypothermia are as follows:

- Remove all wet garments from the victim.

- Protect against heat loss and wind chill (use blankets and insulating equipment).

- Maintain the patient in the horizontal position.

- Avoid rough movement and excessive activity.

- Allow 30 to 45 seconds to assess breathing and at the same time to assess signs of circulation.

- If no breathing is detected, provide rescue breathing, preferably with bag-mask and warm, humidified oxygen (42°C to 46°C [108°F to 115°F]) if available.

- If the victim is not in cardiac arrest, provide passive rewarming if available.

- If the victim is in cardiac arrest, start chest compressions and provide up to 3 shocks with an AED. If the victim does not respond, continue CPR and stabilize for transport.

Successful resuscitation of a hypothermic submersion victim will be more difficult if the submersion produced the cardiac arrest and the hypothermia developed subsequently. When it is not clinically possible to know which event occurred first, the arrest or hypothermia, attempt to stabilize the patient with CPR, and if hypothermia is documented, initiate basic maneuvers to limit heat loss and aid with rewarming. In the hospital physicians should use their clinical judgment to decide when to end resuscitative efforts for a hypothermic arrest victim.

In the field resuscitation may be withheld if the victim has obvious lethal injuries or if the body is frozen so completely that chest compression is impossible and the nose and mouth are blocked with ice. In the hospital physicians should use their judgment to determine when resuscitative efforts should cease. Complete rewarming is not indicated for all victims. Predictors of outcome may be unreliable in the face of injury or other complicating factors. Because severe hypothermia is frequently preceded by other disorders (eg, drug overdose, alcohol use, or trauma), you must look for those underlying conditions and be prepared to treat them.

Submersion/Near-Drowning

The most detrimental consequence of prolonged underwater submersion without ventilation is hypoxia. The duration of hypoxia is the critical factor in determining the victim's outcome.[16] Therefore, oxygenation, ventilation, and perfusion should be restored as quickly as possible. This requires immediate initiation of BLS support and prompt activation of the EMS system. Victims with spontaneous circulation and breathing when they reach the hospital usually recover with a good outcome.[17-19]

Submersion victims may develop primary or secondary hypothermia. If submersion occurs in icy water (less than 5°C [41°F]), hypothermia may develop quickly and provide some protection against hypoxia. Such effects, however, have typically been reported only after submersion of *small* victims in *icy* water.[19] Hypothermia may also develop as a secondary complication of submersion and subsequent heat loss through evaporation during attempted resuscitation. In these victims hypothermia is not protective (see preceding section, "Hypothermia").[11]

Transport all victims of submersion who require resuscitation to the hospital for evaluation and monitoring. The hypoxic insult can produce pulmonary complications that may ultimately require advanced life support. Some victims of submersion will also have a head or spinal cord injury.[20,21]

Rescue From the Water

When attempting to rescue a near-drowning victim, get to the victim as quickly as possible, preferably with a boat, raft, surfboard, or flotation device. Always be aware of your personal safety when attempting a rescue and take precautions to minimize the danger. Treat all submersion victims as potential victims of spinal cord injury, and immobilize the cervical and thoracic spine. Spinal injury is particularly likely after submersion associated with diving or involving recreational equipment, but it should be suspected if the submersion episode was not witnessed.[20,21]

Diving into shallow water can result in cervical spine fracture and paralysis.[20,21] If neck injury is suspected, maintain the victim's neck in a neutral position (without flexion or extension), and float the victim supine onto a horizontal back support before being removed from the water. Rescue the victim from water quickly to ensure timely initiation of CPR. If the victim must be turned, align and support the head, neck, chest, and body and turn them as a unit to the horizontal, supine position. Provide rescue breathing with the head maintained in a neutral position. Open the airway by using either the jaw thrust without head tilt or chin lift without head tilt.

Rescue Breathing

The first and most important treatment of the near-drowning victim is to provide immediate rescue breathing with the mouth-to-mouth technique or use of a barrier device. Prompt initiation of rescue breathing has a positive association with survival.[17-19,22] Start rescue breathing as soon as the victim's airway can be opened and protected and the rescuer's safety ensured.[18] This is usually achieved when the victim is in shallow water or out of the water. If it is difficult for you to pinch the victim's nose, support the head, and open the airway in the water, you may use mouth-to-nose ventilation as an alternative to mouth-to-mouth ventilation.

Appliances (such as a snorkel for the mouth-to-snorkel technique or buoyancy aids) may permit specially trained rescuers to perform rescue breathing in deep water. But do not delay rescue breathing for lack of such equipment if it can otherwise be provided safely. Untrained rescuers should not attempt to use such adjuncts.

Management of the airway and breathing of the submersion victim is similar to that of any victim in cardiopulmonary arrest. BLS airway management with adjuncts, such as bag-mask ventilation and intubation, can be accomplished in the near-drowning victim. There is no need to clear the airway of aspirated water.[22] At most only a modest amount of water is aspirated by the majority of drowning victims, and most water in the lungs is rapidly absorbed into the central circulation.[16,22,23] Furthermore, some victims do not aspirate at all because of laryngospasm or breath-holding.[16] An attempt to remove water from the breathing passages by any means other than suction is usually unnecessary and apt to be dangerous because it is likely to eject gastric contents and cause aspiration.[16,22,23]

The Heimlich maneuver is ***not*** recommended for routine resuscitation of submersion victims.[22] Performance of the Heimlich maneuver may not only delay

Critical Concepts:
BLS Care for Submersion

General BLS principles for the management of submersion are as follows:

■ When possible use a boat, raft, surfboard, or flotation device to rescue the victim from the water.

■ Begin rescue breathing as soon as possible (in shallow water, in a boat, or on shore).

■ If a diving accident or head injury is suspected, maintain the neck in the neutral position, protect the cervical spine, and remove the victim from the water using a spine board if available.

■ Do not attempt chest compressions in the water; if needed, start chest compressions immediately after removal from the water.

■ Do not attempt to drain water from the lungs.

■ Remove foreign bodies in the airway, eg, seaweed, sand, or mud.

■ Transport all submersion victims who require resuscitation to the hospital.

the initiation of ventilation and breathing, which have been shown to improve survival,[18] but also produce injuries (see Chapter 8, "Foreign-Body Airway Obstruction").[22] Use a Heimlich maneuver only if you suspect that foreign matter is obstructing the airway or if the victim does not respond appropriately to mouth-to-mouth ventilation.[22,23] If necessary, resume CPR after the Heimlich maneuver has been performed.

Submersion victims frequently have water or foreign material, such as seaweed or mud, in their mouth.[24] Remove any solid material seen in the mouth or pharynx before rescue breathing to avoid forcing this material into the trachea during the rescue breaths. Vomiting and regurgitation are very common after submersion: 86% in cases with chest compression and 68% in cases with expired air resuscitation.[24-27] You should be prepared to manage the airway appropriately with suction or manual clearance using a gloved hand.

Chest Compressions

Do not attempt chest compressions in the water. It is usually impossible to keep the victim's body horizontal and the head above water in position for CPR.

After removing the victim from the water and delivering rescue breaths, immediately assess for signs of circulation. The pulse may be difficult to appreciate in a hypothermic near-drowning victim. If you cannot feel a pulse, start chest compressions at once.

Cardiac Arrest From Trauma

The survival rate from prehospital cardiac arrest secondary to blunt trauma is uniformly low in children and adults.[28-30] Indeed, some researchers recommend withholding resuscitative efforts in patients who are found in asystole or agonal electrical cardiac activity secondary to trauma.[30] Survival after cardiac arrest resulting from penetrating trauma is only slightly better; rapid transport to a trauma center is associated with better outcome than resuscitative attempts in the field.[31]

BLS for the trauma patient is fundamentally the same as care of the patient with a primary cardiac or respiratory arrest. A Primary Survey is performed, with rapid evaluation and stabilization of airway, breathing, circulation, and neurologic function. The trauma rescuer must anticipate, rapidly identify, and immediately treat life-threatening conditions that will interfere with establishment of effective airway, oxygenation, ventilation, and circulation.

Cardiopulmonary arrest associated with trauma has several possible causes; the

management plan may vary for each. Potential causes of cardiorespiratory deterioration and arrest in the trauma victim include

- Severe central neurologic injury with secondary cardiovascular collapse

- Hypoxia secondary to respiratory arrest resulting from neurologic injury, airway obstruction, large open pneumothorax, or severe tracheo-bronchial laceration or crush

- Direct and severe injury to vital structures, such as the heart, aorta, or pulmonary arteries

- Underlying medical problems or other conditions that led to the injury, such as sudden VF in the driver of a motor vehicle or the victim of electric shock

- Severely diminished cardiac output from tension pneumothorax or pericardial tamponade

- Exsanguination leading to hypovolemia and severely diminished oxygen delivery

- Injuries in a cold environment (eg, fractured leg) complicated by secondary severe hypothermia

If cardiac arrest is associated with uncontrolled internal hemorrhage or pericardial tamponade, survival requires rapid transport to an emergency facility with immediate operative capabilities.[31,32] Respiratory arrest may also be treated successfully with early airway management and ventilatory support. VF may be treated with an AED. Shock resulting from a tension pneumothorax or pericardial tamponade may be successfully treated by ACLS personnel. To be effective, these treatments must be provided at the scene or during transport.

When an injured patient becomes pulseless as a result of intravascular volume loss, functional long-term survival is unlikely unless single-organ hemorrhage can be rapidly identified and controlled and circulation supported with volume resuscitation. Survival has been reported

in a small number of trauma patients with prehospital cardiopulmonary arrest. Characteristics associated with survival are young age, penetrating injuries, prehospital tracheal intubation, and prompt transport by highly skilled paramedics to a definitive care facility.[33,34] Patients with prehospital cardiopulmonary arrest due to multiple-organ hemorrhage will rarely survive neurologically intact.[28-30,33-35]

Prehospital Approaches to Resuscitation

The injured patient without a pulse requires immediate assessment. Despite the bleak outlook, resuscitative efforts should be initiated when the patient appears to have some potential for survival. Resuscitation should not be attempted in patients with obvious, severe blunt trauma who are without vital signs, pupillary response, or an organized or shockable cardiac rhythm at the scene.

Extrication and Initial Evaluation

In resuscitative attempts patients should be quickly extricated and prepared for rapid evacuation to a facility that provides definitive trauma care. If an AED is available, use it to treat VF. Accomplish airway assessment and ventilation as soon as possible, with intubation of the trachea a priority.[32-34] Consider intercept with prehospital ACLS providers. During airway procedures an assistant should immobilize the victim's neck.[30] Lateral neck supports, strapping, and use of backboards are also recommended to minimize exacerbation of an occult neck injury.[36]

Establishing Unresponsiveness

Head trauma or shock may produce loss of consciousness. If spinal cord injury is present, the victim may be conscious but unable to move. Throughout initial assessment and stabilization, the rescuer should monitor patient responsiveness; deterioration could indicate either neurologic compromise or cardiorespiratory failure.

Airway

When multisystem trauma is present or trauma is isolated to the head and neck, the spine must be immobilized throughout BLS maneuvers. To open the airway, use a jaw thrust instead of a head tilt–chin lift. If at all possible, a second rescuer should be responsible for immobilizing the head and neck during BLS and until spine immobilization equipment is attached.

Once the airway is opened with jaw thrust or head tilt–chin lift, clear the mouth of blood, vomitus, and other secretions. Remove this material with a (gloved) finger sweep, or use gauze or a towel to wipe out the mouth. Suction may also be used to clear the airway.

Breathing/Ventilation

Once a patent airway is established, assess for breathing. If breathing is absent or grossly inadequate (eg, agonal or slow and extremely shallow), ventilation is needed. When ventilation is provided with a barrier device, a pocket mask, or a bag-mask system, immobilize the cervical spine. If the chest does not expand during ventilation despite repeated attempts to open the airway with a jaw thrust, a tension pneumothorax or hemothorax may be present. They should be ruled out or treated by ACLS personnel.

Deliver breaths slowly to reduce the development of gastric inflation and possible regurgitation.

Circulation

If the victim has no signs of circulation (no pulse, no breathing, no coughing, no movement) in response to rescue breaths, provide chest compressions until an AED is available and attached.[33,34] The AED will evaluate the victim's cardiac rhythm and advise delivery of a shock if appropriate.[35]

Disability

Throughout all interventions, assess the victim's response. The Glasgow Coma Scale is useful and can be assessed in seconds. Monitor the victim closely for signs of deterioration.

Exposure

The victim may lose heat to the environment through evaporation. Such heat loss will be exacerbated if the victim's clothes are removed or if the victim is covered in blood. Keep the victim warm.

Triage and Treatment of Multiple Critically Injured Patients

When multiple patients receive serious injuries, emergency personnel must establish priorities for care. When the number of patients with critical injuries exceeds the capability of the EMS system, victims without a pulse should be considered the lowest priority for care and triage.[36,37] Most EMS systems have developed guidelines that permit the prehospital pronouncement of death or withholding of cardiac resuscitative efforts in the setting of multiple patients with critical injuries or injuries incompatible with life. EMS personnel should work within such guidelines when available.

Electric Shock

Electric shock accounts for approximately 500 to 1000 deaths annually in the United States and causes injuries sufficient to require emergency treatment for another 5000 patients every year.[38-40] Victims of electric shock experience a wide spectrum of injury, ranging from a transient unpleasant sensation from low-intensity current to instantaneous cardiac arrest from accidental electrocution.

Electric shock may occur by a variety of mechanisms. Most electric shock injuries to adults occur at the worksite.[41] Pediatric electric shock injuries are more likely to occur in the home when a child bites electrical wires, places an object in an electrical socket, or touches a low-voltage wire or appliance or a high-voltage wire outdoors.[42] Electric shock injuries result from the direct effects of current on cell membranes and vascular smooth muscle and the conversion of electric energy into heat energy as current passes through body tissues. Factors that determine the nature and severity of electric trauma include the magnitude of energy delivered, voltage, resistance to current flow, type of current, duration of contact with the current source, and current pathway.

High-tension current generally causes the most serious injuries, although fatal electrocutions may occur with low-voltage household current (110 V).[43] Bone and skin are most resistant to the passage of electric current. Muscle, blood vessels, and nerves conduct with least resistance.[39,40] Skin resistance, the most important factor impeding current flow, can be substantially reduced by moisture, thereby converting what ordinarily might be a minor low-voltage injury into a life-threatening shock.[44] Skin resistance can be overcome with increased duration of exposure to current flow. Contact with alternating current at 60 cycles per second (the frequency used in most household and commercial sources of electricity) may cause tetanic skeletal muscle contractions and prevent the victim from releasing the source of the electricity, thereby leading to prolonged duration of exposure. The repetitive frequency of alternating current also increases the likelihood of current flow through the heart during the vulnerable recovery period of the cardiac cycle. This exposure can precipitate VF.[45]

Transthoracic current flow (eg, a hand-to-hand pathway) is more likely to be fatal than a vertical (hand-to-foot) or straddle (foot-to-foot) current path.[46] The vertical pathway, however, often causes myocardial injury, which has been attributed to the direct effects of current and coronary artery spasm.[47-49]

Cardiac and Respiratory Arrest

Cardiopulmonary arrest is the primary cause of immediate death due to electrical injury.[50] VF or ventricular asystole may occur as a direct result of electric shock. Other serious cardiac arrhythmias, including ventricular tachycardia (VT), that may progress to VF may result from exposure to low- or high-voltage current.[51]

Respiratory arrest may develop with electric shock for several reasons:

- Electric current passing through the brain and causing inhibition of medullary respiratory center function

- Tetanic contraction of the diaphragm and chest wall musculature during current exposure

- Prolonged paralysis of respiratory muscles, which may continue for minutes after the electric shock has ended

If respiratory arrest persists untreated, hypoxic cardiac arrest will develop.

Basic Life Support

Scene Rescue

You must be certain that your rescue efforts will not put you in danger of electric shock. When a rescue involves proximity to live current, only specially trained rescuers who know how to perform this type of rescue should attempt it.

After the power is turned off by authorized personnel or the energized source is safely cleared from the victim, immediately determine the victim's responsiveness and cardiopulmonary status. Immediately after electrocution, respiration or circulation or both may fail. The patient may be apneic, mottled, unresponsive, and in cardiac arrest with VF or asystole.

Vigorous resuscitation is indicated, even for victims who appear dead on initial evaluation. The prognosis for recovery from electric shock is not readily predictable because the amplitude and duration of the charge are usually unknown. However, because many victims are

young and have no preexisting cardiopulmonary disease, they have a reasonable chance for survival if CPR is provided immediately.

Electrical injuries are also likely to result in related trauma, including injury to the spine[52] and muscles as well as fractures caused by the tetanic response of skeletal muscles. If injury is suspected, maintain inline immobilization of the spine on the scene and during transport.[41,52]

Airway, Breathing, and Circulation

If spontaneous respiration or circulation is absent, the BLS techniques outlined in this manual should be initiated, including activation of the EMS system, prompt CPR, and use of the AED. The presenting cardiac ECG rhythm may be asystole or VF.[53]

As soon as possible, secure airway patency and ventilation and provide supplemental oxygen. When electric shock occurs in a location that is not readily accessible, such as on a utility pole, start rescue breathing at once and lower the victim to the ground as quickly as possible. Begin ventilations and chest compressions as soon as feasible for victims of cardiac arrest. Maintain spinal protection and immobilization during extrication and treatment if there is any likelihood of head or neck trauma. Remove smoldering clothing, shoes, and belts to prevent further thermal damage.

Lightning Strike

Lightning strike causes approximately 50 to 300 fatalities per year in the United States, with about twice that number of persons sustaining serious injury.[41,53,54] Lightning injuries have a 30% mortality rate, and up to 70% of survivors sustain significant morbidity.[55]

The presentation of lightning strike injuries varies widely, even among groups of people struck at the same time. In some victims symptoms are mild and may not require hospitalization, whereas others may die of their injuries.[38,56]

The primary cause of death in lightning-strike victims is cardiac arrest, which may be due to primary VF or ventricular asystole.[57] Lightning acts as an instantaneous, massive direct current shock, depolarizing the entire myocardium at once and producing asystole. In many cases cardiac automaticity may restore organized cardiac activity, and sinus rhythm may return spontaneously. However, concomitant respiratory arrest due to thoracic muscle spasm and suppression of the respiratory center may continue after return of spontaneous circulation. Unless ventilatory assistance is provided or spontaneous respirations resume, hypoxic cardiac arrest will develop.

Lightning can produce widespread effects on the cardiovascular system, producing extensive catecholamine release or autonomic stimulation. If cardiac arrest does not occur, the victim may develop hypertension, tachycardia, nonspecific ECG changes (including prolongation of the QT interval and transient T-wave inversion), and myocardial necrosis with release of myocardial enzymes. Reversible myocardial dysfunction may also be observed.

Lightning may produce a wide variety of neurologic injuries. The injuries may be primary, resulting from effects on the brain, or secondary, as a complication of cardiac arrest and hypoxia. The current can produce brain hemorrhages, swelling, and injury to small vessels and nerves.

Those who suffer immediate respiratory or cardiac arrest are most likely to die of lightning injury if no treatment is forthcoming. If the victim in respiratory or cardiac arrest does receive and respond to immediate treatment, however, the prognosis is excellent because subsequent arrests are uncommon. Patients who do not suffer respiratory or cardiac arrest already have an excellent chance of recovery and are unlikely to deteriorate further at the scene. Therefore, when multiple victims are struck simultaneously by lightning, the usual triage priorities should be reversed. Give highest priority to patients in respiratory or cardiac arrest because they require and may respond to treatment.

For victims in cardiopulmonary arrest, begin BLS and ACLS immediately. The goal is to oxygenate the heart and brain adequately until cardiac activity is restored. Victims of respiratory arrest may require only ventilation and oxygenation to avoid secondary hypoxic cardiac arrest. Resuscitative attempts for victims of cardiac arrest caused by lightning may have higher success rates than those for victims of cardiac arrest from other causes.

Pregnancy

Resuscitation of expectant mothers is unique because of dramatic alterations in maternal cardiovascular and respiratory physiology and the relationship of the two victims. During normal pregnancy maternal cardiac output and blood volume increase up to 50%. Maternal heart rate, minute ventilation, and oxygen consumption also increase.[58] Together these changes render the pregnant woman more susceptible to and less tolerant of major cardiovascular and respiratory insults. Also, when the mother is supine, the gravid uterus may compress the iliac vessels, the inferior vena cava, and the abdominal aorta, resulting in hypotension and as much as a 25% reduction in cardiac output.[59]

Potential causes of cardiac arrest during pregnancy are most often associated with events during delivery, including

- Amniotic fluid embolism
- Eclampsia
- Drug toxicity

Cardiac arrest may also be related to changes associated with the pregnancy itself, including

- Congestive cardiomyopathy
- Aortic dissection
- Pulmonary embolism
- Hemorrhage associated with a pregnancy-related pathological condition

Finally, cardiac arrest may be the result of injuries caused by motor vehicle crashes, falls, assault, attempted suicide, or penetrating trauma.[60]

To prevent cardiac arrest in the injured pregnant woman, if possible place the patient in the left lateral position (or gently manually displace the uterus to the left). This will reduce pressure on the inferior vena cava and may improve venous return to the maternal heart and increase cardiac output.

When cardiac arrest occurs in a pregnant woman, standard resuscitative measures and procedures should be performed. If VF is present, treat it with defibrillation according to the VF algorithm. Perform chest compressions slightly higher on the sternum because the uterus has probably pushed the diaphragm up higher than the normal position. Chest compressions may be most effective if performed with the victim propped on her left side, with a hard surface behind her back. If refractory VF or other rhythms are present with a *"no shock indicated"* message from the AED, rapid transport to the hospital may be of value because emergency cesarean section may used in an attempt to save a viable fetus.[61,62]

Allergies

Severe allergic reactions are rare, but when they occur, they may be life-threatening. Exposure to a known allergen (foods, pollens, etc) or a reaction to an insect bite (eg, bee stings) may be the initial inciting event. The most severe consequence of an allergic reaction is upper airway obstruction due to laryngeal edema or anaphylactic shock (life-threatening cardiovascular collapse). Prompt action can limit adverse effects from allergic reactions. After activating the EMS system, place the victim in a supine position (or a position of comfort) and closely monitor the victim's airway. If respiratory or cardiac arrest occurs, initiate rescue breathing or CPR.

Asphyxiation

Asphyxiation (suffocation) is commonly caused by inhalation of a gas other than air or oxygen. It may develop during fires or from chemical spills or gas leaks. It can also be the result of breathing carbon monoxide in an enclosed space. The result of asphyxiation is insufficient oxygen delivery to the body, resulting in loss of consciousness and ultimately cardiopulmonary arrest. Perform appropriate CPR. Scene safety for rescuers should be a priority. Always relocate the victim away from any environment with toxic gases. If the victim is ventilating adequately or regains spontaneous ventilation after resuscitative efforts, administer high-concentration as soon as possible. Victims of severe smoke inhalation may require transport to a regional medical center with a hyperbaric oxygen chamber.

Summary of Special Resuscitation Situations

Special resuscitation situations require the rescuer to carefully assess scene conditions to ensure the safety of the victim and all personnel. Each special situation has one or more important exceptions to the conventional BLS approach to resuscitation. But basic BLS actions remain substantially unchanged.

Summary of Key Concepts

- In special resuscitation situations rescuers must ensure that scene conditions will not put them or other rescuers in danger.

- A period of 30 to 45 seconds may be required to assess breathing and pulse in a severely hypothermic victim.

- In hypothermic cardiac arrest, if the victim's body temperature is less than 30°C (86°F), use of an AED is limited to 3 shocks to determine the victim's response to defibrillation. If 3 shocks are not effective, CPR should be continued and the patient transported to the hospital.

- For hypothermic victims, rescuers should avoid rough movement and excess activity to prevent VF. The patient should be transported in the horizontal position to avoid aggravating hypotension.

- Drowning can occur as a result of diving into shallow water, resulting in cervical spine fracture and paralysis.

- If the submersion victim is not breathing, rescue breathing should be initiated immediately.

- For a drowning victim, the Heimlich maneuver should be used *only* if the rescuer suspects that foreign matter is obstructing the airway or the victim does not respond appropriately to mouth-to-mouth ventilation.

- The prognosis is poor for victims in cardiac arrest caused by blunt trauma.

- If available, an AED should be used for all special situation victims of cardiac arrest.

- For victims of electrocution or lightening strike, vigorous resuscitative efforts are indicated, especially for those who appear to be dead on initial evaluation.

- CPR for expectant mothers should be undertaken without modification except to wedge a pillow under the right abdominal flank and hip to displace the uterus to the left side of the abdomen. This keeps the uterus from interfering with venous return to the heart and cardiac output during CPR.

- Proper CPR technique will lessen the potential for complications from this life-saving procedure.

Review Questions

1. You find an unresponsive 27-year-old man in the woods during the winter. His skin is cold and frozen to the touch, and he is not breathing. You cannot feel a carotid pulse. How long should you take to check the pulse before starting CPR?

   a. 5 to 10 seconds

   b. 10 to 15 seconds

   c. 30 to 45 seconds

   d. 1 to 2 minutes

2. You observe a 12-year-old victim in a lake, 100 feet from shore. The child is struggling in the water, then sinks below the surface. What should you do?

   a. swim to the victim and pull the victim to shore

   b. use a boat to rescue the victim

   c. get an AED

   d. phone first — phone the EMS system

3. You have just removed a 10-year-old girl from a pool and she is unresponsive. You send a bystander to call 911, and you note that the child is not breathing and has vomit in her mouth. You should

   a. quickly sweep the vomit from her mouth and begin rescue breathing immediately

   b. perform the Heimlich maneuver immediately

   c. turn her on her side and allow the water to drain for 1 minute before starting rescue breathing

   d. wait for suction to arrive before beginning rescue breathing

4. You stop to help at the scene of a car crash. You find a 24-year-old man who was thrown from his car. He is in cardio-pulmonary arrest. What is the best method for opening the victim's airway?

   a. head tilt–chin lift

   b. head tilt without jaw thrust

   c. chin lift only

   d. jaw thrust without head tilt

5. While you are visiting friends, their 2-year-old son bites into the electrical wire of a lamp and is having a seizure. His mouth is still in contact with the wire. Your immediate action is to

   a. open the airway and evaluate breathing

   b. disconnect the plug from the outlet and send your friend to call 911

   c. hold the child and protect him from the effects of the seizure

   d. perform CPR and attach an AED

6. A pregnant woman collapses in the office building where you work. She is unresponsive, not breathing, and has no pulse. You start CPR and the security staff arrives with an AED. They note she is pregnant and are not sure if they should use the AED. Your advice to them is

   a. use the AED as you would for any cardiac arrest victim

   b. do not use the AED because it will hurt the fetus

   c. use the AED but attempt only up to 3 shocks

   d. place the AED electrodes higher on the chest to avoid injuring the fetus

How did you do?

Answers: **1,** c; **2,** b; **3,** a; **4,** d; **5,** b; **6,** a.

References

1. Danzl DF, Pozos RS, Hamlet MP. Accidental hypothermia. In: Auerbach PS, Geehr EC, eds. *Management of Wilderness and Environmental Emergencies.* St. Louis, Mo: CV Mosby Co; 1989:35-65.

2. Jones AI, Swann IJ. Prolonged resuscitation in accidental hypothermia: use of mechanical cardiopulmonary resuscitation and partial cardiopulmonary bypass. *Eur J Emerg Med.* 1994;1:34-36.

3. Weinberg AD. Hypothermia. *Ann Emerg Med.* 1993;22:370-377.

4. Mair P, Kornberger E, Schwarz B, Baubin M, Hoermann C. Forward blood flow during cardiopulmonary resuscitation in patients with severe accidental hypothermia: an echocardiographic study. *Acta Anaesthesiol Scand.* 1998; 42:1139-1144.

5. Schneider SM. Hypothermia: from recognition to rewarming. *Emerg Med Rep.* 1992;13:1-20.

6. Steedman DJ, Rainer T, Campanella C. Cardiopulmonary resuscitation following profound immersion hypothermia. *J Accid Emerg Med.* 1997;14:170-172.

7. Ireland AJ, Pathi VL, Crawford R, Colquhoun IW. Back from the dead: extracorporeal rewarming of severe accidental hypothermia victims in accident and emergency. *J Accid Emerg Med.* 1997;14:255-257.

8. Mair P, Schwarz B, Kornberger E, Balogh D. Case 5-1997: successful resuscitation of a patient with severe accidental hypothermia and prolonged cardiocirculatory arrest using cardiopulmonary bypass. *J Cardiothorac Vasc Anesth.* 1997;11:901-904.

9. Sanada T, Ueki M, Tokudome M, Okamura T, Nishiki S, Niimura A, Yabuki S, Watanabe Y. Recovery from out-of-hospital cardiac arrest after mild hypothermia: report of two cases [in Japanese]. *Masui.* 1998;47:742-745.

10. Lamperti M, Croci M, Carboni P, Beverini C, Trazzi R. Cardiopulmonary resuscitation. The effect of severe hypothermia on clinical outcome [in Italian]. *Minerva Anestesiol.* 1998;64: 459-464.

11. Romet TT. Mechanism of afterdrop after cold water immersion. *J Appl Physiol.* 1988;65: 1535-1538.

12. Reuler JB. Hypothermia: pathophysiology, clinical settings, and management. *Ann Intern Med.* 1978;89:519-527.

13. Emergency Cardiac Care Committee and Subcommittees, American Heart Association. Guidelines for cardiopulmonary resuscitation and emergency cardiac care, IV: special resuscitation situations. *JAMA.* 1992;268:2242-2261.

14. Weinberg AD, Hamlet MP, Paturas JL, White RD, McAninch GW. *Cold Weather Emergencies: Principles of Patient Management.* Branford, Conn: American Medical Publishing Co; 1990:10-30.

15. Weinberg AD. The role of inhalation rewarming in the early management of hypothermia. *Resuscitation.* 1998;36:101-104.

16. The National Spinal Cord Injury Statistical Center. *The 1994 Annual Statistical Report for the National SCI Database.* Birmingham, Alabama: The National Spinal Cord Injury Statistical Center; 1994.

17. Rosen P, Stoto M, Harley J. The use of the Heimlich maneuver in near-drowning: Institute of Medicine report. *J Emerg Med.* 1995;13: 397-405.

18. Kyriacou DN, Arcinue EL, Peek C, Kraus JF. Effect of immediate resuscitation on children with submersion injury. *Pediatrics.* 1994;94: 137-142.

19. Kluger Y, Jarosz D, Paul DB, Townsend RN, Diamond DL. Diving injuries: a preventable catastrophe. *J Trauma.* 1994;36:349-351.

20. Quan L, Wentz KR, Gore EJ, Copass MK. Outcome and predictors of outcome in pediatric submersion victims receiving prehospital care in King County, Washington. *Pediatrics.* 1990;86:586-593.

21. Modell JH, Davis JH. Is the Heimlich maneuver appropriate as first treatment for drowning? *Emerg Med Serv.* 1981;10:63-66.

22. Levin DL, Morriss FC, Toro LO, Brink LW, Turner GR. Drowning and near-drowning. *Pediatr Clin North Am.* 1993;40:321-336.

23. Modell JH. Drowning. *N Engl J Med.* 1993; 328:253-256.

24. Manolios N, Mackie I. Drowning and near-drowning on Australian beaches patrolled by life-savers; a 10-year study, 1973-1983. *Med J Aust.* 1988;148:165-167, 170-171.

25. Quan L. Drowning issues in resuscitation. *Ann Emerg Med.* 1993;22:366-369.

26. Bross MH, Clark JL. Near-drowning. *Am Fam Physician.* 1995;51:1545-1551, 1555.

27. Szpilman D. Near-drowning and drowning classification: a proposal to stratify mortality based on the analysis of 1,831 cases. *Chest.* 1997;112:660-665.

28. Fisher B, Worthen M. Cardiac arrest induced by blunt trauma in children. *Pediatr Emerg Care.* 1999;15:274-276.

29. Hazinski MF, Chahine AA, Holcomb GW III, Morris JA Jr. Outcome of cardiovascular collapse in pediatric blunt trauma. *Ann Emerg Med.* 1994;23:1229-1235.

30. Battistella FD, Nugent W, Owings JT, Anderson JT. Field triage of the pulseless trauma patient. *Arch Surg.* 1999;134:742-745.

31. Bickell WH, Wall MJ Jr, Pepe PE, Martin RR, Ginger VF, Allen MK, Mattox KL. Immediate versus delayed fluid resuscitation for hypotensive patients with penetrating torso injuries. *N Engl J Med.* 1994;331;1105-1109.

32. Pepe PE, Copass MK. Prehospital care. In: Moore EE, Ducker TB, American College of Surgeons, Committee on Trauma, eds. *Early Care of the Injured Patient.* 4th ed. Philadelphia, Pa: BC Decker; 1990:34-55.

33. Copass MK, Oreskovich MR, Bladergroen MR, Carrico CJ. Prehospital cardiopulmonary resuscitation of the critically injured patient. *Am J Surg.* 1984;148:20-26.

34. Durham LA III, Richardson RJ, Wall MJ Jr, Pepe PE, Mattox KL. Emergency center thoracotomy: impact of prehospital resuscitation. *J Trauma.* 1992;32:775-779.

35. Rozycki G, Adams C, Champion HR, Kihn R. Resuscitative thoracotomy: trends in outcome. *Ann Emerg Med.* 1990;19:462.

36. American College of Surgeons Committee on Trauma. *Advanced Trauma Life Support Course Student Manual.* 6th ed. Chicago, Ill: American College of Surgeons; 1997.

37. Pepe PE. Emergency medical services systems and prehospital management of patients requiring critical care. In: Carlson R, Geheb M, eds. *Principles and Practice of Medical Intensive Care.* Philadelphia, Pa: WB Saunders Co; 1992:9-24.

38. Browne BJ, Gaasch WR. Electrical injuries and lightning. *Emerg Med Clin North Am.* 1992;10:211-229.

39. Cooper MA. Electrical and lightning injuries. *Emerg Med Clin North Am.* 1984;2:489-501.

40. Kobernick M. Electrical injuries: pathophysiology and emergency management. *Ann Emerg Med.* 1982;11:633-638.

41. Cooper MA. Emergent care of lightning and electrical injuries. *Semin Neurol.* 1995;15: 268-278.

42. Zubair M, Besner GE. Pediatric electrical burns: management strategies. *Burns.* 1997;23: 413-420.

43. Budnick LD. Bathtub-related electrocutions in the United States, 1979 to 1982. *JAMA.* 1984; 252:918-920.

44. Wallace JF. Electrical injuries. In: Wilson JD, Braunwald E, Isselbacher KJ, et al, eds. *Harrison's Principles of Internal Medicine.* 12th ed. New York, NY: McGraw-Hill Book Co, Health Professions Division; 1991:2202-2204.

45. Geddes LA, Bourland JD, Ford G. The mechanism underlying sudden death from electric shock. *Med Instrum.* 1986;20:303-315.

46. Thompson JC, Ashwal S. Electrical injuries in children. *Am J Dis Child.* 1983;137:231-235.

47. Chandra NC, Siu CO, Munster AM. Clinical predictors of myocardial damage after high voltage electrical injury. *Crit Care Med.* 1990; 18:293-297.

48. Ku CS, Lin SL, Hsu TL, Wang SP, Chang MS. Myocardial damage associated with electrical injury. *Am Heart J.* 1989;118:621-624.

49. Xenopoulos N, Movahed A, Hudson P, Reeves WC. Myocardial injury in electrocution. *Am Heart J.* 1991;122:1481-1484.

50. Homma S, Gillam LD, Weyman AE. Echocardiographic observations in survivors of acute electrical injury. *Chest.* 1990;97:103-105.

51. Jensen PJ, Thomsen PE, Bagger JP, Norgaard A, Baandrup U. Electrical injury causing ventricular arrhythmias. *Br Heart J.* 1987;57: 279-283.

52. Arevalo JM; Lorente JA; Balseiro-Gomez J. Spinal cord injury after electrical trauma treated in a burn unit. *Burns.* 1999;25:449-452.

53. Duclos PJ, Sanderson LM. An epidemiological description of lightning-related deaths in the United States. *Int J Epidemiol.* 1990;19: 673-679.

54. Epperly TD, Stewart JR. The physical effects of lightning injury. *J Fam Pract.* 1989;29: 267-272.

55. Cooper MA. Lightning injuries: prognostic signs for death. *Ann Emerg Med.* 1980;9: 134-138.

56. Patten BM. Lightning and electrical injuries. *Neurol Clin.* 1992;10:1047-1058.

57. Kleiner JP, Wilkin JH. Cardiac effects of lightning strike. *JAMA.* 1978;240:2757-2759.

58. Lee W, Cotton DB. Cardiorespiratory changes during pregnancy. In: Clark SL, Cotton DB, Hankins GDV, Phelan JP, eds. *Critical Care Obstetrics.* 2nd ed. Boston, Mass: Blackwell Scientific Publications; 1991:2-34.

59. Kerr MG. The mechanical effects of the gravid uterus in late pregnancy. *J Obstet Gynecol Br Commonw.* 1965;72:513-529.

60. Satin AJ, Hankins GDV. Cardiopulmonary resuscitation in pregnancy. In: Clark SL, Cotton DB, Hankins GDV, Phelan JP, eds. *Critical Care Obstetrics.* 2nd ed. Boston, Mass: Blackwell Scientific Publications; 1991:579.

61. Luppi CJ. Cardiopulmonary resuscitation: pregnant women are different. *AACN Clin Issues.* 1997;8:574-585.

62. Parker J, Balis N, Chester S, Adey D. Cardiopulmonary arrest in pregnancy: successful resuscitation of mother and infant following immediate caesarean section in labour ward. *Aust N Z J Obstet Gynaecol.* 1996;36:207-210.

Case Scenario 1

You are working the night shift in the Emergency Department. An EMS ambulance team notifies you that it is transporting a 72-year-old woman from a nursing home. She is having difficulty breathing and has an advance DNR directive.

The patient soon arrives in the ED in obvious respiratory distress. She is cyanotic with ineffective respiratory efforts and a low blood pressure. She is unable to speak. The nursing home papers contain no advance directives that indicate the patient's choices for healthcare decisions. When you phone the nursing home, the night nurse says she thinks the patient has an advanced directive requesting DNR, but she cannot find any paperwork in the patient's chart. The patient still has a pulse but is in respiratory failure with impending respiratory arrest. What do you do?

Case Scenario 2

You are working in the ED and have been involved in the attempted resuscitation of 3 members of a single family whose car was struck by a drunk driver. Despite heroic efforts on the part of the prehospital and ED providers, all 3 victims — a father and his 2 children — died. The man's wife (the children's mother) arrives in the ED and is told of the deaths of her husband and children. You are with her as she says her goodbye to her family and then leaves. For days after the experience you have trouble sleeping, and you relive the attempts to save the lives of that family, wondering what you could have done better. What are some steps you can take to help you deal with this experience?

CPR and Defibrillation: The Human Dimension

Outcomes of Resuscitation: Definitions of "Success"

Since 1973 more than 70 million people have learned CPR. Many public health experts consider CPR training to be the most successful public health initiative of modern times. Millions of people have been willing to learn how to take action to save the life of a fellow human being.

Until recently the outcome of out-of-hospital resuscitation attempts was predictably poor.[1-3] Of all patients with sudden cardiac arrest, only approximately 70% to 80% have witnessed VF arrest. Victims with *witnessed VF* arrest are most likely to respond to resuscitative efforts, and it is the outcome of resuscitative efforts in these victims that is reported as the "gold standard" for comparison of resuscitative efforts from one community to another. In Seattle (King County), Washington, where there is a high rate of bystander CPR and a short EMS call-to-shock interval, approximately 50% of patients with witnessed VF arrest are successfully resuscitated and survive to hospital *admission*, and about half of those admitted to the hospital survive to hospital *discharge*.[4,5] Survival rates vary widely in reports around the country. In large metropolitan cities such as Chicago and New York, which have a low rate of bystander CPR and longer call-to-shock intervals, the survival

Learning Objectives

At the end of this chapter you will be able to

1. Discuss the reported survival-to-hospital discharge rate after resuscitation from cardiac arrest and variables that affect survival

2. List the signs of a stress reaction

3. Describe the purpose of a critical incident stress debriefing (CISD)

4. List psychological barriers to action during cardiorespiratory emergencies

5. Define the ethical values of autonomy, beneficence, non-maleficence, and justice

6. List examples of advance directives

7. Define the term *DNAR* (also called *No CPR*)

8. List criteria for discontinuing basic life support out-of-hospital and in-hospital

9. Discuss DNAR policies out-of-hospital, in-hospital, and in nursing homes

10. Explain the purpose of Good Samaritan laws

rate averages less than 5%.[1,2] These reports are somewhat discouraging, because even in a community with a strong Chain of Survival, 3 of every 4 out-of-hospital resuscitative efforts would be expected to fail.[4,5]

Reports of resuscitation within the past few months and years, however, provide reason for more optimism about the outcome of resuscitative efforts. These reports suggest that the use of an AED in addition to bystander CPR will dramatically increase the number of survivors of cardiac arrest.[6] In the Heart Save program at Chicago airports, 75% of the first 12 victims with witnessed VF arrest in O'Hare and Midway airports survived to hospital discharge.[7] Improved survival rates have also been documented in public access defibrillation (PAD) programs in airplanes,[8] with police in Rochester, Minnesota,[9] in several casinos,[10] and at sporting events.[11]

No matter how exciting the new developments in resuscitation, the reality is that many resuscitative efforts will fail. The effect of this failure on the rescuer can be profound.

Stress Reactions

A cardiac arrest is a dramatic and emotional event, especially if the victim is a friend or loved one. The emergency may involve disagreeable physical details, such as bleeding, vomiting, or poor hygiene. Any emergency can be emotionally charged, especially if the rescuer is closely involved with the victim. The emergency can produce strong emotional reactions in bystanders, lay rescuers, and healthcare professionals alike. Failed attempts at resuscitation can impose even more stress on rescuers. This stress can result in a variety of emotional reactions and physical symptoms that may last long after the original emergency. These reactions are frequent and quite normal.

It is common for a person to experience emotional aftershocks when he or she experiences an unpleasant event. Usually stress reactions occur immediately or within the first few hours after the event. Sometimes the emotional response occurs later.[12]

Psychologists who work with professional emergency personnel have learned that rescuers may experience grief, anxiety, anger, and sometimes guilt.[13] Typical physical reactions include difficulty sleeping, fatigue, irritability, changes in eating habits, and confusion.[14] Many people say that they are unable to stop thinking about the event.[14]

Remember that these reactions are common and normal. Strong reactions simply indicate that a particular event had a powerful impact. With understanding and the support of loved ones, stress reactions usually pass quickly.

Critical Incident Stress Debriefings

Psychologists have learned that the most successful way to reduce stress after rescue efforts is very simple: *Talk about it*.[15] Sit down with other people who witnessed the event and talk it over. EMS personnel are encouraged to offer emotional support to lay rescuers and bystanders. More formal discussions should include not only lay rescuers but also professional responders.

In these discussions participants should be encouraged to describe what happened and to relive the event. It is natural and healthy to do this. Most reactions will diminish within a few days. Sharing thoughts and feelings with companions at work, fellow rescuers, EMS personnel, friends, or clergy will prevent stress reactions and help with recovery.[15]

In some locations EMS leaders may conduct more formal discussions or debriefings after resuscitation attempts. Such sessions have been called *critical incident stress debriefings,* or CISDs.[15]

Specially trained teams are available to organize and conduct CISDs. These teams are usually associated with EMS services, employee assistance programs, community mental health centers, or public school systems. Other sources of psychological and emotional support are local clergy, police chaplains, fire service chaplains, or hospital and ED social workers.[12-15]

CISDs are confidential. Participants agree that they will not discuss what was said during the meeting. The facilitator leads and encourages persons involved in a stressful situation to express their thoughts and feelings about the event. Such discussion may help and reassure others. Rescuers and witnesses to an event can express and discuss shared feelings they experienced during and after a resuscitative attempt. These may include feelings of guilt, anxiety, or failure, especially if the resuscitative attempt had a negative outcome.[12-15] Ideally the rescuers who were most involved in the resuscitation should be present for the debriefing. In some PAD programs EMS personnel visit lay rescuers who were involved in the resuscitative effort.

Psychological Barriers to Resuscitation

Both students and healthcare professionals may express concerns about performing CPR and using an AED.[16,17] Concerns include fear of imperfect performance, fear of responsibility, anxiety, guilt, and fear of infection.[18] Training programs should incorporate information about willingness to perform CPR and encourage students to develop an individualized action plan in the event of an emergency.[19]

Even healthcare professionals may express a fear of performing mouth-to-mouth ventilation.[16,17] Those with a duty to respond to a cardiac emergency have a responsibility to provide timely CPR, including ventilations and chest compressions. Professional rescuers should carry a barrier device or positive-pressure ventilation device with them at all times. Having a barrier device immediately available is likely to increase rescuers' confidence and willingness to provide timely interventions.

Fear of lawsuits is sometimes a concern for rescuers faced with performing CPR in a nonprofessional setting.[20] The likelihood of litigation arising from a CPR attempt is extremely low. There has never been a successful lawsuit against a lay rescuer who attempted to provide CPR for a victim of cardiac arrest. Although professional rescuers are held to a higher standard than lay rescuers, many states provide Good Samaritan protection for professional rescuers performing CPR in a nonprofessional setting. Furthermore, approximately 70% of all cardiac arrests occur in the home, where the victim is likely to be a friend or relative.[21]

Both CPR and defibrillation require that the rescuer remove clothing from the victim's chest. For example, defibrillation electrodes cannot be attached unless the pads are placed directly on the skin of the chest. The rescuer must open the cardiac arrest victim's shirt or blouse and remove (or cut) the person's undergarments. Common courtesy and modesty may inhibit the rescuer from removing the clothing of a stranger, especially in front of other people in a public location. Rescuers should anticipate these possible feelings and not let courtesy or modesty delay immediate lifesaving interventions for a victim of cardiac arrest.[22]

Principles of Ethics and Decisions About Resuscitation

The goal of medical therapy is to preserve life, restore health, relieve suffering, and limit disability. These goals are influenced by society's common values — autonomy, beneficence, nonmaleficence, and justice. CPR is a medical therapy that must be considered within the context of these goals and ethical values. It should be used to preserve life, restore health, and limit disability. Often these goals cannot be achieved.

As for all medical interventions, there are indications and contraindications to the use of CPR. Ethical values should be considered, including the potential benefit to patients and their requests regarding its use. CPR is unique, however, in that there is no time for deliberation before beginning resuscitation, and unlike other medical therapies, CPR is instituted without physician's orders. It is begun on the premise of implied consent.

Because one of the primary goals of medical therapy is to preserve life, there is a strong presumption in favor of the institution of CPR, and the standard of care remains that CPR should be initiated promptly unless specific contraindications exist.

The purpose of this section is to guide healthcare providers in making difficult decisions about starting and stopping CPR. These are guidelines only. Each decision must be individualized and made with compassion and reason.[23]

Beneficence and advocacy are values that encourage the healthcare provider to defend the individual patient's best interest. Sometimes there is disagreement between the physician's view and the patient's view of what is in the patient's best interest, and this should be resolved in favor of the patient's view whenever possible.

Patient autonomy has become a dominant value in medical decision making.

A competent and informed person has a moral right to choose whether to consent to or to refuse medical interventions.[24] The physician has an obligation to determine the patient's decision-making capacity and to provide him or her with enough information to make an informed decision. If the patient cannot make an informed decision about CPR, the attending physician should consider the patient's advance directives or decisions by appropriate surrogates as well as the patient's likely response to CPR.

By using advance directives, competent patients can indicate what interventions they wish to refuse or accept should they lose the capacity to make decisions about their care. Advance directives include conversations, written directives, living wills, and durable powers of attorney for health care.

Advance directives are often vague and require interpretation and development of a care plan with specific physician's orders (ie, "no CPR"). Physicians should endeavor to have each patient clearly state advance directives, even if the patient's health status is good.

The term *no CPR* is used to request that in the event of a cardiac arrest, no cardiopulmonary resuscitative measures will be instituted. If a no-CPR order is in effect when a patient has a cardiac arrest, no further treatment will be provided.

No-CPR orders do not preclude the administration of other forms of beneficial medical therapy (eg, oxygen, IV fluids), nor do they preclude resuscitative efforts (eg, volume therapy or administration of antiarrhythmics) before the development of cardiac arrest.[25] In some communities the term *DNAR (Do Not Attempt Resuscitation)* is used synonymously with *no CPR*.

The physician must obtain informed consent for writing a no-CPR order or provide informed disclosure in cases where it can be shown that CPR is of no physiological benefit.[26] The order should be

discussed with the patient's family, as appropriate.

The right to refuse care does not mean that the patient has the right to demand nonbeneficial treatments. However, it is often difficult to determine if a resuscitative attempt will be futile or of no benefit to the patient. The determination of efficacy or futility should be based on physiological outcome criteria, not quality-of-life criteria.

As far as is reasonably possible, medical decision making should be based on the results of well-designed research trials that include a sufficient number of cases to determine the likelihood of a benefit from CPR.[27]

Instituting and Discontinuing CPR

Determination of Death in the Prehospital Setting

For patients who experience sudden cardiac arrest, prompt initiation of CPR remains the standard of care except when rigor mortis, lividity, tissue decomposition, or obviously fatal trauma are present — because these conditions are reliably used in the determination of death.[25] Unwitnessed death in the presence of serious, chronic, debilitating disease in the terminal stage of a fatal illness may be used as a criterion for not instituting CPR.[28] Successful resuscitation is rarely achieved for patients in traumatic cardiac arrest except under specific clinical conditions.[29-32]

For patients with valid no-CPR orders, CPR should not be initiated in the prehospital setting.[33] Pronouncement of death requires direct communication with physician medical control unless local protocol dictates otherwise.

Brain death cannot be determined by prehospital personnel, and pupil status or other evidence of neurologic activity should not be used to determine death in the prehospital setting.[34] Patients who are hypothermic should be aggressively resuscitated even when long transport times are involved.

Discontinuing BLS

Rescuers who initiate BLS should continue until one of the following occurs:

- Restoration of effective spontaneous circulation and ventilation

- Transfer of care to emergency medical responders or other trained personnel who continue BLS or initiate advanced life support

- Transfer of care to a physician who determines that resuscitation should be discontinued

- Inability to continue resuscitation because of exhaustion, because environmental hazards endanger the rescuer, or because continued resuscitation would jeopardize the lives of others

- Recognition of reliable criteria for determination of death

- Presentation of a valid no-CPR order to the rescuers

There is ongoing debate about the efficacy of BLS beyond 30 minutes in the prehospital setting. Rescuers in remote environments and some BLS ambulance services have long transport times before advanced life support can be instituted. During prolonged resuscitation attempts these providers are not only engaged in a futile effort but also they are unavailable for other calls.

The risk of vehicular accidents during high-speed emergency transport must also be weighed against the likelihood of successful resuscitation after prolonged BLS resuscitative efforts.

State or local EMS authorities should be encouraged to develop protocols for initiation and withdrawal of BLS in areas where advanced life support is not readily available, with appropriate consideration given to local circumstances, resources, and risk to rescuers.

The AHA recommends that defibrillators be included as standard equipment on all ambulances. If a defibrillator or an AED indicates the absence of a shockable rhythm after an adequate trial of CPR, this can provide an additional criterion for withdrawing BLS.[25]

Discontinuing In-Hospital Resuscitation

In-hospital CPR may be withheld or discontinued under the following circumstances:

- No restoration of circulation despite appropriate BLS and an adequate trial of advanced life support

- Deterioration in the patient's vital functions despite maximum therapy, so that no physiological benefit can be expected from basic and advanced life support. For example, CPR would not be expected to restore circulation in a patient who suffered a cardiac arrest despite aggressive vasoactive therapy for septic or cardiogenic shock. Bradycardia and asystole are unlikely to respond to resuscitation in a patient who is receiving high-dose continuous epinephrine infusion at the time of arrest.

- A decline in vital functions in a patient with a terminal condition: large, well-designed studies have shown that these patients do not survive when CPR is provided.[35] For example, when CPR is attempted in patients with metastatic cancer, several large series have reported that no patients survived to hospital discharge.[36]

Often when family members are unwilling to accept an impending death, they will refuse to consent to a no-CPR order. This can create a dilemma for healthcare providers that must be resolved through further interaction with the family. Healthcare providers should not engage in "slow codes" or "sham codes" in which perfunctory CPR is performed. Such deceptive activity will undermine the trust between healthcare providers and patients and should not be attempted. If the family is adamant that resuscitation be attempted and the physician is convinced of its futility, the physician may order an initial attempt at resuscitation to test the responsiveness of the cardiovascular system. This test can be promptly discontinued if it has no benefit.[37-39]

Hospital Policies Regarding CPR

Hospitals are required by the Joint Commission on the Accreditation of Health Care Organizations (JCAHO) to have written policies for no-CPR orders. These policies need to be reviewed periodically to reflect developments in medical technology, changes in guidelines for CPR, or changes in the law.[40,41]

Hospital policies should state that the attending physician is required to write no-CPR orders in the patient's chart. The rationale for the no-CPR order and other specific limits to care should be documented in the progress notes.[42] Oral no-CPR orders can create problems; they may be misunderstood and may place nurses and other healthcare workers in legal jeopardy. If the attending physician is not present, nurses may accept a no-CPR order over the telephone, with the understanding that the physician will sign the order promptly. No-CPR orders should be reviewed periodically, particularly if the patient's condition changes and especially before the patient undergoes anesthesia.[43,44]

A no-CPR order means only that CPR will not be initiated. It does not mean that other care should be limited. These orders should not lead to abandonment of patients or denial of appropriate medical and nursing care. They do not constitute "giving up." For many patients interventions for diagnosis or treatment remain appropriate after a no-CPR order is written.[39]

Hospitals are now required to have advisers, such as ethics committees, that can respond to requests for resolution of ethical questions. Ethics committees traditionally have been consultative and advisory and are effective in organizing educational programs and developing hospital policies and guidelines regarding CPR.[40,41]

CPR in Nursing Homes

Nursing homes should develop and implement institutional guidelines for providing CPR to or withholding CPR from their residents. Care plans for residents should be individualized because CPR may not be indicated for all residents. Guidelines for withholding or initiating CPR should be based on clinical criteria and patient preferences. All patients should be encouraged to state clearly whether they prefer resuscitation should the need arise.[45-47]

Community Systems for Communicating No-CPR Orders

There is often confusion about whether a no-CPR order is transferred from the hospital to the prehospital setting. Prehospital settings include homes, nursing homes, and public places. There are problems with how to identify patients who have a no-CPR order.[48] The most commonly used method is a standard form that is available from health departments, EMS agencies, or physicians. Other methods include the use of a bracelet, an identification card, or a central registry. Healthcare providers and patients should be educated about appropriate documentation and authenticity of various no-CPR orders in their local system.

Sometimes a family may demand CPR despite the presence of a well-documented no-CPR order at the scene of an emergency. It may be appropriate in such cases to begin resuscitation and transport the patient to the hospital. Treatment can be withdrawn when the conflicts are resolved and the authenticity and legitimacy of the no-CPR order are validated.

Sometimes there is confusion about the difference between no-CPR orders and living wills.[49] No-CPR orders are physician orders directed to healthcare personnel specifically to withhold CPR.[25] Living wills are legal documents stating a patient's preference regarding many forms of medical care to be implemented if the patient loses decision-making capacity.[25] Living wills require interpretation and formulation into a medical care plan. Confusion occurs when living wills (not no-CPR orders) are presented to ambulance personnel who provide ECC. Because of their complexity, ambulance personnel often cannot interpret living wills. Living wills often require an assessment of the patient's decision-making capacity, the presence of terminal illness, the identification of proxies, and the formulation of vague requests into specific treatment plans. Generally if a living will is presented to prehospital personnel who are providing resuscitation to a victim of cardiac arrest, prehospital emergency treatment should be initiated or continued, and the patient should be transported to the hospital for interpretation of the living will.

State laws, local ordinances, or EMS policy about the applicability of living wills in the prehospital setting should be reviewed. Advance directives that include written notations by the patient or verbal requests by family members about what the patient would want do not generally meet the procedural requirements for withholding emergency medical care.

Legal Aspects of CPR

While the provision of medical care is guided by the standard of care determined by the medical profession, courts, legislative bodies, and regulatory agencies have increasingly influenced the practice of medicine. State courts have consistently upheld the patient's right to refuse medical care, and state living-will laws provide procedural guidelines for patients who wish to exercise this right to direct their medical care should they lose decision-making capacity. Living wills are statutorily defined documents providing very specific instructions by which people convey their requests in a fashion that is legally enforceable. The Federal Patient Self-determination Act requires various healthcare agencies to inform patients of their rights under state living-will laws.[25,50]

Virtually all 50 states have enacted laws to protect persons who render aid in an emergency from liability. These laws are often termed *Good Samaritan laws* after the biblical story of the Samaritan who stopped to render aid to a stranger while other travelers passed him by (Luke 10: 30-37). These laws are intended to encourage people to render aid in emergencies without fear of litigious consequences.

Good Samaritan laws generally provide that persons who render aid at the scene of an emergency will not be liable for civil damages if they act in good faith and are not specifically compensated for that aid. The persons protected under these laws vary greatly from state to state. In some states the laws apply both to laypersons and healthcare and other professionals who act in an emergency. In other states they apply to only specific healthcare professionals, such as physicians, surgeons, or nurses, or to other professionals, such as firefighters, police officers, school personnel, or lifeguards. In still other states the laws apply to laypersons or emergency service personnel only if they have received certain training in emergency aid.

Some states allow protection only if the aid is provided at the scene of the emergency. In other states protection applies to aid provided at the hospital by persons who are not ED or hospital personnel.

Most Good Samaritan laws provide that the person rendering emergency aid must have provided it in good faith, must not have acted with the expectation of remuneration, must not have been the cause of the emergency, and must not have been willfully or wantonly negligent in providing the aid.

Good Samaritan laws do not generally cover those who teach CPR. But as this manual goes to press, there has not been a successful lawsuit directed against a CPR instructor.

Good Samaritan laws are useful and important tools to encourage the administration of aid in emergencies. As the

Review Questions

1. Two weeks after a difficult and unsuccessful resuscitation, your EMS colleague confides in you that he is unable to stop thinking about the resuscitative effort, is having difficulty sleeping, and appears anxious and depressed. These are most likely signs of

   a. a metabolic abnormality

   b. major psychiatric illness

   c. stress response

   d. a heart attack

2. You are an EMS provider. You receive a 911 call concerning an otherwise healthy 65-year-old man who you confirm has no pulse and is not breathing. Cardiac arrest is estimated to have occurred 3 minutes before your arrival. A family member states that he thinks the patient may have a living will indicating that he has requested DNAR status. However, the family member isn't sure and cannot produce any documents. You should

   a. discuss the case with medical control before intervening

   b. do nothing until ACLS providers arrive

   c. respect the family's wishes and not intervene

   d. initiate CPR and use an AED

3. You are an EMS provider called to the home of a 58-year-old man who does not have a pulse and is not breathing. On further evaluation you note that the victim is cold and has dependent lividity and rigor mortis. Your most appropriate action is to

   a. initiate CPR and use an AED

   b. approach the family to consider DNAR orders

   c. not intervene and confirm your decision with medical control

   d. initiate CPR but withhold AED use

4. You are an emergency physician. BLS transports an 82-year-old woman from the nursing home to the ED. Papers from the nursing home include valid, legal DNAR orders. Shortly after arrival in the ED the patient has a cardiac arrest. Your most appropriate action is to

   a. initiate CPR and use an AED

   b. call the patient's physician and ask advice on how to proceed

   c. not intervene and notify the family of the patient's death

   d. initiate a "slow code"

How did you do?

Answers: **1,** c; **2,** d; **3,** c; **4,** c.

References

1. Becker LB, Ostrander MP, Barrett J, Kondos GT. Outcome of CPR in a large metropolitan area — where are the survivors? *Ann Emerg Med.* 1991;20:355-361.

2. Lombardi G, Gallagher J, Gennis P. Outcome of out-of-hospital cardiac arrest in New York City: the pre-hospital arrest survival evaluation (PHASE) study. *JAMA.* 1994;272:1573-1574.

3. Callaham M, Madsen CD. Relationship of timeliness of paramedic advanced life support interventions to outcome in out-of-hospital cardiac arrest treated by first responders with defibrillator. *Ann Emerg Med.* 1996;27:638-648.

4. Cummins RO, Ornato JP, Thies WH, Pepe PE. Improving survival from sudden cardiac arrest: the "chain of survival" concept; a statement for health professionals from the Advanced Cardiac Life Support Subcommittee and the Emergency Cardiac Care Committee, American Heart Association. *Circulation.* 1991;83:1832-1847.

5. Larsen MP, Eisenberg MS, Cummins RO, Hallstrom AP. Predicting survival from out-of-hospital cardiac arrest: a graphic model. *Ann Emerg Med.* 1993;22:1652-1658.

6. White RD, Vukov LF, Bugliosi TF. Early defibrillation by police: initial experience with measurement of critical time intervals and patient outcome. *Ann Emerg Med.* 1994;23:1009-1013.

7. Willoughby PJ, Caffrey S. Improved survival with an airport-based PAD program. *Circulation.* In press.

8. McKenas DK. On-board defibrillators. *Aviat Space Environ Med.* 1999;70:533.

9. White RD, Hankins DG, Bugliosi TF. Seven years' experience with early defibrillation by police and paramedics in an emergency medical services system. *Resuscitation.* 1998;39:145-151.

10. Valenzuela TD, Roe DJ, Nichol G, Clark LL, Spaite DW. Casino project: implications for public access defibrillation [abstract]. *Academic Emerg Med.* 2000;7:426.

11. Wassertheil J, Keane G, Fisher N, Leditschke JF. Cardiac arrest outcomes at the Melbourne Cricket Ground and Shrine of Remembrance using a tiered response strategy — a forerunner to public access defibrillation. *Resuscitation.* 2000;44:97-104.

12. Ragaisis KM. Critical incident stress debriefing: a family nursing intervention. *Arch Psychiatr Nurs.* 1994;8:38-43.

13. Wong JC, Ursano RJ. Traumatic stress – an overview of diagnostic evolution and clinical treatment. *Ann Acad Med Singapore.* 1997;26:76-87.

14. Bell JL. Traumatic event debriefing: service delivery designs and the role of social work. *Soc Work.* 1995;40:36-43.

15. Curtis JM. Elements of critical incident debriefing. *Psychol Rep.* 1995;77:91-96.

Summary of CPR and Defibrillation: The Human Dimension

Ethical values should guide the initiation and withdrawal of CPR, with patient autonomy and the burden and benefit of treatment considered rather than the threat of legal liability. Patient autonomy is respected by providing appropriate informed consent, allowing surrogate decision making, and honoring valid no-CPR orders. Important differences exist between no-CPR orders, living wills, and other advance directives. Education of physicians, EMS providers, other healthcare personnel, and the public is needed regarding the appropriate indications for instituting, withholding, and withdrawing CPR.[25]

There has never been a lawsuit in which a lay rescuer was found guilty of doing harm in attempting CPR on a victim of cardiac arrest. There has never been a lawsuit in which a professional responder was found guilty of doing harm in using an AED on a victim of cardiac arrest. Almost all states have added AED use to their Good Samaritan laws so that a lay rescuer will be immune from legal action.[52]

Summary of Key Concepts

- Most out-of-hospital CPR attempts are likely to be unsuccessful.

- Very early defibrillation with AEDs may substantially improve rates of successful resuscitation in the prehospital setting.

- Difficulty sleeping, fatigue, irritability, changes in eating habits, and confusion can be signs of a stress reaction.

- Psychologists have learned that the most successful way to reduce stress after rescue efforts is to talk about it.

- Critical incident stress debriefing (CISD) is a confidential group process in which a facilitator encourages persons involved in a stressful situation to express their thoughts and feelings about the event.

- Psychological barriers to CPR may include fear of imperfect performance, fear of responsibility, concerns about modesty, anxiety, guilt, and fear of infection.

- Autonomy is the principle that a person should be free to make his or her own decisions.

- Beneficence is the principle of doing good.

- An advance directive is a legal document stating an individual's healthcare choices or naming someone to make those choices should the individual be unable to do so.

- A living will and durable power of attorney for health care are examples of advance directives. A living will is a document directing healthcare providers to withhold certain life-sustaining procedures in the event of a terminal condition or inability to independently make those choices. Durable power of attorney for health care is a document naming another person to make healthcare decisions if the person is unable to do so.

- The term *DNAR* (also called *no CPR*) means that in the event of a cardiac arrest, no cardiopulmonary resuscitative measures (no CPR attempts) should be instituted.

- Criteria for discontinuing BLS efforts include (1) restoration of effective spontaneous circulation and ventilation, (2) transfer of care to emergency medical responders, (3) the rescuer is physically unable to continue resuscitation (or to do so would jeopardize the life of the rescuer or others), (4) recognition of reliable criteria for determination of death, or (5) presentation of a valid no-CPR order to the rescuers.

- Criteria for discontinuing CPR in-hospital include (1) failure to restore circulation despite appropriate BLS and an adequate trial of ACLS, (2) deterioration in the patient's vital functions despite maximum therapy, with no anticipated benefit from BLS and ACLS, or (3) the patient has a terminal condition for which studies have shown no benefit of CPR.

- CPR and AED use should be promptly instituted for patients in cardiac arrest with these important exceptions: (1) the presence of a no-CPR order, (2) the presence of reliable criteria for determination of death, or (3) the reliable prediction of no benefit.

- Establishing and understanding DNAR policies is important for healthcare providers in the out-of-hospital, in-hospital, and nursing home settings.

- Good Samaritan laws generally provide that persons who render aid at the scene of an emergency will not be liable for civil damages if they act in good faith, and not for remuneration, in rendering aid.

- Most states have changed existing laws and regulations to include use of AEDs under the Good Samaritan law. Because of state-to-state variation, it is important to know the laws in your state for both CPR and AED use and how they apply specifically to you.

- BLS is a fundamental area of medical science that requires sound, scientific investigation to continue to improve the quality, delivery, and outcome of BLS.

Review Questions

1. Two weeks after a difficult and unsuccessful resuscitation, your EMS colleague confides in you that he is unable to stop thinking about the resuscitative effort, is having difficulty sleeping, and appears anxious and depressed. These are most likely signs of

   a. a metabolic abnormality

   b. major psychiatric illness

   c. stress response

   d. a heart attack

2. You are an EMS provider. You receive a 911 call concerning an otherwise healthy 65-year-old man who you confirm has no pulse and is not breathing. Cardiac arrest is estimated to have occurred 3 minutes before your arrival. A family member states that he thinks the patient may have a living will indicating that he has requested DNAR status. However, the family member isn't sure and cannot produce any documents. You should

   a. discuss the case with medical control before intervening

   b. do nothing until ACLS providers arrive

   c. respect the family's wishes and not intervene

   d. initiate CPR and use an AED

3. You are an EMS provider called to the home of a 58-year-old man who does not have a pulse and is not breathing. On further evaluation you note that the victim is cold and has dependent lividity and rigor mortis. Your most appropriate action is to

   a. initiate CPR and use an AED

   b. approach the family to consider DNAR orders

   c. not intervene and confirm your decision with medical control

   d. initiate CPR but withhold AED use

4. You are an emergency physician. BLS transports an 82-year-old woman from the nursing home to the ED. Papers from the nursing home include valid, legal DNAR orders. Shortly after arrival in the ED the patient has a cardiac arrest. Your most appropriate action is to

   a. initiate CPR and use an AED

   b. call the patient's physician and ask advice on how to proceed

   c. not intervene and notify the family of the patient's death

   d. initiate a "slow code"

How did you do?

Answers: **1,** c; **2,** d; **3,** c; **4,** c.

References

1. Becker LB, Ostrander MP, Barrett J, Kondos GT. Outcome of CPR in a large metropolitan area — where are the survivors? *Ann Emerg Med.* 1991;20:355-361.

2. Lombardi G, Gallagher J, Gennis P. Outcome of out-of-hospital cardiac arrest in New York City: the pre-hospital arrest survival evaluation (PHASE) study. *JAMA.* 1994;272:1573-1574.

3. Callaham M, Madsen CD. Relationship of timeliness of paramedic advanced life support interventions to outcome in out-of-hospital cardiac arrest treated by first responders with defibrillator. *Ann Emerg Med.* 1996;27:638-648.

4. Cummins RO, Ornato JP, Thies WH, Pepe PE. Improving survival from sudden cardiac arrest: the "chain of survival" concept; a statement for health professionals from the Advanced Cardiac Life Support Subcommittee and the Emergency Cardiac Care Committee, American Heart Association. *Circulation.* 1991;83:1832-1847.

5. Larsen MP, Eisenberg MS, Cummins RO, Hallstrom AP. Predicting survival from out-of-hospital cardiac arrest: a graphic model. *Ann Emerg Med.* 1993;22:1652-1658.

6. White RD, Vukov LF, Bugliosi TF. Early defibrillation by police: initial experience with measurement of critical time intervals and patient outcome. *Ann Emerg Med.* 1994;23:1009-1013.

7. Willoughby PJ, Caffrey S. Improved survival with an airport-based PAD program. *Circulation.* In press.

8. McKenas DK. On-board defibrillators. *Aviat Space Environ Med.* 1999;70:533.

9. White RD, Hankins DG, Bugliosi TF. Seven years' experience with early defibrillation by police and paramedics in an emergency medical services system. *Resuscitation.* 1998;39:145-151.

10. Valenzuela TD, Roe DJ, Nichol G, Clark LL, Spaite DW. Casino project: implications for public access defibrillation [abstract]. *Academic Emerg Med.* 2000;7:426.

11. Wassertheil J, Keane G, Fisher N, Leditschke JF. Cardiac arrest outcomes at the Melbourne Cricket Ground and Shrine of Remembrance using a tiered response strategy — a forerunner to public access defibrillation. *Resuscitation.* 2000;44:97-104.

12. Ragaisis KM. Critical incident stress debriefing: a family nursing intervention. *Arch Psychiatr Nurs.* 1994;8:38-43.

13. Wong JC, Ursano RJ. Traumatic stress – an overview of diagnostic evolution and clinical treatment. *Ann Acad Med Singapore.* 1997;26:76-87.

14. Bell JL. Traumatic event debriefing: service delivery designs and the role of social work. *Soc Work.* 1995;40:36-43.

15. Curtis JM. Elements of critical incident debriefing. *Psychol Rep.* 1995;77:91-96.

CPR in Nursing Homes

Nursing homes should develop and implement institutional guidelines for providing CPR to or withholding CPR from their residents. Care plans for residents should be individualized because CPR may not be indicated for all residents. Guidelines for withholding or initiating CPR should be based on clinical criteria and patient preferences. All patients should be encouraged to state clearly whether they prefer resuscitation should the need arise.[45-47]

Community Systems for Communicating No-CPR Orders

There is often confusion about whether a no-CPR order is transferred from the hospital to the prehospital setting. Prehospital settings include homes, nursing homes, and public places. There are problems with how to identify patients who have a no-CPR order.[48] The most commonly used method is a standard form that is available from health departments, EMS agencies, or physicians. Other methods include the use of a bracelet, an identification card, or a central registry. Healthcare providers and patients should be educated about appropriate documentation and authenticity of various no-CPR orders in their local system.

Sometimes a family may demand CPR despite the presence of a well-documented no-CPR order at the scene of an emergency. It may be appropriate in such cases to begin resuscitation and transport the patient to the hospital. Treatment can be withdrawn when the conflicts are resolved and the authenticity and legitimacy of the no-CPR order are validated.

Sometimes there is confusion about the difference between no-CPR orders and living wills.[49] No-CPR orders are physician orders directed to healthcare personnel specifically to withhold CPR.[25] Living wills are legal documents stating a patient's preference regarding many forms of medical care to be implemented if the patient loses decision-making capacity.[25] Living wills require interpretation and formulation into a medical care plan. Confusion occurs when living wills (not no-CPR orders) are presented to ambulance personnel who provide ECC. Because of their complexity, ambulance personnel often cannot interpret living wills. Living wills often require an assessment of the patient's decision-making capacity, the presence of terminal illness, the identification of proxies, and the formulation of vague requests into specific treatment plans. Generally if a living will is presented to prehospital personnel who are providing resuscitation to a victim of cardiac arrest, prehospital emergency treatment should be initiated or continued, and the patient should be transported to the hospital for interpretation of the living will.

State laws, local ordinances, or EMS policy about the applicability of living wills in the prehospital setting should be reviewed. Advance directives that include written notations by the patient or verbal requests by family members about what the patient would want do not generally meet the procedural requirements for withholding emergency medical care.

Legal Aspects of CPR

While the provision of medical care is guided by the standard of care determined by the medical profession, courts, legislative bodies, and regulatory agencies have increasingly influenced the practice of medicine. State courts have consistently upheld the patient's right to refuse medical care, and state living-will laws provide procedural guidelines for patients who wish to exercise this right to direct their medical care should they lose decision-making capacity. Living wills are statutorily defined documents providing very specific instructions by which people convey their requests in a fashion that is legally enforceable. The Federal Patient Self-determination Act requires various healthcare agencies to inform patients of their rights under state living-will laws.[25,50]

Virtually all 50 states have enacted laws to protect persons who render aid in an emergency from liability. These laws are often termed *Good Samaritan laws* after the biblical story of the Samaritan who stopped to render aid to a stranger while other travelers passed him by (Luke 10: 30-37). These laws are intended to encourage people to render aid in emergencies without fear of litigious consequences.

Good Samaritan laws generally provide that persons who render aid at the scene of an emergency will not be liable for civil damages if they act in good faith and are not specifically compensated for that aid. The persons protected under these laws vary greatly from state to state. In some states the laws apply both to laypersons and healthcare and other professionals who act in an emergency. In other states they apply to only specific healthcare professionals, such as physicians, surgeons, or nurses, or to other professionals, such as firefighters, police officers, school personnel, or lifeguards. In still other states the laws apply to laypersons or emergency service personnel only if they have received certain training in emergency aid.

Some states allow protection only if the aid is provided at the scene of the emergency. In other states protection applies to aid provided at the hospital by persons who are not ED or hospital personnel.

Most Good Samaritan laws provide that the person rendering emergency aid must have provided it in good faith, must not have acted with the expectation of remuneration, must not have been the cause of the emergency, and must not have been willfully or wantonly negligent in providing the aid.

Good Samaritan laws do not generally cover those who teach CPR. But as this manual goes to press, there has not been a successful lawsuit directed against a CPR instructor.

Good Samaritan laws are useful and important tools to encourage the administration of aid in emergencies. As the above summary illustrates, however, the laws vary significantly from state to state. Healthcare and emergency personnel, as well as others who may require CPR, should determine whether their state has a Good Samaritan law, and if so, determine the persons and activities protected by that law.

Legal Aspects of AED Use

Defibrillators, including AEDs, are restricted medical devices. Most states currently have legislation that permits the use of AEDs by laypeople when prescribed by a physician. These laws vary from state to state, but most have provisions of Good Samaritan protection for the user of an AED. Many states have specifically added the inclusion of Good Samaritan limited immunity to AED owners, physicians who prescribe the use of an AED or provide oversight for AED programs, and educators who train AED providers. AED laws may also provide for requirements associated with implementation of a program, including physician oversight, training, device maintenance, and notification of the EMS system.[51]

In the United States fear of malpractice accusations and product liability lawsuits increases every year. Innovative programs to bring early CPR and early defibrillation into every community have fallen under the shadow of this fear.[51] Physicians, trainers, program directors, corporation heads, and legal counsel for many groups have often refused to support early defibrillation programs for fear of being involved in a lawsuit. Without medical authority lay rescuers cannot use an AED. Yet physicians may be reluctant to support programs that place defibrillators in homes, worksites, and public places if doing so exposes them to legal risk. Likewise, lay rescuers, even with physician authorization, fear being sued if they try to help someone by using an AED and "something goes wrong."

This problem is now being solved because most states are changing existing laws and regulations.[52] Many legislators are amending Good Samaritan laws to include the use of AEDs by lay rescuers.[52] This means that lay rescuers will be considered Good Samaritans when they attempt CPR and defibrillation on someone in cardiac arrest.

As a Good Samaritan the lay rescuer cannot be successfully sued for any harm or damage that occurs during the rescue effort (except in cases of gross negligence).

In most PAD legislation, layperson immunity from lawsuits is granted only when specific recommendations are fulfilled. These recommendations state that the rescuer must

- Have formal training in CPR and use of an AED (a nationally recognized course, such as the AHA Heartsaver AED Course or its equivalent, may be recommended)

- Use treatment protocols such as the CPR-AED algorithm that are approved by a medical authority

- Perform routine checks and maintenance on the AED (or use an AED that has undergone these checks)

- Notify local EMS authorities of AED placement so that EMS personnel, particularly the EMS dispatcher, are aware that the 911 caller is in a setting in which an AED is available

- Report actual use of the AED to EMS authorities (reporting is usually done by phoning 911)

During this course the instructor will briefly discuss the limited legal immunity in your state for performing CPR and using an AED and what you should do to report any clinical event in which an AED was used. You also will need to know who the medical authority is (often the medical director of your EMS system or the medical advisor to your worksite).

BLS Research Initiatives

The ongoing success and improvement of BLS programs require sound scientific research. Because of the lack of scientific data in some areas, many current guidelines are based on a consensus derived from limited published data, some clinical experience, and clinical judgment. Research in BLS is a fertile area for education, public health, and clinical and basic science investigators. A number of potential areas of investigation were identified during the Guidelines 2000 Conference.

Barriers to CPR learning, various educational approaches to training, alternative BLS teaching aids, definition of populations being trained in CPR, and the relation of quality of CPR performance to patient outcome are issues to be addressed by education researchers.

EMS and public health investigators can improve BLS knowledge through studies of public awareness and action in obtaining early access to EMS systems. To facilitate this public awareness, it is important to learn how CPR is perceived and accepted by members of various socioeconomic and cultural groups.

It is important to emphasize the need for controlled scientific studies that evaluate all the current recommendations for ventilation and circulation. The impact and effectiveness of devices presently available for CPR and ventilation should be defined. Only through such studies can educated decisions be made for improvement of CPR.

Although knowledge has grown considerably in the last 25 years, BLS is a fundamental area of medical science with many more questions that remain to be investigated. Future changes and advances in CPR based on sound scientific investigation will likely improve the quality, delivery, and outcome of BLS.

16. Berkowitz LL. Breaking down the barriers: improving physician buy-in of CPR systems. *Health Inform.* 1997;14:73-76.

17. Locke CJ, Berg RA, Sanders AB, Davis MF, Milander MM, Kern KB, Ewy GA. Bystander cardiopulmonary resuscitation: concerns about mouth-to-mouth contact. *Arch Intern Med.* 1995;155:938-943.

18. Rowe BH, Shuster M, Zambon S, Wilson E, Stewart D, Nolan RP, Webster K. Preparation, attitudes, and behaviour in nonhospital cardiac emergencies: evaluating a community's readiness to act. *Can J Cardiol.* 1998;14:371-377.

19. Flint LS Jr, Billi JE, Kelly K, Mandel L, Newell L, Stapleton ER. Education in adult basic life support training programs. *Ann Emerg Med.* 1993;22:468-474.

20. Hamburg RS. Public policy solutions sought for emergency care. *J Cardiovasc Nurs.* 1996;10:85-92.

21. Becker L, Eisenberg M, Fahrenbruch C, Cobb L. Public locations of cardiac arrest: implications for public access defibrillation. *Circulation.* 1998;97:2106-2109.

22. Aufderheide TP, Stapleton ER, Hazinski MF, Cummins RO. *Heartsaver AED: Handbook for the Lay Rescuer.* Dallas, Tex: American Heart Association: 1998.

23. Jonsen AR, Siegler M, Winslade WJ. *Clinical Ethics: A Practical Approach to Ethical Decisions in Clinical Medicine.* 2nd ed. New York, NY: Macmillan Publishing Co Inc; 1986:102-109.

24. The Hastings Center. *Guidelines on the Termination of Life-Sustaining Treatment and the Care of the Dying: A Report.* Briarcliff Manor, NY: The Hastings Center; 1987:16-34.

25. Marco CA. Ethical issues of resuscitation. *Emerg Med Clin North Am.* 1999;17:527-538.

26. Moskop JC. Informed consent in the emergency department. *Emerg Med Clin North Am.* 1999;17:327-340.

27. Tomlinson T, Brody H. Futility and the ethics of resuscitation. *JAMA.* 1990;264:1276-1280.

28. Kellerman AL, Hackman BB, Somes G. Predicting the outcome of unsuccessful prehospital advanced cardiac life support. *JAMA.* 1993;270:1433-1436.

29. Cogbill TH, Moore EE, Millikan JS, Cleveland HC. Rationale for selective application of emergency department thoracotomy in trauma. *J Trauma.* 1983;23:453-460.

30. Bickell WH, Wall MJ Jr, Pepe PE, Martin RR, Ginger VF, Allen MK, Mattox KL. Immediate versus delayed fluid resuscitation for hypotensive patients with penetrating torso injuries. *N Engl J Med.* 1994;331:1105-1109.

31. Rosemurgy AS, Norris PA, Olson SM, Hurst JM, Albrink MH. Prehospital traumatic cardiac arrest: the cost of futility. *J Trauma.* 1993;35: 468-473.

32. Hazinski MF, Chahine AA, Holcomb GW III, Morris JA Jr. Outcome of cardiovascular collapse in pediatric blunt trauma. A*nn Emerg Med.* 1994;23:1229-1235.

33. Guidelines for 'do not resuscitate' orders in the prehospital setting: American College of Emergency Physicians. *Ann Emerg Med.* 1988;17: 1106-1108.

34. Report of a special task force. Guidelines for the determination of brain death in children: American Academy of Pediatrics Task Force on Brain Death in Children. *Pediatrics.* 1987; 80:298-300.

35. Marik PE, Craft M. An outcome analysis of in-hospital cardiopulmonary resuscitation: the futility rationale for do not resuscitate orders. *J Crit Care.* 1997;12:142-146.

36. Faber-Langendoen K. Resuscitation of patients with metastatic cancer: is a transient benefit still futile? *Arch Intern Med.* 1991;151:235-239.

37. Blackhall LJ. Must we always use CPR? *N Engl J Med.* 1987;317:1281-1285.

38. Muller JH. Shades of blue: the negotiation of limited codes by medical residents. *Soc Sci Med.* 1992;34:885-898.

39. Schears RM. Emergency physician's role in end-of-life care. *Emerg Med Clin North Am.* 1999;17:539-559.

40. Teres D. Trends from the United States with end of life decisions in the intensive care unit. *Intensive Care Med.* 1993;19:316-322.

41. Rasooly I, Lavery JV, Urowitz S, Choudhry S, Seeman N, Meslin EM, Lowy FH, Singer PA. Hospital policies on life-sustaining treatments and advance directives in Canada. *CMAJ.* 1994;150:1265-1270.

42. Lo B. Unanswered questions about DNR orders. *JAMA.* 1991;265:1874-1875.

43. Layon AJ, Dirk L. Resuscitation and DNR: ethical aspects for anaesthetists. *Can J Anaesth.* 1995;42:134-140.

44. Lonchyna VA. To resuscitate or not — in the operating room: the need for hospital policies for surgeons regarding DNR orders. *Ann Health Law.* 1997;6:209-227.

45. Levin JR, Wenger NS, Ouslander JG, Zellman G, Schnelle JF, Buchanan JL, Hirsch SH, Reuben DB. Life-sustaining treatment decisions for nursing home residents: who discusses, who decides and what is decided? *J Am Geriatr Soc.* 1999;47:82-87.

46. Low JA, Yap KB, Chan KM, Tang T. Care of elderly patients with DNR orders in Singapore — a descriptive study. *Singapore Med J.* 1998;39:456-460.

47. Teno JM, Branco KJ, Mor V, Phillips CD, Hawes C, Morris J, Fries BE. Changes in advance care planning in nursing homes before and after the patient Self-Determination Act: report of a 10-state survey. *J Am Geriatr Soc.* 1997;45:939-944.

48. Crimmins TJ. The need for a prehospital DNR system. *Prehosp Disaster Med.* 1990;5:47-48.

49. O'Brien LA, Grisso JA, Maislin G, LaPann K, Krotki KP, Greco PJ, Siegert EA, Evans LK. Nursing home residents' preferences for life-sustaining treatments. *JAMA.* 1995;274:1775-1779.

50. Wolf SM, Boyle P, Callahan D, Fins JJ, Jennings B, Nelson JL, Barondess JA, Brock DW, Dresser R, Emanuel L, Johnson S, Lantos J, Mason DCR, Mezey M, Orentlicher D, Rouse F. Sources of concern about the Patient Self- Determination Act. *N Engl J Med.* 1991; 325:1666-1671.

51. Lazar RA. Legal, regulatory issues impact AED (automated external defibrillator) deployment. *J Emerg Med Serv.* 1997;22:S21-S22.

52. Smith SC Jr, Hamburg RS. Automated external defibrillators: time for federal and state advocacy and broader utilization. *Circulation.* 1998;97:1321-1324.

Comparison Across Age Groups of Resuscitation Interventions

CPR/Rescue Breathing	Adult and Older Child	Child (≈1-8 y old)	Infant (<1 y old)	Newly Born
Establish unresponsiveness, activate EMS				
Open airway (Head tilt–chin lift or jaw thrust	Head tilt–chin lift (If trauma is present, use jaw thrust)	Head tilt–chin lift (If trauma is present, use jaw thrust)	Head tilt–chin lift (If trauma is present, use jaw thrust)	Head tilt–chin lift (If trauma is present, use jaw thrust)
Check for breathing: (Look, listen, feel) If victim is breathing: place in recovery position If victim is not breathing: give 2 effective slow breaths				
Initial	2 effective breaths at 2 sec/breath (unless oxygen available)	2 effective breaths at 1 to 1½ sec/breath	2 effective breaths at 1 to 1½ sec/breath	2 effective breaths at ≈1 sec/breath
Subsequent	12 breaths/min (approximate)	20 breaths/min (approximate)	20 breaths/min (approximate)	30 to 60 breaths/min (approximate)
Foreign-body airway obstruction	Abdominal thrusts	Abdominal thrusts	Back blows and chest thrusts (no abdominal thrusts)	Back blows and chest thrusts (no abdominal thrusts)
Signs of circulation: Check for breathing, coughing, movement, or pulse If signs of circulation are present: provide airway and breathing support If signs of circulation are absent: begin chest compressions interposed with breaths	Pulse check (healthcare providers)* Carotid	(Healthcare providers)* Carotid	(Healthcare providers)* Brachial	(Healthcare providers)* Umbilical
Compression landmarks	Lower half of sternum	Lower half of sternum	Lower half of sternum (1 finger's width below intermammary line)	Lower half of sternum (1 finger's width below intermammary line)
Compression method	Heel of one hand, other hand on top	Heel of one hand	2 fingers or 2 thumb–encircling hands for 2-rescuer trained providers	2 fingers or 2 thumb–encircling hands for 2-rescuer trained providers
Compression depth	≈1½ to 2 in (4 to 5 cm)	≈⅓ to ½ the depth of the chest	≈⅓ to ½ the depth of the chest	≈⅓ the depth of the chest for newly born
Compression rate	≈100/min	≈100/min	≥100/min	≈120 events/min (90 compressions/ 30 breaths)
Compression-ventilation ratio	15:2 (1 or 2 rescuers, unprotected airway) 12 to 15 breaths/min asynchronous with compressions (2 rescuers, protected airway)	5:1 (1 or 2 rescuers)	5:1 (1 or 2 rescuers)	3:1 (1 or 2 rescuers)

*Pulse check is performed as one of the signs of circulation assessed by healthcare providers. Lay rescuers check for other signs of circulation (breathing, coughing, movement).

Skills Performance Sheets

The skills performance sheets serve two purposes. First and most important, the participant should use them to prepare and reinforce essential skills. Second, they are used to evaluate participant performance for satisfactory course completion.

Integrated Skills Evaluation Sheets are preferred for evaluation of healthcare providers. *Note that the healthcare provider should be able to demonstrate rescue breathing with mouth-to-mouth (or mouth-to–nose-and-mouth) ventilation, mouth-to–barrier device ventilation (with and without oxygen), and bag-mask ventilation.* Healthcare providers should use the ventilation devices used in their healthcare settings to increase their familiarity and facility with that device.

For AED skills performance sheets, ask 1 participant to act as timekeeper. This participant should time the collapse-to-shock interval (should be less than 3 minutes for healthcare providers) and the AED arrival–to-shock interval (should be less than 90 seconds). An interval of less than 90 seconds from arrival at the victim's side to delivery of a shock confirms that the rescuer is able to operate the AED efficiently.

The Integrated Skills Performance Sheets are designed to create a streamlined approach to evaluation. To demonstrate successful course completion, the healthcare provider must be able to perform 17 skills (including rescue breathing: mouth-to-mouth, mouth-to–barrier device, and bag-mask ventilation). Evaluation of each individual skill would require excessive time and thus detract from the practice of skills. For this reason integrated skills checklists have been developed as evaluation tools for the healthcare provider. These checklists are used to document the following skills demonstrations:

1. Integrated adult 1- and 2-rescuer CPR

2. Integrated rescue breathing and relief of adult FBAO in the responsive and unresponsive victim

3. Integrated mouth-to-mask ventilation and CPR with use of an AED

4. Adult bag-mask ventilation (to be demonstrated during the integrated scenario)

5. Integrated relief of child FBAO in the responsive and unresponsive victim, CPR, and rescue breathing

6. Integrated relief of infant FBAO in the responsive and unresponsive victim, CPR, and rescue breathing

7. Child bag-mask ventilation (can be demonstrated during the integrated scenario)

8. Infant bag-mask ventilation (can be demonstrated during the integrated scenario)

The instructor should copy and distribute these simple skills performance sheets at each class for use during participant preparation and peer practice sessions. Participants will benefit from a review of important skills before the class to establish mental imagery and sequencing before skills practice. The checklists can also reinforce skills after the CPR course.

American Heart Association®

Learn and Live sm

Appendix B
BLS Performance Criteria

Healthcare Provider Skills Performance Sheet
Adult 1-Rescuer CPR
Performance Criteria

Participant Name _____ Date _____

Performance Guidelines	Performed
1. Establish unresponsiveness. Activate the emergency response system.	
2. Open the airway (head tilt–chin lift or jaw thrust). Check breathing (look, listen, and feel).*	
3. If breathing is absent or inadequate, give 2 slow breaths (2 seconds per breath),† ensure adequate chest rise, and allow for exhalation between breaths.	
4. Check for carotid pulse and other signs of circulation (breathing, coughing, or movement in response to the 2 rescue breaths). If signs of circulation are present but breathing is absent or inadequate, provide rescue breathing (1 breath every 5 seconds, about 10 to 12 breaths per minute).†	
5. If no signs of circulation are present, begin cycles of 15 chest compressions (rate of about 100 compressions per minute) followed by 2 slow breaths.†	
6. After 4 cycles of compressions and ventilations (15:2 ratio, about 1 minute), recheck for carotid pulse and other signs of circulation. If no signs of circulation are present, continue 15:2 cycles of compressions and ventilations, beginning with chest compressions. If signs of circulation are present but breathing is absent or inadequate, continue rescue breathing (1 breath every 5 seconds, or about 10 to 12 breaths per minute).*†	

*If the victim is breathing or resumes adequate breathing and no trauma is suspected, place in the recovery position.

†If mouth-to-mask or bag-mask ventilation is provided **with supplementary oxygen,** smaller tidal volumes can be used but the chest should still rise. If ventilation is provided and there is a pulse, monitor oxygen saturation (if available).

Comments _____

_____

_____

_____

Instructor _____

Circle one: Complete   Needs more practice

Appendix B
BLS Performance Criteria

American Heart
Association®

Learn and Live sm

Healthcare Provider Skills Performance Sheet
Adult Bag-Mask Ventilation
Performance Criteria

Participant Name _____ Date _____

Performance Guidelines	Performed
1. Establish unresponsiveness. Activate the emergency response system.	
2. Open the airway (head tilt–chin lift or jaw thrust). Check breathing (look, listen, and feel).*	
3. If breathing is absent or inadequate, properly position the mask to achieve an effective seal while holding the airway open.	
4. Give 2 slow breaths (2 seconds per breath), ensure adequate chest rise, and allow for exhalation between breaths.*	
5. Check for carotid pulse and other signs of circulation (breathing, coughing, movement in response to the 2 rescue breaths). If signs of circulation are present but breathing is absent or inadequate, provide rescue breathing (1 breath every 5 seconds, about 10 to 12 breaths per minute).† If signs of circulation are absent, begin cycles of 15 chest compressions (rate of about 100 compressions per minute) with 2 rescue breaths.	

*If the victim is breathing or resumes adequate breathing and no trauma is suspected, place in the recovery position.

†If mouth-to-mask or bag-mask ventilation is provided **with supplementary oxygen,** smaller tidal volumes can be used but the chest should still rise. If ventilation is provided and a pulse is present, monitor oxygen saturation (if available).

Comments _____

_____

_____

Instructor _____

Circle one: Complete   Needs more practice

American Heart Association®

Learn and Live sm

Appendix B
BLS Performance Criteria

Healthcare Provider Skills Performance Sheet
Adult 2-Rescuer CPR
Performance Criteria

Participant Name _____ Date _____

Performance Guidelines	Performed
1. Establish unresponsiveness. One rescuer should activate the emergency response system.	
Rescuer 1	
2. Open the airway (head tilt–chin lift or jaw thrust). Check breathing (look, listen, and feel).*	
3. If breathing is absent or inadequate, give 2 slow breaths (2 seconds per breath), ensure effective chest rise, and allow for exhalation between breaths.†	
4. Check for carotid pulse and other signs of circulation (breathing, coughing, or movement in response to the 2 rescue breaths). If signs of circulation are present but breathing is absent or inadequate, provide rescue breathing 1 breath every 5 seconds, about 10 to 12 breaths per minute).†	
Rescuer 2	
5. If no signs of circulation are present, give cycles of 15 chest compressions (rate of about 100 compressions per minute) followed by 2 slow breaths given by Rescuer 1.* Start compressions after chest rise (inspiration) from second breath.	
6. After 4 cycles of compressions and breaths (15:2 ratio, about 1 minute), Rescuer 1 delivers 2 rescue breaths and rechecks for signs of circulation (carotid pulse, normal breathing, cough, movement, or response to stimulation).* If no signs of circulation are present, continue 15:2 cycles of compressions and ventilations, beginning with chest compressions until an AED or emergency medical response team arrives.	

*If the victim is breathing or resumes adequate breathing and no trauma is suspected, place in the recovery position.

†If mouth-to-mask or bag-mask ventilation is provided **with supplementary oxygen,** smaller tidal volumes can be used but the chest should still rise. If ventilation is provided and a pulse is present, monitor oxygen saturation (if available).

Comments _____

_____

Instructor _____

Circle one: Complete   Needs more practice

Appendix B
BLS Performance Criteria

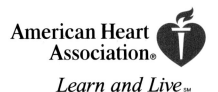

American Heart Association®

Learn and Live ℠

Healthcare Provider Skills Performance Sheet
Adult FBAO in Responsive Victim
(and Responsive Victim Who Becomes Unresponsive)
Performance Criteria

Participant Name _____ Date _____

Performance Guidelines	Performed
1. Ask "Are you choking?" If yes, ask "Can you speak?" If no, tell the victim you are going to help.	
2. Give abdominal thrusts with proper hand position (chest thrusts for victim who is pregnant or obese), avoiding compressions on the lower sternum (xiphoid).	
3. Repeat thrusts until the object is expelled (obstruction relieved) or the victim becomes unresponsive.	

Adult Foreign-Body Airway Obstruction — Victim Becomes Unresponsive	
4. Activate the emergency response system.	
5. Open the airway with a tongue-jaw lift; perform a finger sweep to remove the foreign object.	
6. Open the airway and try to ventilate; if it is still obstructed (chest does not rise), reopen the airway (reposition head and chin) and try to ventilate again.	
7. If ventilation is unsuccessful, provide 5 abdominal thrusts with the victim supine. Ensure proper hand position, avoiding the lower sternum (xiphoid).	
8. Repeat steps 5 through 7 until rescue breathing is effective, then continue the steps of CPR as needed.*	

*If the victim is breathing or resumes adequate breathing and no trauma is suspected, place in the recovery position.

Comments _____

_____

_____

_____

Instructor _____

Circle one: Complete   Needs more practice

Appendix B
BLS Performance Criteria

American Heart Association®

Learn and Live sm

Healthcare Provider Skills Performance Sheet
Adult FBAO in Unresponsive Victim
Performance Criteria

Participant Name _____ Date _____

Performance Guidelines	Performed
1. Establish unresponsiveness. Activate the emergency response system. If a second rescuer is available, send that rescuer to activate the emergency response system while you remain with the victim.	
2. Open the airway (head tilt–chin lift or jaw thrust) and check breathing. If breathing is absent or inadequate, go to step 3.	
3. Attempt to ventilate; if unsuccessful (chest does not rise), reopen the airway (reposition head and chin) and try to ventilate again.	
4. If ventilation is unsuccessful, perform up to 5 abdominal thrusts with the victim supine. Ensure proper hand position, avoiding the lower sternum (xiphoid).	
5. Open the airway with a tongue-jaw lift followed by a finger sweep to attempt to remove the object.	
6. Repeat steps 3 through 5 until ventilation is effective (chest rises), then continue the steps of CPR as needed.*	

*If the victim is breathing or resumes adequate breathing and no trauma is suspected, place in the recovery position.

Comments _____

_____

_____

_____

Instructor _____

Circle one: Complete   Needs more practice

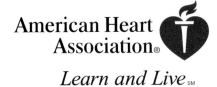

Appendix B
BLS Performance Criteria

Healthcare Provider Skills Performance Sheet
Infant 1-Rescuer CPR
Performance Criteria

Participant Name _____ Date _____

Performance Guidelines	Performed
1. Establish unresponsiveness. If a bystander is available, send that person to activate the emergency response system.	
2. Open the airway (head tilt–chin lift or jaw thrust). Check breathing (look, listen, and feel).*	
3. If breathing is absent or inadequate, give 2 slow effective rescue breaths (1 to 1½ seconds per breath), ensure adequate chest rise, and allow for exhalation between breaths.	
4. Check for brachial pulse and other signs of circulation (breathing, coughing, or movement in response to the 2 initial rescue breaths). If signs of circulation are present but breathing is absent or inadequate, provide rescue breathing (1 breath every 3 seconds, about 20 breaths per minute).*	
5. If no signs of circulation are present or heart rate is less than 60 bpm with signs of poor perfusion, begin cycles of 5 chest compressions (2-finger technique, rate of at least 100 compressions per minute) followed by 1 slow breath.	
6. After about 1 minute of rescue support, check for signs of circulation.* If rescuer is alone, activate the emergency response system. If no signs of circulation are present (or heart rate is less than 60 bpm with poor perfusion), continue 5:1 cycles of compressions and ventilations. If signs of circulation are present but breathing is absent or inadequate, continue rescue breathing (1 breath every 3 seconds, about 20 breaths per minute).	

*If the victim is breathing or resumes adequate breathing and no trauma is suspected, place in the recovery position.

Comments _____

_____

_____

_____

Instructor _____

Circle one: Complete   Needs more practice

Appendix B
BLS Performance Criteria

Healthcare Provider Skills Performance Sheet
Infant Bag-Mask Ventilation
Performance Criteria

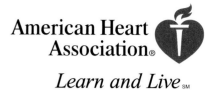

American Heart
Association®

Learn and Live sm

Participant Name _____ Date _____

Performance Guidelines	Performed
1. Establish unresponsiveness. If a bystander is available, send that person to activate the emergency response system.	
2. Open the airway (head tilt–chin lift or jaw thrust). Check breathing (look, listen, and feel).*	
3. If breathing is absent or inadequate, properly position the mask to achieve an effective seal while holding the airway open.	
4. Give 2 slow breaths (1 to 1½ seconds per breath), ensure adequate chest rise, and allow for exhalation between breaths.	
5. Check for brachial pulse and other signs of circulation. If signs of circulation are present but breathing is absent or inadequate, provide rescue breathing (1 breath every 3 seconds, about 20 breaths per minute).	
6. If signs of circulation are absent or heart rate is less than 60 bpm with signs of poor perfusion, provide 5:1 cycles of chest compressions and ventilations. If rescuer is alone, activate the emergency response system after approximately 1 minute.	

*If the victim is breathing or resumes adequate breathing and no trauma is suspected, place in the recovery position.

Comments _____

_____

_____

_____

Instructor _____

Circle one: Complete   Needs more practice

Appendix B
BLS Performance Criteria

American Heart Association®

Learn and Live sm

Healthcare Provider Skills Performance Sheet
Infant FBAO in Responsive Victim
(and Responsive Victim Who Becomes Unresponsive)
Performance Criteria

Participant Name _____ Date _____

Performance Guidelines	Performed
1. Check for serious breathing difficulty, ineffective cough, *no* strong cry. Confirm signs of severe or complete airway obstruction.	
2. Give up to 5 back blows and 5 chest thrusts.	
3. Repeat step 2 until the object is expelled (obstruction relieved) or the victim becomes unresponsive.	
Infant Foreign-Body Airway Obstruction — Victim Becomes Unresponsive	
4. If a second rescuer is available, send that rescuer to activate the emergency response system while you remain with the victim.	
5. Open the airway with a tongue-jaw lift. If you see the object, remove it *(no blind finger sweeps)*.	
6. Open the airway and try to ventilate; if still obstructed (chest does not rise), reopen the airway (reposition head and chin) and try to ventilate again.	
7. If ventilation is unsuccessful, give 5 back blows and 5 chest thrusts.	
8. Repeat steps 5 through 7 until ventilation is effective, then continue the steps of CPR as needed.*	
9. If the rescuer is alone and the airway obstruction is not relieved after about 1 minute, activate the emergency response system.	

*If the victim is breathing or resumes normal breathing and no trauma is suspected, place in the recovery position.

Comments _____

_____

_____

Instructor _____

Circle one: Complete   Needs more practice

Appendix B
BLS Performance Criteria

Healthcare Provider Skills Performance Sheet
Infant FBAO in Unresponsive Victim
Performance Criteria

American Heart
Association®

Learn and Live sm

Participant Name _____ Date _____

Performance Guidelines	Performed
1. Establish unresponsiveness. If a second rescuer is available, send that rescuer to activate the emergency response system while you remain with the victim.	
2. Open the airway, check for breathing. If breathing is absent or inadequate, go to step 3.	
3. Attempt to ventilate if unsuccessful (chest does not rise), reopen the airway (reposition head and chin), and try to ventilate again.	
4. If ventilation is unsuccessful, give up to 5 back blows with heel of hand and 5 chest thrusts (use 2-finger technique).	
5. Open the airway with a tongue-jaw lift. If you see the object, remove it *(no blind finger sweeps).*	
6. Repeat steps 3 through 5 until ventilation is effective, then continue the steps of CPR as needed.*	
7. If the rescuer is alone and airway obstruction is not relieved after about 1 minute, activate the emergency response system.	

*If the victim is breathing or resumes normal breathing and no trauma is suspected, place in the recovery position.

Comments _____

_____

_____

_____

_____

Instructor _____

Circle one: Complete   Needs more practice

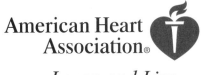

Appendix B
BLS Performance Criteria

Healthcare Provider Skills Performance Sheet
Infant and Child 2-Rescuer CPR
Performance Criteria

Participant Name _____ Date _____

Performance Guidelines	Performed
1. Establish unresponsiveness. One rescuer activates the emergency response system.	
Rescuer 1	
2. Open the airway (head tilt–chin lift or jaw thrust). Check breathing (look, listen, and feel).*	
3. If breathing is absent or inadequate, give 2 slow breaths (1 to 1½ seconds per breath), ensure adequate chest rise, and allow for exhalation between breaths.	
4. Check for pulse (brachial in infants, carotid in children) and other signs of circulation (breathing, coughing, or movement in response to 2 rescue breaths). If signs of circulation are present but breathing is absent or inadequate, provide rescue breathing (1 breath every 3 seconds, about 20 breaths per minute).	
Rescuer 2	
5. If no signs of circulation are present, or heart rate is less than 60 bpm with signs of poor perfusion, begin cycles of 5 chest compressions and 1 breath. Pause to allow Rescuer 1 to provide 1 slow breath after 5 compressions.* Start compression at end of chest rise from rescue breath. • *Infants: use 2 thumb–encircling hands compression technique, compression rate of at least 100 per minute.* • *Child: typically use 1-hand compression technique, compression rate of about 100 compressions per minute.*	
6. After 20 cycles of 5:1 (about 1 minute), Rescuer 1 provides 1 breath and rechecks for signs of circulation (pulse, breathing, cough, movement, response to stimulation).* If no signs of circulation are present, continue cycles of compressions and ventilations (5:1 ratio), beginning with chest compressions.	

*If the victim is breathing or resumes normal breathing and no trauma is suspected, place in the recovery position.

Comments _____

Instructor _____

Circle one: Complete   Needs more practice

Appendix B
BLS Performance Criteria

American Heart Association®
Learn and Live ﹰﹰﹰ

Healthcare Provider Skills Performance Sheet
Child 1-Rescuer CPR
Performance Criteria

Participant Name _____ Date _____

Performance Guidelines	Performed
1. Establish unresponsiveness. If a bystander is available, send that person to activate the emergency response system.	
2. Open the airway (head tilt–chin lift or jaw thrust). Check for normal breathing (look, listen, and feel).*	
3. If breathing is absent or inadequate, give 2 slow effective rescue breaths (1 to 1½ seconds per breath), ensure adequate chest rise, and allow for exhalation between breaths.	
4. Check for carotid pulse and other signs of circulation (breathing, coughing, or movement in response to initial 2 rescue breaths). If signs of circulation are present but breathing is absent or inadequate, provide rescue breathing (1 breath every 3 seconds, about 20 breaths per minute).*	
5. If no signs of circulation are present or heart rate is less than 60 bpm with signs of poor perfusion, begin cycles of 5 chest compressions (typically 1-hand compression technique, rate of about 100 compressions per minute) and 1 slow breath.	
6. After about 1 minute of rescue support, check for signs of circulation.* If rescuer is alone, activate the emergency response system. If no signs of circulation are present, continue 5:1 cycles of compressions and ventilations. If signs of circulation are present but breathing is absent or inadequate, continue rescue breathing (1 breath every 3 seconds, about 20 breaths per minute).	

*If the victim is breathing or resumes normal breathing and no trauma is suspected, place in the recovery position.

Comments _____

_____

_____

_____

Instructor _____

Circle one: Complete   Needs more practice

American Heart Association®

*Learn and Live*sm

Healthcare Provider Skills Performance Sheet
Child Bag-Mask Ventilation
Performance Criteria

Participant Name _____ Date _____

Performance Guidelines	Performed
1. Establish unresponsiveness. If a second rescuer is available, send that person to activate the emergency response system.	
2. Open the airway (head tilt–chin lift or jaw thrust). Check breathing (look, listen, and feel).*	
3. If breathing is absent or inadequate, properly position mask to achieve an effective seal while holding the airway open.	
4. Give 2 slow effective breaths (1 to 1½ seconds per breath), ensure adequate chest rise, and allow for exhalation between breaths.	
5. Check for carotid pulse and other signs of circulation (breathing, coughing, or movement in response to 2 breaths). If signs of circulation are present but breathing is absent or inadequate, provide rescue breathing (1 breath every 3 seconds, about 20 breaths per minute).	
6. If signs of circulation are absent or heart rate is less than 60 bpm with signs of poor perfusion, begin 5:1 cycles of compressions and ventilations. If the rescuer is alone, activate the emergency response system after approximately 1 minute.	

*If the victim is breathing or resumes normal breathing and no trauma is suspected, place in the recovery position.

Comments _____

_____

_____

_____

_____

Instructor _____

Circle one: Complete   Needs more practice

Appendix B
BLS Performance Criteria

American Heart Association®

Learn and Live SM

Healthcare Provider Skills Performance Sheet
Child FBAO in Responsive Victim
(and Responsive Victim Who Becomes Unresponsive)
Performance Criteria

Participant Name _____ Date _____

Performance Guidelines	Performed
1. Ask "Are you choking?" If yes, ask "Can you speak?" If no, tell child you are going to help.	
2. Give abdominal thrusts using proper hand position (avoid xiphoid).	
3. Repeat thrusts until object is expelled (obstruction removed) or victim becomes unresponsive.	
Child Foreign-Body Airway Obstruction — Victim Becomes Unresponsive	
4. If a second rescuer is available, send that rescuer to activate the emergency response system while you remain with the victim.	
5. Open the airway with a tongue-jaw lift. If you see the object, remove it *(no blind finger sweeps)*.	
6. Open the airway (head tilt–chin lift or jaw thrust), attempt rescue breathing; if no chest rise, reopen the airway (reposition head and chin) and try to ventilate again.	
7. If ventilation is unsuccessful, provide 5 abdominal thrusts with the victim supine (use proper hand position, avoiding the xiphoid).	
8. Repeat steps 5 through 7 until effective, then provide additional steps of CPR as needed.*	
9. If rescuer is alone and airway obstruction is not relieved after about 1 minute, activate the emergency response system.	

*If the victim is breathing or resumes normal breathing and no trauma is suspected, place in the recovery position.

Comments _____

_____

Instructor _____

Circle one: Complete   Needs more practice

American Heart Association®

Learn and Live SM

Healthcare Provider Skills Performance Sheet
Child FBAO in Unresponsive Victim
Performance Criteria

Participant Name _____ Date _____

Performance Guidelines	Performed
1. Establish unresponsiveness. If a second rescuer is available, send that rescuer to activate the emergency response system while you remain with the victim.	
2. Open the airway (head tilt–chin lift or jaw thrust) and check for breathing. If breathing is absent or inadequate, go to step 3.	
3. Attempt to ventilate; if unsuccessful (chest does not rise), reopen the airway (reposition head and chin) and try to ventilate again.	
4. If ventilation is unsuccessful, perform up to 5 abdominal thrusts with the victim supine (use proper hand position, avoid the xiphoid).	
5. Open the airway with a tongue-jaw lift. If you see the object, remove it *(no blind finger sweeps).*	
6. Repeat steps 3 through 5 until ventilation is effective, then continue the steps of CPR as needed.*	
7. If rescuer is alone and airway obstruction is not relieved after about 1 minute, activate the emergency response system.	

*If the victim is breathing or resumes normal breathing and no trauma is suspected, place in the recovery position.

Comments _____

_____

_____

_____

_____

Instructor _____

Circle one: Complete   Needs more practice

Appendix B

BLS for Healthcare Provider Course
CPR and AED for Victims 1 to 8 Years of Age
Performance Criteria

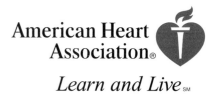

American Heart
Association®

Learn and Live sm

Participant Name _____ Date _____

Performance Guidelines	Performance	
CPR Skills	**Satisfactory**	**Remediate**
1. Establish unresponsiveness — direct coworker to activate the emergency response system and get the AED.		
2. Open the airway (head tilt–chin lift or, if trauma is suspected, jaw thrust) — check breathing (look, listen, and feel).		
3. If breathing is absent or inadequate, give 2 slow breaths (1 to 1½ seconds per breath) that cause the chest to rise (if chest does not rise, reposition, reattempt). Allow for adequate exhalation time.		
4. Check carotid pulse and other signs of circulation **(no signs of circulation).** Start chest compressions (ratio of 5 compressions to 1 breath at about 100 compressions per minute).		
AED Skills (AED arrives after CPR skills have been adequately assessed. Assume that 1 minute of CPR was provided.)		
5. Place the AED next to the victim. POWER ON the AED and note time.		
6. Attach electrode pads in the proper position (sternal-apex or as pictured on each of the AED electrodes) with proper contact and no overlap of pads.		
7. Clear the victim and press the ANALYZE button, if present. **(AED advises shock and charges electrodes.)**		
8. Clear the victim and press the SHOCK button, if advised. Stop timing for collapse-to-shock interval. (May repeat 1 to 2 more analyze-shock cycles. Stop when AED gives *"no shock indicated"* message.)		
9. Check carotid pulse and other signs of circulation. **(Pulse, breathing, coughing, movement present.)**		
10. Continue to monitor breathing and signs of circulation until advanced life support rescuers arrive. (If trauma is not suspected, place in a recovery position with AED attached.)		

(continued on next page)

CPR and AED Performance Criteria
for Victims 1 to 8 Years of Age (continued)

Critical Actions	Performance	
	Satisfactory	Remediate
• Assess responsiveness.		
• Activate the emergency response system (or send second rescuer); get the AED.		
• Open the airway, check breathing.		
• If breathing is absent or inadequate, provide 2 breaths (must cause chest to rise).		
• Check pulse and other signs of circulation.		
• Begin chest compressions (must have proper hand placement). Provide chest compressions and rescue breathing in a 5:1 ratio for 1 minute.		
• After 1 minute of CPR when AED arrives: POWER ON the AED.		
• Attach electrode pads to patient's bare chest in proper location with adequate skin contact and no overlap of pads.		
• "Clear" victim before ANALYZE and SHOCK.		
• Push SHOCK button (if not automated) to attempt defibrillation		
• Check breathing and signs of circulation after *"no shock indicated"* message.		
• Interval from collapse to first shock is less than 3 minutes, interval from AED arrival to first shock is less than 90 seconds		
• Rescuer should be prepared to continue CPR if nonshockable rhythm is present.		

Comments _____

Instructor _____

Circle one:　　Complete　　Needs more practice

Appendix B
Performance Evaluation
BLS for Healthcare Providers Course

Integrated Adult FBAO and Rescue Breathing
Skills Performance Sheet

American Heart Association®

Learn and Live sm

Instructions to Rescuer: You and a colleague enter a waiting room to find an adult man who appears to be in distress. He is clutching his throat. You have a mask or barrier device, but there is no other equipment in the room.

Participant Name _____ Date _____

Performance Guidelines *(Instructor cues to rescuers are in bold italics.)*	**Performed**
Responsive Victim	
1. Asks "Are you choking?" *(He nods yes.)* Asks "Can you speak?" *(He cannot speak.)* Tells the victim "I am going to help."	
2. Gives abdominal thrusts using the proper hand position (avoids the xiphoid). *(The victim is not pregnant or obese.)*	
3. Repeats thrusts until the foreign body is expelled or the victim becomes unresponsive. *(The foreign body is not expelled.)*	
Victim Becomes Unresponsive — Airway Remains Obstructed	
4. Eases the victim to the ground. Sends colleague to activate the emergency response system and bring the AED.	
5. Opens the airway with a tongue-jaw lift and looks for the object *(no object seen)*. Performs a finger sweep *(no object found)*.	
6. Opens the airway (head tilt–chin lift) and tries to ventilate *(chest does not rise)*. Repositions the head and tries to ventilate again *(chest does not rise)*.	
7. Performs 5 abdominal thrusts with the victim on his back (uses proper hand position, avoids the xiphoid).	
8. Opens the airway with a tongue-jaw lift and looks for the object *(object seen)*. Performs a finger sweep *(object removed)*.	
9. Opens the airway and attempts to provide 2 ventilations *(chest rises)*.	
10. Checks carotid pulse and other signs of circulation *(pulse present, no breathing)*.	
11. Performs mouth-to-mask (or barrier device) rescue breathing for several breaths.	
Colleague returns bringing a code cart with AED. The code team is on the way. Rescuers demonstrate each of the following skills for several breaths:	
12. One-rescuer bag-mask ventilation with oxygen.	
13. Two-rescuer bag-mask ventilation with oxygen. (One student is evaluated holding the mask in position with head tilt–chin lift and forming an effective seal while the second student compresses the bag.*)	
Victim Begins Breathing Normally	
14. Because there was no trauma, place the victim in the recovery position.	

*If there is only one student, instructor acts as colleague/Rescuer 2 and compresses the bag.

Comments _____

Instructor _____ **Circle one:** Complete   Needs more practice

Appendix B
Performance Evaluation
BLS for Healthcare Providers Course

Integrated Infant FBAO, CPR, and Rescue Breathing
Skills Performance Sheet

American Heart Association®

Learn and Live ℠

Instructions to Rescuer: You and a colleague hear a call for help from the hospital cafeteria. You find a woman holding an infant who is clearly in distress. He is making frantic attempts to breathe and his face is turning blue, but he is making no noise. You suspect that he is choking. The cafeteria is equipped with a standard CPR kit, which includes pediatric barrier devices.

Participant Name _____ Date _____

Performance Guidelines *(Instructor cues to rescuers are in bold italics.)*	Performed
Responsive Victim	
1. Confirms severe or complete airway obstruction with poor air exchange, ineffective cough, and a weak cry. *(Infant is silent and trying to breathe.)*	
2. Gives up to 5 forceful back blows with the heel of hand while holding the infant in the correct position (face down over arm, the head supported and lower than the torso). *(The infant is still struggling silently; no object is expelled.)*	
3. Turns the infant face up in the correct position (face up over arm, the head supported and lower than the torso) and provides 5 chest thrusts using the 2-finger chest compression technique. *(The infant is still struggling silently; no object is expelled.)*	
4. Repeats 5 back blows followed by 5 chest thrusts until the object is expelled or infant becomes unresponsive. *(The object is not expelled; infant stops struggling and goes limp.)*	
Victim Becomes Unresponsive — Airway Remains Obstructed	
5. Sends colleague to activate the emergency response system.	
6. Opens the airway with a tongue-jaw lift, looks for the object, and removes it if seen *(no object seen—no blind finger sweeps).*	
7. Opens the airway and attempts to provide a rescue breath *(chest does not rise).* Repositions the head and tries to ventilate again *(chest does not rise).*	
8. Provides 5 back blows, followed by 5 chest thrusts.	
9. Performs a tongue-jaw lift, looks for object, and removes it if seen *(object is seen and removed).*	
10. Opens the airway using head tilt–chin lift or jaw thrust and attempts to provide 2 rescue breaths *(chest rises).*	
11. Checks brachial pulse and other signs of circulation *(no signs of circulation).*	
Airway Open. No Signs of Circulation *(Colleague has not yet returned.)*	
12. Begins cycles of 5 chest compressions (at least 100 compressions per minute) and 1 slow breath.	
13. After about 1 minute of rescue support, checks for signs of circulation *(pulse present)* and breathing *(breathing absent).*	
Pulse Present — No Breathing	
14. Performs rescue breathing for several breaths (1 breath every 3 seconds for 4 to 6 breaths).	

Performance Guidelines	Performed
Colleague returns bringing an oxygen set-up with bag-mask device.	
15. Provides bag-mask ventilation with oxygen for several breaths.	
Colleague assesses the infant and finds a weak, slow pulse at a rate of 20 beats per minute.	
16. Performs 2-rescuer CPR using the 2-thumbs–encircled hands technique.	

Comments _____

Instructor _____

Circle one: Complete   Needs more practice

Performance Evaluation
BLS for Healthcare Providers Course

Integrated Child FBAO, CPR, and Rescue Breathing
Skills Performance Sheet

American Heart Association®

Learn and Live ℠

Instructions to Rescuer: You and a colleague enter a waiting room and find a 4-year-boy who is responsive and appears to be in distress. He is clutching his throat. You have a mask or barrier device, but there is no other equipment in the room.

Participant Name _____ Date _____

Performance Guidelines *(Instructor cues to rescuers are in bold italics.)*	**Performed**
Responsive Victim	
1. Ask "Are you choking?" *(Child nods yes.)* Asks "Can you speak?" *(He cannot speak.)* Tells the child "I am going to help."	
2. Stands or kneels behind the child with arms encircling the child's abdomen. Gives abdominal thrusts using the proper hand position (avoids the xiphoid) and supports the body.	
3. Repeat thrusts until the object is expelled or the child becomes unresponsive *(object is not expelled)*.	
Victim Becomes Unresponsive — Airway Remains Obstructed	
4. Lowers the child to the ground and sends colleague to activate the emergency response system and bring the AED.	
5. Opens the airway with a tongue-jaw lift. Looks for the object to remove it *(no object seen—no finger sweeps)*.	
6. Opens the airway and attempts rescue breathing *(chest does not rise).* Reopens the airway with head tilt–chin lift (repositions head and chin) and tries to ventilate again *(chest does not rise).*	
7. Gives 5 abdominal thrusts with the victim on his back (uses proper hand position, avoids xiphoid).	
8. Performs a tongue-jaw lift, looks for the object, and removes it if seen *(object is seen and removed).*	
9. Opens the airway using head tilt–chin lift or jaw thrust and attempts to provide 2 rescue breaths *(chest rises).*	
No Signs of Circulation	
10. Checks carotid pulse and other signs of circulation *(no signs of circulation).*	
11. Begins cycles of 5 chest compressions (1-hand compression technique, about 100 compressions per minute) and 1 slow breath.	
12. After about 1 minute of CPR, checks for signs of circulation *(signs of circulation present)* and breathing *(breathing absent).*	
Pulse Present — No Breathing	
13. Performs rescue breathing for several breaths *(1 breath every 3 seconds for 4 to 6 breaths).*	

Performance Guidelines	Performed
Colleague returns bringing the AED and an oxygen set-up with bag-mask device. Rescuers demonstrate each of the following skills for several breaths:	
14. One-rescuer bag-mask ventilation with oxygen.	
15. Two-rescuer bag-mask ventilation with oxygen. (One student is evaluated holding the mask in position with head tilt–chin lift and forming an effective seal while the second student compresses the bag.*)	
Victim Begins Breathing Normally	
16. Because there was no trauma, rescuer places the victim in the recovery position.	

*If there is only one student, the instructor acts as colleague/Rescuer 2.

Comments _____

Instructor _____

Circle one: Complete   Needs more practice

Appendix B
Performance Evaluation
BLS for Healthcare Providers Course

Adult 1- and 2-Rescuer CPR With AED
Skills Performance Sheet

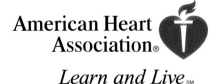

American Heart
Association®

Learn and Live sm

Instructions to Rescuer: You and a colleague enter a room to find an adult man who appears to be unresponsive. There are no signs of trauma. You have a face mask or barrier device, but there is no other equipment in the room. The nearest AED is down the hall near the phone.

Participant Name _____ Date _____

Performance Guidelines *(Instructor cues to rescuers are in bold italics.)*	**Performed**
1. Checks responsiveness *(unresponsive)*.	
2. Sends colleague to activate the emergency response system and get the AED.	
3. Opens the airway (head tilt–chin lift) and assesses for breathing (look, listen, and feel) *(no breathing)*.	
4. Gives 2 slow breaths (2 seconds per breath) that cause the chest to rise. If the chest does not rise, reposition the head and try again *(chest rises)*.	
5. Checks for carotid pulse and other signs of circulation *(no signs of circulation)*.	
1-Rescuer CPR	
6. Starts 1-rescuer CPR at a ratio of 15 compressions to 2 ventilations.	
Colleague Arrives With AED	
7. Rescuer 1 continues with 1-rescuer CPR until directed to stop by Rescuer 2 (AED Rescuer).* Rescuer 2 places AED near the patient's head, turns it on (if necessary), and applies the electrodes. *(If the AED is fully automated, stay clear of the victim while the AED performs steps 8 and 9).*	
8. Follows AED prompts. If directed to press analyze, Rescuer 2 clears the victim and presses the analyze button.	
Shock Advised	
9. Follows AED prompts. If directed to provide a shock, Rescuer 2 clears the victim and presses the shock button. Then if so directed, analyzes again.	
AED Analyzes, No Shock Advised, No Signs of Circulation— 2-Rescuer CPR	
10. Rescuer 1 checks for a carotid pulse and other signs of circulation *(no signs of circulation)*.	
11. Rescuers begin 2-rescuer CPR using the 15:2 compression-to-ventilation ratio. *Continue until AED signals a pause for analysis and assessment (no signs of circulation)*.	
12. Code Team arrives and assumes care of the patient.	

Note: If there is only 1 student, Rescuer 1 uses the AED and the instructor provides compressions during 2-rescuer CPR.

Comments _____

Instructor _____

Circle one: Complete   Needs more practice

Abdominal thrust: A thrust applied to the abdomen just above the navel and well below the xiphoid to expel a foreign-body airway obstruction. Also called the Heimlich maneuver.

Active compression-decompression CPR (ACD-CPR): An alternative form of CPR using a hand-held mechanical device to augment chest relaxation between compressions. The device uses a type of suction cup attached to the chest. The device provides positive pressure to the chest on the compression downstroke and negative pressure to lift the anterior chest on the upstroke. Use of this device appears to augment venous return to the heart during CPR.

Acute coronary syndromes: A term that encompasses symptomatic conditions resulting in an inadequate blood supply to the heart, including angina and acute myocardial infarction.

Adhesive electrode pads: Pads that adhere directly to the skin of the patient's chest. These electrodes can be used to capture the surface ECG, and they can be used as a contact medium for conducting electric current from an automated external defibrillator (AED) or transcutaneous pacer to the patient.

Advance directive: A medical order written by a physician in response to the expressed wishes of the patient. The advance directive should state the level of care the patient desires at the end of life. An advance directive may name a surrogate decision maker to make those choices if the patient is unable to do so. In common usage this term includes living wills, but it is preferable that these terms are not interchanged. A living will contains an expression of the patient's wishes. An advance directive, in contrast, is a physician order that is based on the patient's wishes.

Advanced cardiovascular life support (ACLS): A group of interventions used to treat and stabilize adult victims of life-threatening cardiorespiratory emergencies and to resuscitate victims of cardiac arrest. These interventions include CPR, basic and advanced airway management, tracheal intubation, medications, electrical therapy, and intravenous (IV) access. ACLS also refers to a training course sponsored by the American Heart Association that instructs healthcare providers in the basic and advanced techniques of resuscitation.

Advocacy: Acting in the best interest of the patient.

Aerosol transmission: Transmission of disease by the inhalation of micro-organisms suspended in droplets in the air.

Agonal electrical cardiac activity: A cardiac arrest rhythm characterized by occasional wide complexes on the electrocardiogram (ECG).

Agonal respirations: Ineffective, reflex, gasping respiratory efforts that may occur at the moment of cardiac arrest.

Alveoli: Small, saclike outpouchings in the lungs where gas exchange takes place between alveolar gas and pulmonary capillary blood.

Amniotic fluid embolism: Arterial obstruction caused by amniotic fluid in the bloodstream.

Aneurysm: An abnormal localized dilation of a blood vessel wall, which weakens it, often causing sudden rupture and bleeding.

Angina: Transient pain, pressure, or discomfort resulting from a temporary lack of adequate blood supply to the heart muscle.

Antiplatelet agents: Platelets are small disc-shaped structures in the blood that adhere together or aggregate to form clots. Platelet aggregate activity serves an important function by stopping bleeding (hemostasis), but it also may contribute to the formation of harmful blood clots (thrombosis) in the coronary arteries or brain. Antiplatelet agents block this action. Aspirin is a well-known and effective antiplatelet agent.

Apneic: May refer to either a pause (of 20 seconds or longer) in breathing or complete cessation of breathing.

Arrhythmia: Abnormal heart rhythm.

Arteries: Muscular blood vessels that carry blood away from the heart.

Arterioles: Very small muscular blood vessels located throughout the body that regulate blood pressure.

Arteriosclerosis: Commonly called "hardening of the arteries," arteriosclerosis includes a variety of conditions that cause the artery walls to thicken and lose elasticity.

Asphyxia: A life-threatening condition caused by a lack of oxygen (ie, carbon monoxide poisoning).

Asymptomatic coronary artery disease (CAD): The phase of CAD in which the patient has not yet experienced symptoms.

Asystole: Cardiac standstill or an absence of any electrical cardiac rhythm; also called *flat line*.

Atherosclerosis: A process that leads to a group of diseases characterized by a thickening of artery walls. Atherosclerosis is a leading cause of death from heart attack and stroke.

Atrial fibrillation: An abnormal, irregular heart rhythm that results in quivering of the atria so that they no longer contract. This arrhythmia can lead to stasis of blood in the atria and formation of clots. These clots can embolize to other parts of the body.

Automated external defibrillator (AED): An external computerized defibrillator designed for use in unresponsive victims with no breathing and no signs of circulation. The AED captures the victim's ECG signal through adhesive electrodes placed on the victim's chest and analyzes the victim's heart rhythm, identifying shockable rhythms. Once a shockable rhythm is identified, the AED automatically charges to a preset energy level and provides voice prompts for the operator. When activated by the rescuer, the AED will deliver a shock through the adhesive electrodes.

Automaticity: The ability of cardiac tissue to generate its own electrical impulse.

Autonomy: The principle that a person should be free to make his or her own decisions.

Bag-mask (device): A mechanical aid used to deliver positive-pressure ventilation. The device consists of a bag with an oxygen inlet and a mask. Many bags contain a unidirectional valve to divert the patient's exhaled air into the atmosphere; a bag, unidirectional valve, and mask can be referred to as a bag-mask system.

Barrier device: Any number of devices used in rescue breathing (including face shields and masks) that create a physical barrier between a rescuer and a victim to decrease the small chance of disease transmission.

Basic life support (BLS): A group of actions and interventions used to treat, stabilize, and resuscitate victims of cardiac or respiratory arrest. These BLS actions and interventions include recognition of a cardiac or respiratory emergency or stroke, activation of the emergency response system, cardiopulmonary resuscitation (CPR), use of an AED, and relief of foreign-body airway obstruction. BLS also refers to a training course sponsored by the American Heart Association that instructs healthcare providers in the basic techniques of resuscitation.

Beneficence: The principle of doing good.

Biphasic: Having 2 phases or variations.

Biphasic waveform defibrillator: A defibrillator that delivers a current that flows in a positive direction for a specified duration and then reverses and flows in a negative direction for the remaining milliseconds of electrical discharge.

Bradycardia: Slow heart rate (usually less than 60 beats per minute in an adult).

Capillaries: Minute, thin-walled blood vessels in which there is an interchange of various substances between the blood and tissue, including gases.

Cardiac arrest: The cessation of a functional heartbeat.

Cardiopulmonary resuscitation: In the broadest sense, attempting any maneuvers or techniques designed to restore circulation, or a technique combining artificial ventilation and chest compressions designed to perfuse vital organs or restore circulation to a victim of cardiopulmonary arrest.

Cardiovascular: Pertaining to the heart and blood vessels.

Cardioversion: Typically referred to as synchronized cardioversion. This is the delivery of a shock to the heart in an attempt to terminate a rapid supraventricular arrhythmia. Cardioversion uses lower energy than defibrillation. Unlike defibrillation, the shock used for cardioversion is *timed* to coincide with the patient's R wave.

Cerebral: A term referring to the cerebrum, the main portion of the brain occupying the upper part of the cranial cavity.

Cerebral thrombosis: Formation of a blood clot in an artery in the brain. This is a common cause of an ischemic stroke.

Cerebrovascular: A term referring to the brain and the vessels that supply the brain with blood.

Chain of Survival: An American Heart Association metaphor that uses the links in a chain to describe the actions needed to save a victim of sudden cardiac arrest. The links in the adult Chain of Survival are early access to 911, early CPR, early defibrillation, and early advanced care. The links in the pediatric Chain of Survival are prevention of injury and arrest, early CPR, early access to 911, and early advanced care.

Cholesterol: A fatlike substance in the blood that contributes to the formation of atherosclerosis.

Cincinnati Stroke Scale: A focused physical exam designed to rapidly detect patients with stroke. This scale is designed to detect facial droop, arm drift (the patient's eyes are closed and the arms held out), and abnormal speech.

Computed tomography (CT) scan: A series of x-rays (radiographs) that are analyzed and reconstructed by a computer into a pictorial image of a part of the body. CT scans can be used to visualize a variety of disorders, including tumors, hemorrhages, and abscesses, and they may reveal areas of abnormal blood flow or injury. A CT scan of the brain is required to rule out the presence of hemorrhagic stroke before administration of fibrinolytics.

Coronary artery disease (CAD): A group of diseases, including angina and myocardial infarction, caused by the development of arteriosclerotic plaques that narrow the artery walls and obstruct distal blood flow to part of the heart.

Coronary artery spasm: Severe, usually localized constriction of a coronary artery resulting in a lack of blood supply to the heart.

Coronary care unit: A specialized intensive care unit in a hospital that treats victims of heart disease during the critical or unstable phase of their illness.

Coronary reperfusion: Restoration of some blood flow to an area of the heart. This may be accomplished by administration of fibrinolytics, angioplasty with or without stent placement, or coronary revascularization (coronary artery bypass grafting).

Coronary revascularization: The restoration of blood flow to the heart by means of blood vessel grafting.

Cricothyroidotomy (cricothyrotomy): A surgical procedure opening the cricothyroid membrane (in the windpipe of the neck) to provide an airway.

Critical incident stress debriefing (CISD): A group meeting of rescuers involved in a resuscitation attempt designed to educate and to ease the psychological and emotional impact of the incident.

Cyanosis: Bluish discoloration of the skin (most often around the lips and nail beds) caused by a severe lack of oxygen in the blood.

Deciliter: One tenth of a liter.

Defibrillation: The untimed (asynchronous) depolarization of the myocardium that *successfully* terminates ventricular fibrillation (VF) or pulseless ventricular tachycardia (VT). In defibrillation and defibrillation attempts, a shock is delivered to the myocardium, most often through the chest wall (although internal defibrillation may be accomplished if the chest is open). The goal of defibrillation is to enable resumption of a perfusing rhythm, but the shock may convert the rhythm to asystole. In common usage the term *defibrillation* is used interchangeably with the term *shock*. However, the shock is used to *attempt* defibrillation, and the term *defibrillation* should be reserved for the successful termination of VF/VT.

Defibrillator: A device used to deliver a shock to the heart. A defibrillation shock depolarizes the heart in an effort to suppress ventricular fibrillation (VF) or pulseless ventricular tachycardia (VT) and allow a perfusing rhythm to return. Defibrillators may be manual or automated (see Automated external defibrillator). Manual defibrillators often have the capacity to perform synchronized cardioversion (see Cardioversion).

Diabetes: A general term referring to persistent elevations of blood sugar in the bloodstream.

DNR (No CPR, DNAR): The terms *DNR ("do not resuscitate"), No CPR,* and *DNAR ("do not attempt resuscitation")* are used to indicate that in the event of a cardiac arrest, no cardiopulmonary resuscitative measures should be instituted.

Durable power of attorney for health care: An advance directive naming another person to make healthcare decisions if a patient is unable to do so.

Electrical therapy: Interventions used to convert, resuscitate, or stabilize a cardiac rhythm, including defibrillation, cardioversion, and pacing.

Embolic stroke: A stroke caused by an embolism.

Embolism: The sudden blockage of an artery by a clot, that has traveled through the bloodstream from another location.

Emergency cardiovascular care (ECC): A system including all interventions to manage emergencies related to the heart, blood vessels, and brain. These interventions include BLS, PALS, and ACLS assessments and interventions performed by bystanders, trained responders, healthcare professionals, and allied health personnel.

Emergency medical dispatchers (EMDs): EMS personnel who answer 911 calls and dispatch EMS responders to the scene of an emergency. EMDs also provide telephone instructions to bystanders at the scene while the responders are en route.

Emergency medical services (EMS): The planned configuration of community resources and personnel designed to respond to medical emergencies and provide immediate care to persons who have suffered an unexpected illness or injury. The EMS system includes EMS dispatchers and EMS responders.

Emergency medical technicians (EMTs): Prehospital emergency care providers trained in a program using the structure and guidelines set forth by the Department of Transportation (DOT).

EMS responders: A group of EMTs-basic, EMTs-intermediate, and EMTs-paramedic who respond with specialized equipment and resources to emergencies in the community.

Enhanced 911: An emergency medical dispatch system (911) that allows the dispatcher to identify the location and telephone number of incoming telephone calls. This system allows the dispatcher to send responders to the scene of an emergency even if the caller cannot provide the address or other information.

Epiglottis: A lidlike structure attached to the base of the tongue overhanging the entrance to the larynx. This structure normally prevents food from entering the larynx.

Epiglottitis: Inflammation (usually with swelling) of the epiglottis. This inflammation can lead to severe upper airway obstruction, particularly in young children who have relatively small upper airways.

Evidence based: The conscientious, explicit, and judicious use of current best medical and scientific evidence in determining recommendations for medical care or policy or decisions about patient care.

Exsanguination: Drainage or massive loss of blood from the body.

Face shield: A barrier device placed over the mouth and nose of a cardiac arrest victim (or manikin) during rescue breathing.

Fat emboli: Arterial obstruction caused by fat droplets in the bloodstream (usually the result of long bone fractures).

Fibrinolytic: A term referring to "clot-busting" medications administered to heart attack and stroke victims. If given within the recommended time, these drugs dissolve the blood clot that is causing the heart attack or stroke. The benefit of these medications is time-dependent.

First responders: A group including police officers and firefighters trained in a nationally recognized program to respond to emergencies with resources such as oxygen and an AED.

Focal neurologic dysfunction: Loss of function of part of the body caused by localized damage to the brain controlling that area.

Foreign-body airway obstruction (FBAO): An obstruction of the airway in any location from the mouth to the bronchioles, caused by food, toys, or other external objects.

Genetic: Related to heredity.

Glasgow Coma Scale: A reliable scale used to quickly assess the severity of neurologic dysfunction in patients with altered consciousness. The scale is based on the best responses for eye opening (1 to 4), verbal responses (1 to 5), and movement (1 to 6). The total score ranges from 3 to 15.

Good Samaritan laws: Laws (which vary from state to state) that generally protect a person who renders emergency aid from civil damages if the person acts in good faith and not for remuneration.

HDL: High-density lipoprotein ("good" cholesterol).

Heimlich maneuver: An abdominal thrust performed in children or adults (not infants) to relieve FBAO.

Hemorrhagic stroke: Localized brain damage caused by bleeding resulting from the rupture of a blood vessel in the brain.

Hemothorax: Bleeding within the pleural cavity (the space between the lung and chest wall).

Hyperbaric oxygen chamber: A compartment capable of delivering oxygen at pressures many times higher than barometric pressure. Hyperbaric oxygen may be used to treat carbon monoxide poisoning, decompression sickness, and anaerobic infections.

Hypercholesterolemia: High levels of cholesterol in the bloodstream.

Hypertension: High blood pressure. Systolic pressure, diastolic pressure, or both may be elevated.

Hypertriglyceridemia: High levels of triglycerides (fats) in the bloodstream.

Hypoglycemia: Low blood sugar.

Hypothermia: An abnormally low body temperature caused by exposure to environmental extremes or physiological factors that affect mechanisms of heat production and heat loss.

Hypothermic: Referring to a low body temperature.

Hypovolemia: Low blood volume caused by hemorrhage, burns, metabolic disorders, or other causes of loss of body fluid. Hypovolemia may be absolute (caused by intravascular volume loss) or relative (caused by expansion of the vascular space)

Hypoxia: Reduced oxygen supply (delivery) to the body's tissues. When hypoxia is present, tissues must switch to anaerobic metabolism, and lactic acid is generated (lactic acidosis).

Implanted cardioverter defibrillator (ICD): A biomedical device (slightly larger than a pacemaker) implanted under the skin of the chest or upper abdomen and joined to the heart by wire electrodes. An ICD detects abnormal ("shockable") heart rhythms (ventricular tachycardia or fibrillation) and automatically defibrillates the heart if required.

Incontinence: Loss of urinary or bowel control.

Infectious disease: A classification of disease in which the causative agent can be transmitted from one person to another directly or indirectly.

Interposed abdominal compression CPR (IAC-CPR): A 2- or 3-person CPR technique that includes manual compression of the abdomen during the relaxation phase of chest compression. This alternative form of in-hospital CPR requires an additional rescuer to press on the abdomen in the midline, halfway between the xiphoid process and the umbilicus.

Intracerebral hemorrhage: Bleeding into brain tissue caused by rupture of a blood vessel. Hypertension is the most common cause of intracerebral hemorrhage.

Intravascular: Within the blood vessels.

Ischemia: Inadequate blood supply to an organ such as the heart or brain.

Ischemic stroke: Localized brain damage caused by blockage of a blood vessel supplying the brain. A blood clot is the most common cause of blood vessel blockage. The blood clot may form at the site of the blockage (thrombotic stroke) or originate elsewhere in the body (usually the heart) and travel to the blood vessel in the brain (embolic stroke).

Justice: The principle of fairness in the allocation of resources and the physician's obligation to patients.

Laryngeal edema: Swelling of the larynx and surrounding tissues. This swelling can result in airway obstruction.

Laryngospasm: Severe constriction of the larynx.

Larynx: The structure in the neck formed by rings of cartilage guarding the entrance to the trachea and functioning secondarily as the organ of voice. Commonly called the *voice box.*

LDL: Low-density lipoprotein ("bad" cholesterol).

Living will: An expression of an individual's wishes regarding healthcare issues at the end of life. It should be enforced by a formal advance directive that comes from a physician.

Los Angeles Prehospital Stroke Screen (LAPSS): A focused physical exam designed to quickly identify patients with stroke.

Medullary respiratory center: The portion of the medulla in the brainstem that is responsible for monitoring and controlling respiration.

Microorganisms: Microscopic organisms, including bacteria, fungi, and viruses.

Mobile life support unit: An intensive care transport vehicle that treats victims of a wide variety of illnesses and injuries using specialized equipment and personnel.

Modifiable: Changeable.

Monomorphic: Existing in only 1 form.

Monophasic: Exhibiting only 1 phase or variation.

Morphology: Form and structure.

Mouth-to-nose ventilation: An alternative form of rescue breathing in which the rescuer provides positive-pressure ventilation through the victim's nose. This technique is recommended when it is impossible to ventilate through the victim's mouth, when the mouth cannot be opened, or when a tight mouth-to-mouth seal is difficult to achieve.

Myocardial infarction (MI): Death of heart tissue commonly caused by a blockage of a coronary artery owing to an arteriosclerotic plaque, thrombus, embolus, or spasm.

Myocardial ischemia: Inadequate delivery of oxygen to the heart muscle. This ischemia may create pain, called *angina.*

Needle cricothyroidotomy (needle cricothyrotomy): Placement of a needle through the cricothyroid membrane (in the windpipe) to provide an airway. This is used as a temporary measure (by a trained and qualified rescuer) until a foreign object can be removed or a cricothyroidotomy can be performed.

Neurologic dysfunction: Abnormal function caused by neurologic insult or injury.

Nicotine: A poisonous, colorless chemical obtained from tobacco.

Nonmaleficence: The principle that encompasses the ethical principle of "first do no harm."

Normothermic: Normal core body temperature.

Percutaneous coronary interventions (PCIs): A variety of cardiac procedures using a catheter in combination with other devices to open a blocked coronary artery and maintain patency. PCIs include angioplasty and stent placement.

Percutaneous transluminal coronary angioplasty (PTCA): The process of clearing a blocked coronary artery with a balloon that dilates and compresses an arteriosclerotic plaque against the artery wall.

Pericardial tamponade: A collection of blood or fluid in the pericardial sac around the heart, which can impair cardiac function and obstruct venous return to the heart.

Peripartum: Pertaining to the period immediately before, during, and after the birth of a baby.

Pharynx: The musculomembranous area between the mouth and nares and the esophagus. It communicates with the esophagus, the larynx, the mouth, the nasal passages, and the auditory tubes.

Platelets: Disc-shaped structures in the blood that aggregate (stick together or adhere) to stop bleeding. These platelets can exert a protective effect because they protect from bleeding (hemostasis), but they can also contribute to clot formation (thrombosis) that can lead to myocardial infarction or ischemic stroke.

Pneumatic antishock garment (PASG): Pneumatic trousers used to control hemorrhage in the legs and pelvis, thereby increasing peripheral vascular resistance.

Pneumatic vest CPR: An alternative form of CPR using an inflatable vest that fits completely around the patient's chest. The vest cyclically inflates and deflates, producing an increase in intrathoracic pressure.

Pocket mask: A device that consists of a mask and 1-way valve used to give rescue breaths and provide a physical barrier between the rescuer and the victim.

Polymorphic: Existing in more than 1 form.

Positive-pressure ventilation: The act of delivering air into the lungs under pressure (ie, bag-mask ventilation).

Postmenopausal: Occurring after menopause (cessation of menstruation in the female, usually by the age of 48 to 50).

Prearrival instructions: Instructions given by a dispatcher to a layperson at the scene of an emergency before the arrival of EMS. Instructions may include how to perform chest compressions and rescue breathing, how to assist with childbirth, etc.

Primary hypertension (essential hypertension): High blood pressure of unknown cause.

Primary prevention: A number of changes in behavior or lifestyle designed to prevent disease or injury.

Psychomotor: Pertaining to physical actions, which are the end result of mental activity.

Public access defibrillation (PAD): A healthcare initiative sponsored by the American Heart Association and other organizations that places AEDs throughout the community in the hands of trained lay rescuers. The goal of PAD programs is to shorten the interval between collapse due to sudden cardiac arrest and defibrillation. This should improve survival from sudden cardiac arrest.

Pulmonary embolism: An embolism that causes arterial obstruction in the lung.

Pulseless electrical activity (PEA): A cardiac arrest rhythm characterized by organized electrical activity of the heart but without a palpable pulse.

Quality assurance: An ongoing process of continuous evaluation and assessment of a program with feedback of information to participants. The purpose is to maintain and continually improve quality in the service delivered.

Recurrent VF: Ventricular fibrillation that occurs again.

Refibrillation: The reoccurrence of VF after conversion to an organized rhythm.

Regurgitation: To vomit partially digested food. This term can also be used to indicate backward flow of blood, such as occurs from the left ventricle to the left atrium through an insufficient mitral valve.

Reperfusion: The process of restoring blood flow to a tissue bed. Coronary reperfusion can involve techniques such as fibrinolysis (use of "clot-busters") or angioplasty. Reperfusion can also occur when circulation is restored (eg, to the brain) following cardiac arrest.

Respiratory arrest: Cessation of breathing.

Respiratory failure: The state that exists when the respiratory system can no longer support life. If an intervention is not provided, the victim will become progressively more hypoxic or hypercarbic, or both, and will ultimately die.

Respiratory insufficiency: Respiratory function that is inadequate to maintain normal levels of oxygen and carbon dioxide in the blood.

Secondary hypertension: High blood pressure caused by a condition such as kidney disease.

Secondary prevention: Actions taken to prevent further complications after an injury or illness.

Silent ischemia: An instance in which a patient experiences an ischemic event in the absence of chest pain, making diagnosis of acute MI more difficult. Women, persons with diabetes, and the elderly are more prone to silent ischemia than others.

Stroke: A disruption in blood supply to a region of the brain that causes acute neurologic impairment.

Stroke Chain of Survival and Recovery: The term used to describe the actions for survival and recovery from stroke, which are (1) early recognition, (2) early activation of the EMS system and dispatch instruction, and (3) early EMS response, treatment, and transport.

Subarachnoid hemorrhage: Bleeding into the surface of the brain caused by rupture of a blood vessel. The most common cause of a subarachnoid hemorrhage is rupture of a cerebral aneurysm.

Subdiaphragmatic: A term indicating the area below the diaphragm (the muscular partition separating the abdominal and thoracic cavities).

Sudden cardiac arrest: Sudden or unexpected cessation of heart function, most often caused by a sudden arrhythmia, such as VF or pulseless VT.

Suffocation: Cessation of respiration, most often resulting from obstruction to air flow, such as occurs with obstruction to air passages in victims of avalanche.

Supine: A term used to describe someone who is lying down with the face upward.

Supraventricular tachycardia (SVT): An abnormally rapid cardiac rhythm generated from an electrical focus in the heart that is above the ventricles. SVT typically produces a heart rate greater than 140 beats per minute in the adult and greater than 180 to 220 beats per minute in the infant or child.

Syncope: A temporary loss of consciousness due to cerebral ischemia.

Tension pneumothorax: Air trapped in the pleural space (the space between the lung and the chest wall) caused by a 1-way valve effect. A tension pneumothorax results in increased intrathoracic pressure, respiratory failure, decreased blood return to the heart, and shock.

Tidal volume: Volume of air inspired and expired during 1 respiratory cycle; normal tidal volume at rest is 500 mL.

Tracheobronchial: Pertaining to the trachea (windpipe) or bronchi within the lung.

Tracheostomy: The surgical creation of an opening into the trachea through the neck.

Transient ischemic attack (TIA): A reversible episode of focal neurologic dysfunction.

Transthoracic impedance: The resistance to transmission of electrical current represented by the skin, fat, muscle, and lung of a patient's chest.

Tympanic membrane: The eardrum.

Universal choking sign: The sign in which a victim clutches his neck with both hands, indicating a foreign-body airway obstruction.

Universal precautions: Steps taken to prevent potential contact with body substances that may carry the human immunodeficiency virus (HIV) or hepatitis B virus (HBV). This approach is designed to prevent the transmission of disease by using gloves, goggles, masks, and gowns.

Utstein style: A method of data collection that includes a uniform definition of terms and time intervals related to the discovery, assessment, and management of prehospital and in-hospital cardiac arrest. The Utstein guidelines have been developed to guide collection, publication, and comparison of data in human and laboratory resuscitation research.

Veins: Blood vessels that return blood to the heart.

Vena cava: The largest vein in the body, which returns blood to the right side of the heart.

Ventricular fibrillation (VF): A chaotic and disorganized heart rhythm that results in cardiac arrest.

Ventricular tachycardia (VT): An abnormally rapid heart rhythm generated within the ventricles. VT by itself or by its degeneration into VF can result in cardiac arrest.

Waveform: The form and structure of an electrically conducted impulse.

Xiphoid process: The bony protuberance at the base of the sternum.